the
HORIZONS
of HEALTH

the
HORIZONS
of HEALTH

EDITED BY

Henry Wechsler

Joel Gurin

George F. Cahill, Jr.

Harvard University Press

Cambridge, Massachusetts, and London, England   1977

Library of Congress Cataloging in Publication Data

Main entry under title:

The Horizons of health.

    Bibliography: p.
    Includes index.
    1. Medical research.   2. Medical research—United
States.   I. Wechsler, Henry, 1932–   II. Gurin, Joel,
1953–   III. Cahill, George Francis, 1927–
[DNLM: 1. Research—Popular works.   W20.5 H811]
R850.H67   610'.7'2   76–47012
ISBN 0–674–40630–3

Preface

Medical research encompasses many diverse areas of investigation that overlap in complex ways. Any attempt to organize such a vast body of information must almost inevitably draw certain arbitrary divisions between different areas of research. Nevertheless, we hope that the organization of this book will make it easier for the reader to appreciate the types of research that are now going on in many related medical fields.

The first part, "The Scope of the Problem," contains two chapters that should give the reader a basic idea of the major health problems in America today, and the ways that researchers are attacking them. Chapter 1 deals with the general problems of deciding which research areas are most important to the public health, carrying out the research, and applying it. Chapter 2 describes the epidemiological data used to estimate the impact of different diseases on the health of the nation and hence to help researchers develop some idea of which diseases may be the most urgent to study.

"Basic Processes in Disease," the second part, describes research into certain processes—such as infection and genetic disorders—that can lead to disease affecting many different organs of the body. Most research into these illnesses focuses on the underlying processes rather than on the specific diseases they may cause.

Of all the biological processes that may manifest themselves as disease, those involved in the behavioral disorders—like psychosis, mental retardation, and alcohol and drug abuse—may have been the hardest to define. But now the biology of the mind is beginning to be understood, and whole new ways of looking at behavioral disorders are developing as a result. The four chapters that make up "Biomedical Approaches to Behavioral Disorders" explore the ways in which social and psychological problems have begun to fall into the province of medical research.

"Diseases of Organs and Systems" is the longest section in the book; it comprises research into the large number of abnormalities that restrict themselves primarily to specific organs or biological systems in the body. While research in these areas has generally had more specific goals than some of the more basic research, the study of specific diseases has often clarified more general problems. For instance, several of the chapters, which examine the possible environmental factors that may lead to cancer of a specific organ system, illuminate the general problem of the environmental causes of cancer. And diseases of specific organs—notably diabetes, which is caused by dysfunction of the pancreas—often affect the health of the entire body in fundamental ways. (It should also be noted that neurological problems are technically disorders of a single organ system; but because of the profound effects they may have on the individual's psychological functioning, they have been considered in the part on behavioral disorders.)

Three fields—orthopedics, surgery, and radiology—have applied increasingly sophisticated techniques from physics and engineering to the diagnosis and treatment of disease. These new techniques of diagnosis and intervention have also developed through the theoretical understanding of biological processes in health and disease; the study of joint function has been central to orthopedics, and surgeons have learned a great deal from the study of metabolism. But the main impact of these three fields has been in the application of new diagnostic and treatment techniques, and for that reason they are grouped together.

Finally, basic pragmatic problems must be considered in the planning and application of biomedical research. Even the most promising approaches to the understanding and ultimate treatment of disease can yield results only if the researchers are adequately funded and if communication within the medical profession fosters the application of research results. But there are serious limitations to the amount of money that is available for medical research; and new research findings arise so rapidly that the dissemination of information has become a real problem. The two chapters in "The Implementation of Research" examine these issues and propose some solutions.

Acknowledgments

This book has been assembled under the aegis of The Medical Foundation, Inc., of Boston, which has supported biomedical and community health research since 1957. The foundation's noncategorical approach to research—the "whole person" concept—formed the basis for this collection of information about research into all the major diseases to which the body and mind are subject. Most important, the Foundation's position as a community health agency and as a coordinator of research resources enabled us to assemble these chapters by nationally recognized researchers in the Boston area.

Many thanks are due to Merle W. Mudd, Executive Director of The Medical Foundation, for his continuing encouragement and support; and to Susan Martin, whose tireless efforts in the preparation of the various manuscripts brought this project to the printed page. We also wish to acknowledge Harriet Greenfield's valuable contribution as illustrator.

Finally, we are especially grateful to William Bennett, Science and Medicine Editor for Harvard University Press. His investment in this book has gone beyond the professional duty of a publisher; he has been deeply committed to this project, and his advice and help at every stage have been absolutely invaluable.

Contents

Foreword

DONALD S. FREDRICKSON

Health care today is one of the most complex of human endeavors. It involves all kinds of practitioners, diverse in their organization and modes of delivery, facilities of special design, and a constantly proliferating array of instruments, techniques, devices, and therapies. At the base of it all is biomedical research.

Biomedical knowledge, like scientific knowledge generally, has been accumulating at an exponential rate, as reflected in the output of scientific literature. One sampling of biomedical publications suggests an average annual increase in scientific papers of between 4 and 5 percent for each year from 1965 to 1973. It has become very difficult even for physicians to keep up with developments in their own and related fields; and it has become virtually impossible for the layman to understand and appreciate recent advances in medical knowledge. This book has been designed to help fill the need for collected, accessible information about medical research.

Biomedical research, which unfortunately has usually been seen as the province only of the laboratory scientist or the health care professional, is a field that ultimately affects everyone. Medicine is still empirical enough; without research it would be medieval. We might still be relying

Note: The substance of this foreword was presented at the annual meeting of the American Association for the Advancement of Science in February 1976. In somewhat different form it was published in *American Society for Microbiology News* (1976) 42:266–269, © 1976 by the American Society for Microbiology, and is reprinted here by permission.

on leeches and the purge, be resigned to periodic outbreaks of devastating plagues, and have to endure calamity with uncontrolled anxiety and pain. Modern research results have often been directly translated into social action, such as mass fluoridation, mandatory sanitation practices, and pollution control. Sometimes the individual can directly participate in research application, by changes in life style, for example, in improving nutrition and stopping smoking. When biomedical knowledge becomes a part of daily living, however, we tend to forget its origins in the processes of discovery and development.

Some claim can be made, of course, that the disappearance of small-pox should also mean an end of proclaiming our debt to William Jenner's experiments. The near end of measles and polio will soon make allusions to these achievements boring as well. But the benefits will continue to be enjoyed by succeeding generations, while the fear and memory of the holocausts that once were will disappear with time.

Research continues to provide tangible improvements in health care. In 1975, for the first time since adequate statistics have been prepared, there was a decline in the death rate from cardiovascular diseases. Just which of the discoveries leading to changes in treatment or prevention should take credit for this is not clear, but there is little question that better knowledge rather than chance was the major determinant. The outlook for other diseases has continued to improve, although the results are sometimes less dramatic. Research has had a revolutionary effect on life styles by making it possible for couples to plan the timing and number of their children. Moreover, an increasing number of serious defects are now detectable *in utero,* and safer abortion procedures allow parents the option of not having a child incapable of a reasonably normal life. The world is on the threshold of getting effective vaccines against hepatitis and better ones against influenza. And new knowledge concerning the immune system and tissue compatibilities may soon allow us to identify innate factors in the development of certain diseases.

Obviously, research is but one of the factors that have contributed to gains against mortality and morbidity. The knowledge had to be orga-nized, applied, and delivered; and both the public and private sectors were involved in these processes. Social and economic factors have also figured heavily in the improvement of national health.

Recently there has been an increasingly negative tone in economic analyses of the impact of medical care on health status. Fingers are pointed at the fact that increases in life expectancy appear to be leveling off. Another, more rational criticism is directed toward seeming inattention to accidents, homicide, and crime, which are more important causes of death in youth than is disease. A serious disadvantage of such analyses is their inability to assess the benefits of medical care in terms of relief of the disability, fear, or discomfort that can drastically change the quality of life without appearing in the scores kept of mortality or productivity.

To a certain extent, the criticisms of medical care extend to a questioning of the value of continuing research. This is not anti-intellectualism but part of a national anxiety to commit finite public resources first toward immediate social ends, rather than to a long-term investment in acquiring useful information. This demand for some justification in *economic* terms of the return on research is fair but not always easy to satisfy.

In seeking to appraise the impact of research and technological development in general, economists have examined the factors that account for growth in national output. After allowing for such things as the number and quality of workers and the accumulation of capital, they have concluded that at least 30 percent of U.S. growth nationally has been the result of technological change. The average national economic rate of return for expenditures on research and development activities that generate technical change has been set at substantially more than 13 percent per year. This is a higher rate of return than the 10 percent per year associated with investment in a college education, for example. Historically the rate of return to capital investment generally has been much lower—in the range of 2 to 4 percent.

The return from some kinds of biomedical research may far exceed the general rate of return for research and development. A recent study of the economic impact of surgical research concluded that in the single year of 1970, the United States had benefited to the extent of 2.8 billion dollars from 16 surgical advances that reduced death and disability from 20 disease conditions. According to this study, the expenditure for the research which gave rise to those advances was but one sixtieth of the benefit observed in the single year. In fact, the estimated gains associated with these discoveries exceeded the entire national expenditure for all bio medical research in 1970. Since these gains not only continue but increase each year, one could even argue that they alone "pay" in social terms for the entire national biomedical research effort each year.

The 60/1 ratio of benefit to cost in this case undoubtedly overstates the rate of return to investment in biomedical research generally. All research is proposed with high hopes of significant application to human health, but the route linking basic discovery to the patient is often long and indirect. Some research produces negative findings; hypotheses are discarded. Many experiments lead to no hypotheses. Many potential innovations prove unworkable or unmarketable. The gains from striking successes in research must, in an economic sense, "carry the cost" of blind alleys and modest achievements.

But the potential benefits of biomedical research in both economic and human terms are certainly great enough to warrant generous funding. Federal funds not only are essential to researchers but are a good economic investment for the federal government; as the government begins to take on increasing responsibility for providing health services, it makes economic sense to fund research programs that may lead to improved and more efficient methods of health care. But private foundations, too, play a vital role in research funding. These foundations can generally be more flexible and take more risks than the federal government. They can focus attention on health problems that might otherwise be undersupported and can back innovative ideas that are not yet established but that offer a large potential payoff.

Any attempt to plan biomedical research and allocate funds effectively must begin with a solid review of the modern history of biomedical research, and of the areas that seem to hold the greatest promise for the future. This volume should help provide the necessary perspective that has long been overdue.

The Scope
of the Problem

PART ONE

Biomedical Research:
An Overview

HENRY WECHSLER
JOEL GURIN
GEORGE F. CAHILL, JR.

1

No applied science affects our lives as directly and personally as medicine. It is not too difficult to conceive of a world without nuclear power; but where would we be without penicillin? Without the medical advances of the last century, those of us lucky enough to survive would live under the constant threat of diseases that no one understood and for which only ineffective remedies were available.

The distance between the physician of 1877 and today's doctors is as great as the gap between the Wright brothers and Neil Armstrong. Medicine was a rugged profession a hundred years ago, when the physician had to rely on ingenuity, persuasion, luck, and improvisation to overcome the great technical obstacles he faced. An early doctor's bag contained few effective tools. Heart disease could be treated with digitalis, malaria with quinine, and pain with opium; but for most other disorders, the physician could just prescribe a variety of useless potions and salves that were nonetheless used in desperation and blind faith. The stethoscope and the reflex hammer were the major available diagnostic instruments. One can imagine the awe that the physician of a century ago would feel at today's sophisticated tools for visual diagnosis. What would he think of the computerized radioscanning techniques that can locate tiny areas of damaged tissue in inaccessible organs like the pancreas and brain and can display those tissues on a television screen? How would he like to use a fiberoptic tube to look directly at an ulcer in the patient's stomach, search for a site of bleeding, or examine a small lung tumor?

Medical science, like the other sciences, progresses at an ever-accelerating rate; and revolutionary changes in the diagnosis and treatment of disease have taken place within the professional lifetimes of most doctors practicing today.

The analysis of substances in the blood did not even become a major method of diagnosis until around the time of World War II; and even twenty years ago, no one could have imagined the automatic multichannel analyzers now used to study blood samples. These machines measure the levels of minerals, enzymes, and waste products in the blood and indicate which of these fall outside the normal healthy range. Some machines can even be programmed to give different possible diagnoses based on blood sample data, indicate the probability of each diagnosis, and request further information from the physician.

In the past few years, all sorts of devices have been invented to take over the function of faulty parts of the body. Synthetic heart valves, blood vessels, hip and knee joints, and teeth can all be used to replace their natural counterparts when they fail; and scientists are even working on mechanical glands to supply missing hormones just as the body needs them. Electronic pacemakers can keep the heart beating regularly, and people who suffer kidney failure can live their lives, albeit restricted, with the aid of a dialysis machine.

Surgeons can now perform operations long thought to be technically impossible. The heart-lung machine has given us open-heart surgery; laser beams are used to correct abnormalities in the back of the eye; and organ transplants are no longer in the realm of science fiction.

Chemical approaches to treatment have also advanced at an incredible rate. The therapeutic drugs in use today are radically different from those prescribed just a decade ago; and with the important exceptions of aspirin, insulin, digitalis, some antibiotics and a few other very useful standbys, the physician's pharmacopoeia has changed completely since the 1950s. These advances in drug therapy have been intimately connected to progress in our theoretical understanding of biology at the molecular level.

Molecular biology and biochemistry are probably the youngest and fastest growing of the modern sciences. As recently as 1953 James Watson and Francis Crick first outlined the structure of DNA, which codes the body's genetic information; virtually all of modern biochemistry has stemmed from this revolutionary insight. Researchers now have the theoretical tools to begin answering questions that could not have been raised before. Even the deadly mystery of cancer may soon be solved by modern biochemical research. Cancer cells are characterized primarily by their ability to multiply almost indefinitely, gradually taking over larger and larger areas of the body. This disease process is gradually beginning to be understood as scientists study the very basic biochemical processes that control normal cell division in growth, wound healing, and the replenishment of blood cells.

Since a great deal of knowledge and expertise is required to do research in any disease process on the molecular level, medical researchers have become increasingly specialized; and as a result, communication has become a major problem. Most doctors find it very difficult to keep up with the most recent discoveries and technological innovations in any field of medicine but their own specialty; and many remain ill informed even of advances in their own chosen field. Formal and informal programs have been developed to help physicians continue their medical education (Franz J. Ingelfinger discusses these in Chapter 27). Doctors are finding it hard to understand all of modern medicine, and the layman is truly at a loss. Medical research has taken on an air of mystification that is nearly impossible for an intelligent person without special training to penetrate. Of course, news of sudden "breakthroughs" does filter down through the popular press; but these bits of information, frequently distorted, can hardly give even the most avid newspaper reader a sense of the interrelationship of different research discoveries or any concept of the way in which research priorities are and should be determined.

This volume is intended to further communication between medical researchers and the people they serve by presenting past, present, and future research developments in a context, and in language, that the layman can understand. Part of the impetus for this collection has been the realization that medical researchers must be accountable to the public. Nearly three billion dollars of federal money is now spent on medical research every year; and while this is only 10 percent of the annual federal budget for health, it is still a sizable sum. In addition, medical research often has human as well as financial costs; ethical problems abound in any study of human subjects. The examination of children with an extra Y chromosome for possible behavioral abnormalities has become a central controversy in genetic research. Serious ethical questions were also raised by a much publicized study carried out by the University Group Diabetes Project to determine whether or not certain antidiabetic drugs actually shorten the life span of patients using them. These two groups of studies demonstrate the sensitive issues involved in much medical research and underscore the need for public accountability.

But the most important aim of publicizing research information is not to put limitations on medical research; rather, it is to ensure that medical investigators can work effectively. Health care cannot progress unless ample resources are allocated to the research projects that are likely to lead to the greatest benefits. (Allocation of public funds, a complex issue, is discussed in greater detail in Chapter 26.) Ideally, federal funding should be used not only to support existing research programs that are crucial to national health care, but also to attract talented scientists to areas of research that might otherwise be neglected. Individual researchers are not necessarily the best people to judge the relative importance of different kinds of medical research. For many years it was unfashionable to study alcoholism or mental retardation; consequently, we have remained largely ignorant of the factors involved in these conditions. One way to correct such imbalances of research activity is to allocate substantial amounts of public money to important areas that are being inadequately investigated; once the money is available, qualified scientists will certainly be attracted to the field.

A well-informed and careful approach to research funding is not an idealistic goal; it is an absolute necessity. Yet the people who control the distribution of funds—administrators, legislators, and ultimately the general public—have had little sound basis for deciding between competing claims for the little research funding that is available. This unfortunate state of ignorance has not been anyone's fault; it has simply been a natural by-product of growing specialization in medical science. The situation can be corrected by making research information more accessible, and we hope this volume helps serve that purpose. While this book does not attempt to outline a set of research programs to meet all the nation's health care needs, the following chapters should provide information that can be used to allocate resources for research more rationally and less politically than has been done in the past.

Competition for resources, as everyone knows, is becoming more intense every year. Many different kinds of public programs, such as welfare and education, are laying a claim to some of the money that might otherwise go to health. And even within the field of health care and research, competition for funding is fierce. Virtually every medical researcher can argue convincingly that he is inadequately funded. To give just one example, the annual expenditure for research into heart disease is only 1 percent of the amount that such disease costs the nation every year.

Since resources are limited, the basic problem is to ensure that adequate support goes to those diseases that are deemed the most serious.

But it is very difficult to determine exactly how much money is being spent on research into a given disease area or how serious a health problem that disease poses. Funding for basic research may not be counted as money spent to combat a given disease, although such basic research may ultimately lead to the understanding and control of an illness. Statistics on the prevalence of disease—one measure of seriousness—can also be confusing, because there is a great deal of overlap between different diseases. When one type of disease leads to another, the patient may suffer from different conditions simultaneously. There are thus more cases of disease than there are sick people, and a single patient with one complicated condition may be counted in a health survey as suffering from many different illnesses. When statistics on disease prevalence are examined in ignorance of the relationships between diseases, it may become difficult to determine how many people are actually ill and to assess the relative importance of different diseases to the public health.

Even when studies of disease prevalence and causes of death take these factors into account, they do not automatically indicate which diseases should be the first to be studied. Everyone agrees that research into cancer and heart disease must have a high priority because these two types of disorder are the major causes of death in the United States today. But how much money should go to combat dental disease, a universal, if nonfatal, cause of human suffering? Many diseases that are not major causes of death may cause a great deal of pain and substantial loss of productivity for a long period of time, either directly or through their complications. Diabetics can be maintained with insulin injections, and people who have suffered kidney failure can usually be kept alive and productive through dialysis. But diabetics still frequently develop circulatory problems or become blind; and dialysis is an extremely expensive procedure that keeps many patients alive but cannot necessarily keep them healthy. Finally, causes of death that predominate among the young cause a greater loss of "life years" than those that strike older people and from this point of view may be considered particularly important. For example, automobile accidents may be responsible for the loss of more years of life than any other cause, largely because teenagers are prone to car accidents. (Some of these considerations are discussed in Chapter 2.)

Even if the decision is made to allocate a certain amount of money to research on a given disease, it remains to be decided what type of research should be funded. The fundamental distinction that has been made in the past has been between basic and applied research. The goal of basic research is the investigation and evaluation of theoretical principles. Hypotheses are tested again and again until the results of a number of different experiments all agree to support one theoretical concept. The process of basic research is one of continual probing, questioning, and examining; theories that seem sound at one time may be totally revised a few years later. Applied research, in contrast, makes use of theories that are well enough established to be regarded as fact. The task of the applied researcher is not to break new theoretical ground but to integrate what is already known and thus come up with a new technique for preventing, diagnosing, or treating sickness.

Applied research has yielded dramatic new methods of health care. The truly impressive technological innovations that have come about in the last few decades—advances in radiology, orthopedics, and surgical technique—have come about primarily through the engineering skill of applied researchers. Careful application of theoretical knowledge has also made possible the development of hundreds of new drugs for the treatment of specific diseases.

Since the results of applied research are often so dazzling and since they can come into practical use almost at once, a research program aimed at finding a specific treatment for a certain disease may be funded more readily than a program whose goal is a more general theoretical understanding of the biological processes that lead to illness. This is unfortunate, because such basic research has proven to be absolutely necessary to medical progress. In Chapter 9 Jack Mendelson and Nancy Mello point out quite accurately that the polio vaccine would never have been developed if all available funding had gone to support the applied goal of building iron lungs for polio victims. The concepts used to develop the life-saving vaccine came from years of basic medical research, much of which appeared on the surface to be unrelated to the clinical problem of polio.

Obviously, neither basic nor applied research is better than the other; both are appropriate approaches to different diseases at different times. Rather than blindly championing one method or the other, medical researchers—and the people who support them—must develop a sense of what type of research is needed if they are to use their time and resources as efficiently as possible. In the 1950s, dozens of scientists were intent on finding a chemical cause, and a chemical cure, for schizophrenia; but the vast majority of the theories and remedies proposed at that time turned out to be worthless. In Chapter 8 Seymour Kety attributes this record of failure to the desire to find applications before anyone had basic theoretical principles to apply. Many investigators were ready to propose chemical theories and cures for mental illness at a time when no one even knew that the transmission of signals between neurons took place through chemical (rather than electrical) processes. Such heroic theorizing in the face of ignorance demonstrates the strong prejudice that exists in favor of any research that offers the hope—however spurious—of providing an immediate cure for a major disease.

Today, the value of basic research in certain cases seems to be better appreciated. It is generally acknowledged, for example, that the problems of cancer and atherosclerosis will almost certainly remain insoluble until we have a better theoretical appreciation of the processes underlying these disorders; and a large proportion of funding for the study of these diseases is directed to scientists engaged in basic research. In other areas, however, investigators are still strongly pressured to find cures and immediate solutions, while the most basic theoretical problems remain unsolved. This has certainly been true in the study of alcoholism and the addictions. Vast amounts of money have been spent to treat these disorders, yet it has been impossible to develop any really effective treatment programs as long as the actual nature of these conditions remains poorly understood. This is not to deny the importance of treatment programs for alcoholics and drug addicts; obviously it is vital to help such suffering people in whatever way possible. But basic research into these disorders is essential if their treatment is ever to become truly curative rather than palliative.

In many ways, it is more difficult to begin to study the fundamental processes underlying a given disease than it is to devise treatments for that disease; until the illness is understood at some theoretical level, one simply does not know what to look for.

Careful epidemiological studies can be invaluable in helping the researcher focus on probable causes of disease. The hardest diseases to study are those that develop years or even decades after the individual has been exposed to the causative agent; but with careful epidemiology, even these disorders can be linked to their causes. Different types of cancer have been shown to be associated with a number of environmental agents, ranging from sunlight to asbestos, by studies of their prevalence in groups of people preferentially exposed to these environmental stimuli at some point in their lives. And recently, a number of serious neurological disorders have been attributed to the presence of slow-acting viruses that remain in the body for decades after the initial period of infection is over. The time lag between cause and effect in these diseases is so great that the actual causes might never be suspected without long-range studies that demonstrate the relationship of the agent to the disease that appears years later.

"Targeted" research programs represent another approach to understanding the origins of disease and devising methods of treatment. These are highly organized programs, usually of applied rather than basic research, that are directed toward specific goals. Some recent targeted programs have been aimed at the improvement of drug treatments for cancer, at the development of better artificial kidneys, and at determining whether or not viruses are involved in human cancer.

It would be fairly easy to plan research if breakthroughs always came as a result of long-range, careful, directed programs. But things do not work so rationally. Many of the most valuable insights into specific diseases have come from totally unexpected sources. The drugs chlorpromazine and iproniazid revolutionized the treatment of schizophrenia and depression, respectively, and studies of the chemical action of these agents have provided much of the basis for our understanding of the chemistry of severe mental illness. But when these drugs were introduced, no one had the slightest idea that they would have important psychological effects; chlorpromazine was first used in the treatment of surgical shock, and iproniazid, as therapy for tuberculosis. Even the most apparently esoteric research may lead to important clinical applications in the treatment of major diseases. The virus that causes hepatitis, for example, was discovered by a geneticist examining blood constituents in a tribe of Australian aborigines.

Obviously, medical research should not be done at random in the hope that somebody studying an obscure process somewhere will accidentally come up with a cure for cancer. But the major "accidental" discoveries that have occurred serve as an important reminder that apparently dissimilar areas of medical research can actually be very closely related. As researchers have developed more and more sophisticated methods, the reasons behind these apparently fortuitous relationships have become clearer. Different clinical phenomena may actually originate in identical or closely analogous processes that take place at the cellular, if not the molecular, level.

Since the Second World War, it has become possible to study these fundamental biochemical processes and their relationships to different diseases. Some of the most important research now going on is concerned not with the clinical manifestations of any given illness but with the study of basic biological mechanisms, still incompletely understood, that are involved in a wide range of disorders. Although viral infection has been studied and combated for some time, many serious effects of this infectious process are just beginning to come to light. In addition to the slow-acting viruses that can cause fatal damage to the nervous system, it now appears that diabetes in youth, rheumatoid arthritis, certain types of mental retardation, and even some kinds of cancer (particularly the leukemias) may all have viral origins. Immunologists, who have long been concerned with the body's response to infection and the abnormal response seen in allergic reactions, are now beginning to study the immunological problems involved in organ transplants and cancer, as well as the autoimmune processes that may form the basis of a number of different diseases. And fundamental studies of the genetic code in bacteria have formed the cornerstone for our growing understanding of the biochemistry of hereditary human illnesses.

In view of its central importance, it is certainly strange that basic research has often been seen as a luxury that the public cannot afford. When available funds become scarce, it is usually the basic rather than applied research that suffers the first budgets cuts. Probably the primary reason for this is the often considerable time lag before the knowledge gained through basic research actually leads to improvements in health care. The action of heart muscle has been largely understood at the biochemical level, but this understanding has still not made it any easier to treat heart disease. In contrast, new drugs can be used to control disease as soon as they have been approved by the Food and Drug Administration. Drug research, technological innovation, and other applied approaches thus often seem a better investment than basic research in terms of the probable short-term payoff.

Unfortunately, research planners have tended to ignore the fact that a short-term boon can turn into a long-term disaster. In recent years, it has become all too obvious that new agents introduced before their effects are completely understood can lead to health problems worse than those they were originally intended to prevent. Diethylstilbestrol (DES) was given to pregnant women for many years to prevent miscarriages; but the daughters of women who were given DES during pregnancy are now known to run a risk of vaginal cancer. Nitrates have found long use as meat preservatives that prevent the growth of bacteria that cause botulism; now these chemicals, too, have been shown to be cancer-causing agents. Even antibiotics are no longer seen as the miracle cures they once appeared to be. When improperly given, these drugs can dangerously upset the natural balance of the microorganisms that normally live within the body. Worse, certain kinds of antibiotics may literally poison people who are especially sensitive to them.

Even when a new therapeutic agent or technique is basically safe and effective, there is no guarantee that it will be used beneficially as soon as it is introduced. The applicability of some treatments is limited by their substantial cost. Very few patients suffering from kidney failure would be able to afford dialysis without the government funding programs that have made this life-saving treatment more accessible. Other individuals irrationally turn down the opportunity to become healthy, even when they might actually save money at the same time. Cigarettes have been known to be a primary cause of respiratory disease for at least twenty years, yet the American tobacco industry continues to prosper. (Federal support is even given to tobacco agronomy, at the same time that the law requires the Surgeon General's warning to appear on every cigarette package.) And many patients simply act as if they did not know what was good for them. Diabetes can be effectively treated in many by strict dietary control, and the individual suffering from hypertension can reduce his high blood pressure by taking certain prescribed drugs; but physicians have found that it is often very difficult to get their patients to follow these prescribed treatments on a regular basis.

Advances in medical care do not automatically follow discoveries made in the laboratory. Psychosocial research is clearly necessary if biomedical research findings are to be translated into improved medical care more quickly and effectively. This book primarily describes the process of discovery in medical research; but the problem of implementation is just as complex and important and could well be the subject of another book.

The issues involved in planning medical research are as complex as the actual medical problems that researchers try to solve. As our understanding and control of disease has become increasingly sophisticated, it has become more and more difficult to develop a sense of the interrelationship of research in different fields and to estimate the value of different approaches. This major communication problem must be solved if research is to be planned rationally and carried out efficiently. We hope that this book will help improve the situation by providing the public and its representatives with tangible examples of the current and potential benefits of biomedical research.

Health of the United States Population

BRIAN MacMAHON
JOYCE E. BERLIN

2

What does it mean to talk about the health of a population? To measure or even define something as elusive as good health is extremely difficult and what is actually measured is usually ill health. Specifically, the numbers of people suffering different types of death and illness can be counted. If the same measures are used over a period of time and in different populations, changes in the degree and kind of ill health can be assessed and populations can be compared.

The science of measuring health in populations is epidemiology. In the past the word epidemic (and the science of epidemics) was used only in the context of infectious diseases, but the term literally describes excessive disease prevalence, regardless of the type of disease. For example, the United States is currently suffering epidemics of heart disease and cancer that are as truly epidemic as were the great plagues of infectious diseases of the past.

Several kinds of rates are used to describe the frequency of disease in a population, and it is important to keep their different implications in mind. For example, when enquiring about the health of an individual, we often ask "How are you?" or "How have you been?" In the social context the two questions may be used interchangeably, but interpreted rigorously they have different implications. The first question asks about the individual's health at this particular point in time; the second, about health-related events that the individual may have experienced over some recent time period.

A similar distinction must be made when describing the frequency of disease in a population. Prevalence rates describe what pattern of disease one would find if one were able to examine the entire population at a single point in time—how many people would be found to be ill, to what degree, and with what diseases. Incidence rates, in contrast, describe the frequency of health-related events (onset of illness or death) that occurred in the population over a fixed period of time, commonly a year. Estimates of the frequency of death have the basic characteristics of incidence rates, since they are counts of events during a fixed period of time (incidence of death), but these are usually referred to as mortality rates to specify that they refer to rates of death from, rather than occurrence of, a particular disease.

Why is it important to distinguish between these types of rate? The answer is that no single rate can paint an adequate picture of the significance of any disease in a population. A disease with a very high incidence but short duration, like the common cold, will appear as a minor cause of disease prevalence at any one point in time (unless the data happen to be collected during a severe epidemic). On the other hand, a disease which can occur only once to an individual (and of which incidence rates will therefore be low) but which has long-lasting consequences—such as multiple sclerosis—will make a major contribution to disease prevalence. Consumption of medical and social resources is generally a function of disease prevalence rather than incidence, while the emotional, economic, and social trauma associated with acute illness (and death) relate more directly to disease incidence and mortality. One's purposes and values therefore determine which types of rate one chooses to consider most relevant in a particular context.

Mortality

Death is unequaled as an objective and readily ascertainable index of health status or lack thereof. For this reason, as much as for its intrinsic significance, the frequency of death has long been studied around the world. A common way of summarizing the effect of different levels of mortality is in terms of expectation of life. This is the average duration of life that a population would experience if the observed age-specific death rates were to continue throughout the population's life span.

The annual death rate in the United States is now about 7 per 1,000 population, less than half the rate at the beginning of the century. In 1900 the average expectation of life in the United States was about 48 years for men and 51 years for women. Now the value for men is about 68 years, and for women, 75 years. Death rates for males stabilized between 1955 and 1970; the rates for females are still declining, but at a slower rate than in previous decades.

This historical increase in average life expectancy is due primarily to the decline in mortality rates in infancy and childhood. Death rates are relatively high during the first year of life, particularly during the first 28 days, and then decrease until around age 15. After that there is a steady increase; the rates approximately double with each decade of age. While infants still have a higher death rate than young adults, newborns now have a vastly better chance of survival than they did at the turn of the century. The present infant mortality rate—about 18 deaths under one year of age per 1,000 liveborn infants—is less than one fifth of what it was 60 years ago. During this time, the life expectation for an infant has increased by approximately 22 years. In contrast, the life expectancy for a person of 40 has increased by only six years.

Despite these improvements, death rates in the United States—particularly among males—do not compare favorably with those in many other developed countries. In 1960, for females, New Zealand, the Netherlands, Norway, and Sweden had lower age-adjusted mortality rates than the United States; Canada, New Zealand, and six European countries had lower mortality rates for males.

There have been tremendous changes in the causes of death during this century. In 1900 the leading causes of death were influenza and pneumonia, with tuberculosis a close second. By 1970 influenza and pneumonia had dropped to fifth place and tuberculosis had so diminished that it was no longer among the leading causes of death. In general, over the century, mortality rates due to infectious disease have declined dramatically. At the same time, deaths due to chronic degenerative diseases—ischemic heart disease (caused by inadequate blood flow to heart muscle), malignant neoplasms (cancer), cerebrovascular disease—have increased. Table 2-1 lists the ten leading causes of death in the United States. Together, these causes account for 80 percent of all deaths in this country. Heart disease and cancer lead the list; these two disorders now account for more than half of all American deaths. At least 75 percent of all deaths are now attributable to noninfectious diseases.

Changes in the causes of infant mortality have been as dramatic as the overall changes in causes of death. While infectious diseases 60 years ago accounted for about 70 percent of infant deaths, they now account for only about 10 percent. The most common cause of infant death is now prematurity, and congenital malformations (which cause 15 percent of

Table 2–1. Percentage of deaths attributed to the
ten leading causes, United States, 1970

Ischemic heart disease	34.7
Malignant neoplasm	17.2
Cerebrovascular disease	10.8
Accident	6.0
Influenza and pneumonia	3.3
Diabetes mellitus	2.0
Arteriosclerosis	1.6
Cirrhosis of the liver	1.6
Bronchitis, emphysema, and asthma	1.6
Suicide	1.2

Source: Vital Statistics of the United States,
part A, vol. II, Mortality (Washington, D.C.: National Center for Health Statistics, 1970).

infant deaths) have become more significant than the infectious diseases.

At all ages, death rates are higher for males than for females. The excess is particularly marked in the younger years (ages 15 to 29) and in the later years (ages 55 to 69), when death rates for men are nearly double those for women. Males have had higher death rates than females in nearly all times, places, and races, but the extent of the difference is greatest in modern times in the industrialized nations. The greater mortality for males in the young adult ages is due primarily to accidents, especially automobile accidents. Many of the twentieth-century epidemics like heart disease and lung cancer also affect men more than women. The increasing frequency of early and prolonged widowhood is just one social consequence of this difference in death rates between males and females.

Mortality rates vary not only with respect to sex and age but also according to race and geographic location. Death rates for nonwhites are higher than those for whites, except at the oldest ages. The nonwhite mortality rate is lowest in the Pacific and Mountain states (where much of the nonwhite population is of Oriental or American Indian ancestry) and highest in the South Atlantic division (where the majority are black). Overall, age-adjusted mortality rates are higher by about 5 percent in metropolitan areas than in nonmetropolitan areas of the United States.

One final, important variable closely related to mortality is socio-economic status. The highest socioeconomic groups have the lowest mortality. This relationship, although also seen in adults, is particularly marked in infancy. The lower socioeconomic groups have infant death rates almost 50 percent higher than those of higher socioeconomic groups.

Acute Illness

There are many difficulties in attempting to measure the frequency of illness, particularly illnesses of limited duration. In the United States the most useful information comes from the Health Interview Survey of the National Health Survey. In this program, representative samples of the population are asked about illnesses that have occurred during the two weeks prior to the interview. Acute conditions are defined as those that lasted less than three months, involved either medical attention or restricted activity, and do not appear on a list of conditions defined as chronic (including, for example, arthritis, heart disease, and mental illness).

In 1974, the average person surveyed suffered about two acute illnesses; these conditions caused an average of nine days of restricted activity (including four days in bed), and nearly three days lost from work for each employed person. Respiratory illnesses, especially the common cold and flu, made up the largest number of acute conditions; second to respiratory diseases were injuries. The incidence of acute illnesses varies according to age and sex, as seen in Table 2-2.

The study of acute conditions gives a very different picture of national health than do the observed mortality rates. In contrast to deaths,

Table 2–2. Number of acute conditions per 100 persons per year by sex, age, and condition group, United States, 1974

Condition	Total	Male	Female	<6	6–16	17–44	45+
Respiratory conditions	94.4	92.2	96.5	172.6	131.3	92.5	47.5
Injuries	30.4	36.0	25.2	33.9	38.1	33.8	19.9
Infective and parasitic diseases	19.5	18.1	20.9	47.4	30.3	16.0	8.0
Digestive system conditions	7.8	6.0	9.5	7.3	10.6	8.8	4.8
All other acute conditions	23.5	19.2	27.5	47.8	26.4	24.1	13.3

Source: P. W. Ries, "Current Estimates from the Health Interview Survey, United States—1974," *Vital and Health Statistics,* series 10, no. 100 (Washington, D.C.: National Center for Health Statistics, September 1975).

acute illnesses decline in frequency with age and, except for injuries, tend to be more frequent in females than in males. It is a curious paradox that women are more likely to suffer acute or chronic disease, but death rates are higher in men. John Graunt noted this paradox in London in 1636 and suggested that "men, being more intemperate than women, die as much by reason of their vices, as the women do by the Infirmities of their sex." Though this suggestion is somewhat inconsonant with present views of the differences between the sexes, no better resolution of the paradox has yet been offered.

Chronic Illness

The impact of chronic illness is best seen through prevalence, rather than incidence, rates. The best sources of data are the same Health Interview Survey and the Health Examination Survey, also part of the National Health Survey. In the Health Interview Survey, chronic conditions are defined as those which appear on a special list, or which lasted more than three months. In the Examination Survey, participants are actually examined by physicians; the diagnosis of disease is thus more accurate than in the Interview Survey. But the Examination Survey also has disadvantages. It uses a much smaller sample and does not permit examination of changes over time, since, to date, no age group in the population has been examined more than once. A limitation of both surveys that is particularly important in the context of chronic illness is that the samples are drawn from the noninstitutionalized population.

In spite of these drawbacks, these surveys have provided valuable estimates of the impact of chronic disease on the American population. In 1974 approximately 26 million persons (13 percent of the population)—and almost half of people aged 65 or over—reported some limitation of activity due to one or more chronic conditions (Figure 2-1). The leading causes of activity limitation in persons aged 17 to 64 were heart conditions, arthritis and rheumatism, impairments of the back and spine, and mental and nervous conditions. In persons aged 65 and over, the first two conditions remained the most frequent, but visual impairments and hypertension were third and fourth.

Chronic illness may impair the individual's ability to function or may call for continuous medical care to such an extent that institutionalization becomes necessary. At any given time, approximately 1 percent of the U.S. adult population is in a long-stay medical institution of some kind. For persons aged 65–74, the figure is approximately 2 percent, and for

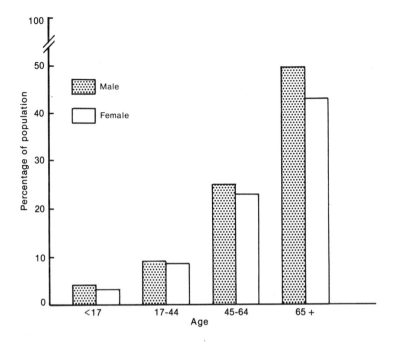

Figure 2–1. Percentage of population with limitation of activity due to chronic conditions, by age and sex, United States, 1974. From P. W. Ries, "Current Estimates from the Health Interview Survey, United States—1974," *Vital and Health Statistics*, series 10, no. 100 (Washington, D.C.: National Center for Health Statistics, September 1975).

those 75 and older it is over 7 percent. Almost half of these institutionalized persons are in mental hospitals, almost half in nursing homes, and the remainder are in geriatric and chronic disease hospitals. Among residents of nursing homes more than 60 percent have some form of cardiovascular problem, over 30 percent have arthritis or rheumatism, and close to 30 percent have had a stroke. In recent years, the number of elderly people in mental hospitals has decreased substantially; but the number in nursing and personal care homes—which are assuming an increasing proportion of the care of the aged mentally ill—has increased.

The impact of a chronic disease is measured not only in terms of its effect on the individual but also in terms of its prevalence in the population. The diseases of the mouth (particularly dental caries and periodontal disease) do not make their presence felt in measures either of reported activity limitation or institutionalization; yet they are the most widespread diseases in the United States. Estimates of the extent of dental disease were made in the Health Examination Survey. The average DMF score—the number of permanent teeth that are "decayed, filled, and either missing or indicated for extraction"—was 18.7 for white adults and 12.2 for blacks. The difference between whites and blacks was largely accounted for by a higher prevalence of filled teeth among whites.

Implications

Patterns of disease and death have changed greatly in the past several decades. The infectious diseases still account for a large number of acute illnesses in the United States, particularly among the young. However, they are rapidly disappearing as causes of mortality. Ischemic heart disease, cancer, and stroke are now the major causes of death; heart disease and stroke also frequently disable those they do not kill. Among the nonfatal though disabling chronic diseases, mental illness and dental conditions are now the most prevalent.

As the most widespread and serious diseases are identified, effective ways of preventing them are also being sought. Cigarette smoking plays a major role in some prominent diseases, notably cardiovascular disease and certain cancers; if everyone stopped smoking, between 100,000 and 200,000 deaths could be prevented each year. The social use and abuse of alcohol also contributes, to an unknown extent, to the nation's burden of disease. But beyond paying attention to these two sources of illness, there is relatively little that can be done in disease prevention that is not already being done. The great majority of deaths and the great preponderance of disability are due to diseases of unknown cause for which preventive measures have not been developed and for which therapy is often ineffective. It appears, therefore, that research into causation should have a high priority in efforts to improve the health of the population.

The studies discussed in this chapter give some picture of the magnitude of the problems facing us and of the relative importance of the major disease categories. In determining research directions, the frequency of a disease is only one factor to be considered. Also required is an estimate of the likelihood that a particular approach to a particular disease will be successful. The originality of the approach, the competence and resources of the investigator, and many other factors all affect the chances that research will succeed. Research support should not be withheld simply because the disease involved is uncommon. But at the same time, prevalent diseases are important to study simply because they affect the greatest numbers of people. The data indicate that cardiovascular disease, cancer, stroke, mental illness, dental disorders, and prematurity and congenital malformations in infants are types of diseases that are certainly widespread enough to warrant more research into their causation.

Basic Processes
in Disease

PART TWO

Cancer

EMIL FREI, III

3

Cancer is a cause of death second only to heart disease in the United States. Current incidence rates indicate that one quarter of all Americans can expect to develop some form of cancer more serious than superficial skin cancer; and three fifths of those who do develop such cancer now die from the illness. And yet the actual disease process involved in cancer, and the factors that may lead to its development, remain a mystery to most Americans.

Cancer begins as a biological alteration (or transformation) in a single cell in one of the body's organs. A transformed cell is biologically different from a normal cell in some very important ways. Cancer cells multiply faster than ordinary cells and cause accelerated tumor growth that is not held in check by the mechanisms that usually regulate cellular growth. Cancer cells are less responsive to the various control mechanisms that make normal cells behave; they continue to spread unless stopped by therapeutic intervention.

Experimental studies indicate that transformation initially occurs in a single cell, which forms tumors by dividing repeatedly. When a growing tumor reaches three to four millimeters in diameter, it must become connected to blood vessels before it can continue to proliferate. There is evidence that tumor cells actually stimulate their own blood supply by producing a substance that stimulates the growth of capillaries. Tumors tend to invade through soft tissue, along the line of least resistance, and produce substances that help them spread. Some tumors, for example, produce enzymes that degrade collagen and other structural proteins and thus help the tumor spread through soft tissue. A myeloma (tumor of the bone marrow) may produce molecular substances that stimulate the dissolution of bone. And recently, breast tumors that have spread to invade the bone have been shown to be associated with increased production of prostaglandins (biologically active lipids) that also act to dissolve bony structures (see Chapter 20).

Thanks largely to improved methodology, our understanding of the process of tumor growth has advanced greatly in the past few years; and that understanding may soon be used to improve the treatment of cancer. Tumor growth may eventually be controlled, for example, through interference with the tumor's production and secretion of chemical substances that stimulate its blood supply and degrade the tissue surrounding it. Studies of tumor growth also have important clinical implications for existing methods of cancer treatment, particularly radiotherapy and chemotherapy.

Arresting the growth of malignant tumors is clearly a central concern of cancer research. But even under optimum circumstances, the methods used to prevent the spread of an already existing cancer may often be costly and dangerous to the patient; worse, there is no guarantee that they will succeed. Since it is axiomatic in medicine that an ounce of prevention is worth a pound of cure, cancer research has focused primarily on identifying those factors that lead a cell to become cancerous in the first place. In addition to studying the biochemical processes that are the direct cause of cellular transformation, many researchers have investigated the environmental and familial factors that may lead to the development of cancer.

The Epidemiology of Cancer

It has been estimated that as many as three quarters of all cases of cancer are caused by contact with harmful agents in the environment. There is a high correlation between exposure to solar ultraviolet light and skin cancer; increasing evidence indicates that dietary factors may affect the development of gastrointestinal cancer; and lung cancer has been linked to cigarette smoking. Both the intensity and duration of exposure to these environmental agents are important variables; many substances do not lead to cancer until the individual has been exposed to them for at least twenty years. This fact explains why the risk of developing cancer increases with age (Figure 3-1). The observed time lag also implies that cancer-causing substances (carcinogens) may remain in the environment

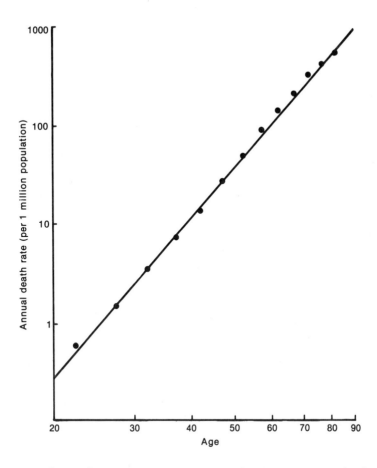

Figure 3–1. The incidence of cancer increases with advancing age. The figures in this graph represent death rates for cancer of the large intestine, but the general correlation of death rates with age holds for many other types of cancer as well. Redrawn from "The Cancer Problem" by John Cairns, *Scientific American,* November 1975, p. 67. Copyright © 1975 by Scientific American, Inc. All rights reserved.

for long periods of time before their effects can be detected by classical epidemiologic techniques.

The identification of carcinogenic agents in the environment is made still more difficult by the interaction of genetic and environmental factors. If members of a given population all show an especially high risk for a certain type of cancer, it may be hard to determine whether that cancer is caused by hereditary or environmental traits shared by that population.

But careful epidemiologic studies can often determine which of these influences is the more important.

Recent surveys of Japanese groups have yielded new insight into the causation of different types of gastrointestinal cancer (see Chapter 16). Japanese populations living in Japan show a higher incidence of gastric cancer and a much lower incidence of colorectal cancer (cancer of the colon and rectum) than Caucasian populations living in the United States; but studies of Japanese immigrants in the United States have shown these differences to be environmental rather than genetic in origin. After arriving in the United States, Japanese populations generally adopt American dietary habits within two to three generations. But these people rarely marry outside their ethnic group, at least through the first several generations. Japanese immigrants (and several other migrant populations) thus provide an excellent opportunity to disassociate the relative effects of genetic and environmental factors on the incidence of disease. Epidemiologic studies have now shown that migrant Japanese populations develop the same pattern of gastrointestinal cancer as American Caucasians once they begin to eat like them. Environmental factors thus seem to predominate in the causation of gastrointestinal cancer.

To treat and prevent the gastrointestinal cancers effectively, it is still necessary to determine what specific dietary factors are involved in these diseases. Epidemiologic studies have also begun to answer this question. We now know that the incidence of colorectal cancer, one of the most common types of gastrointestinal cancer, is generally high in affluent societies and low in underdeveloped countries; this difference remains when one takes into account the average age differences between the populations of rich and poor nations. The incidence of colorectal cancer appears to be linked to specific dietary factors: people living in affluent societies consume much more meat and fat and much less roughage (cellulose and fiber) than do members of poorer countries.

Some investigators have suggested that dietary fiber may be important in preventing the development of cancer of the colon and rectum because dietary fiber increases stool bulk and speeds its transit through the bowel. Carcinogenic agents present in the bowel would theoretically be diluted and more rapidly excreted in individuals whose diets are high in fiber (see Chapter 16).

The possible carcinogenic effects of meat are more difficult to evaluate. Certain foods, but particularly meat, contain nitrates and nitrites; these chemicals were originally added to some cured foods to prevent the growth of bacteria, and especially to prevent botulism, a lethal disease.

These chemicals did prevent bacterial disease effectively and constituted a major public health advance at the time they were introduced. Now, however, there is evidence that under certain circumstances nitrates and nitrites may be converted to nitrosamines, which have been shown to be potent carcinogens in experimental systems. These and other chemicals that may cause cancer are under intensive study epidemiologically, clinically, and in the laboratory.

More recently, investigators have also suggested that high meat intake may cause colorectal cancer through the effects of meat on the bile salts. Bile salts, which different individuals produce in varying amounts, do not cause cancer themselves; however, they do resemble certain carcinogenic substances in chemical structure. Some people who eat a lot of meat may develop a large population of a specific strain of anaerobic bacteria in the large bowel. These bacteria can biologically transform bile acids in a way that may render them capable of producing cancer. While evidence for this theory of cancer causation is limited, it is an important hypothesis that integrates external factors (particularly meat) and internal factors (bile acid production), and which would explain the long suspected importance of bacteria in causing cancer of the colon. (It has been suggested that the reason that cancer of the large bowel is much more common than cancer of the small bowel may be the much greater bacterial population of the large bowel.)

The study of gastrointestinal cancer has advanced through a multidisciplinary approach—one combining epidemiological with chemical, biochemical, microbiological, and clinical studies—that exemplifies the type of research program needed to unravel the causative factors in all forms of cancer.

But epidemiologic studies have one important limitation; they can only be used to determine the distribution and causation of a disease after that disease has spread significantly through the population. The epidemiologic study of cancer poses special problems. Because of the time lag observed in the effects of many carcinogens, population studies may not be able to link certain substances to cancer until they have been in the environment for many years. And the number of new chemicals, pollutants, and other materials introduced into the environment is growing at an ever increasing rate. Epidemiologic surveillance is still valuable, in fact, essential, but it is not an ideal method for detecting carcinogenic substances and, ultimately, for preventing cancer.

Clearly, the ideal must be to determine the potential health hazard posed by various substances before they are introduced into the environment. Basic and applied research is now becoming increasingly directed toward the goal of identifying the chemical carcinogens experimentally. Carcinogenic properties may be suggested by a substance's chemical structure; but a better test is the effect of the agent on experimental cultures of cells. Most known chemical carcinogens are mutagens, that is, they cause mutations; they can alter the genetic apparatus of bacteria and mammalian cells in a way that changes the cell's biochemical or biological behavior. A first step in determining whether or not a given material is carcinogenic is to discover whether or not it is mutagenic. This can now be accomplished by studying the effects of chemicals in bacterial systems.

Studies of the biological effects of many different chemicals have indicated that a large and increasing number of mutagens have in fact been introduced into the environment since the Second World War; but the real risk posed by these substances is difficult to evaluate. In spite of the introduction of these mutagens, the overall incidence of cancer (except for lung cancer) has not increased in the thirty years since the Second World War. How can these conflicting observations be reconciled?

In the first place, not all mutagens are carcinogenic; and second, even those that do produce cancerous transformation of cells in an experimental situation may not do so in real life. Some chemicals may alter animal cells in culture to produce all the cellular characteristics of cancer, and these transformed cells may actually cause cancer when injected back into the animal from which they were originally taken; and yet many of these apparent carcinogens will not induce cancer when administered directly to experimental animals. These substances may be chemically modified, and inactivated, in the animal's body (usually by enzymes in the liver).

Conversely, some chemicals may have carcinogenic effects in life that are not readily apparent from experimental studies. Certain agents that are themselves harmless in the laboratory may be transformed by the liver into substances capable of causing cancer. Furthermore, chemicals that have a low but significant carcinogenic effect are very difficult to identify experimentally. An agent capable of producing cancer in only 1 percent of the population could cause up to two million cases of cancer in the United States if it were widely introduced into the environment; but it is enormously complex and difficult to design an experiment to identify agents that can cause cancer in 1 percent or less of the experimental animals tested. One major problem is that the background incidence of cancer, and the ability to induce cancer with known chemical carcinogens, varies widely among animal species.

Even when agents suspected of causing cancer have been identified, the regulation of those agents is a complicated task that must take political, industrial, moral, and cultural factors into account. Progress in civilization has resulted largely from environmental manipulation and control and has always exacted some price. The relative merits and debits of any environmental change must be carefully considered and balanced, both in terms of the effect on society and the effect on the individual.

A sobering observation in cancer research and health research generally is that identification of a health hazard does not automatically lead to its elimination, even when this could be accomplished through individual choice. It has been known for at least twenty years that smoking is a major cause of cancer and of heart, lung, and other diseases. And yet the absolute incidence of cigarette smoking has not diminished over that period of time. A growing field of research is the study of the organic and psychological factors involved in motivation, habituation, and other fundamental determinants of the individual's life style.

Although they are certainly very important, chemical mutagens may be only one source of human cancer. Of special interest to researchers has been the theory that certain types of cancer in man may actually be due to viral infection.

Tumor Viruses

Viruses have been known since the turn of the century to be capable of causing cancer in experimental animals. Many forms of experimental cancer in animals, particularly leukemias and lymphomas in a variety of species, are induced by viruses. Agents which can cause cancer in such a large variety of subhuman species might reasonably be expected to be the cause of at least some forms of human cancer. Although extensive studies have not yet been able to demonstrate conclusively that any form of human cancer is virus-induced, the indirect evidence for several types of tumors is compelling. If viruses do play a role in human cancer, it is very likely that the epidemiology and pathogenesis of these diseases differ markedly from the pattern seen in classical virus infections.

Basic research has helped to clarify the biochemical mechanism by which tumor viruses may cause cancer. Many studies have focused on relatively simple viruses, such as SV40, that can produce tumors in animals and transform cells in culture. The genetic material of SV40 (coded in deoxyribonucleic acid, or DNA) is small; at most, the virus contains only five or six genes. The virus reproduces itself by attaching to a mammalian cell and injecting its DNA into the cell itself. The viral

DNA may then either replicate within the host cell and form new viruses, or it may become integrated into the DNA of the infected cell; in the latter case, every daughter cell of the host cell will also contain a complete copy of the genetic information contained in the virus. When the viral DNA is integrated into the host cell's DNA, the cell undergoes transformation and becomes cancerous. Most of SV40's genes control the production of proteins essential to the reproduction of the virus and to its integration into the host cell's DNA. Presumably, the remaining one or two genes must control the all-important process of cellular transformation. Research into the function of this part of the viral DNA has begun to uncover the mechanism behind transformation; a viral protein produced by these genes seems to play a central role in the process.

Many known tumor viruses contain not DNA, but RNA (ribonucleic acid). For a long time it was unclear how RNA viruses could effect the changes in the cell's DNA that lead to transformation. After James Watson and Francis Crick developed their model of DNA, molecular biologists came to accept what was dubbed the "central dogma": DNA makes RNA makes protein. The basic idea was that DNA serves as a template for the synthesis of RNA, which in turn directs protein synthesis within the cell; in this way the genetic code of DNA is expressed. The central dogma described no mechanism whereby RNA could direct the synthesis of DNA or change the information coded in a DNA strand; and the effects of RNA-containing tumor viruses on cellular DNA thus remained mysterious. This mystery was solved fairly recently when H. M. Temin and David Baltimore demonstrated the enzyme complex known as reverse transcriptase, which can produce DNA from the RNA of certain tumor viruses. It now appears that DNA formed from tumor virus RNA in this manner can be integrated into the DNA of the host cell and cause transformation.

It is clear that the factors controlling the action of tumor viruses are highly complex; hereditary factors, chemicals, and radiation may all affect the invasion and replication of a tumor virus. But current studies in tumor virology are making major progress in fundamental areas, and this basic research will certainly produce observations that will be useful in the treatment of cancer and possibly of other diseases as well.

The study of cancer causation is obviously essential if cancer is ever to be prevented effectively. Equally important are areas of basic research that may indicate ways to arrest the progress of cancer once the initial tumor has formed. One key area has been the study of immunological mechanisms that may be important in the destruction of tumors.

Tumor Immunology

Tumor cells contain unique antigenic material that is not found in normal cells. This fundamental observation has been confirmed by investigators studying a number of different experimental systems with a variety of techniques; extensive research has involved special inbred strains of mice, while other studies have been carried out in human subjects.

The presence of special antigens on the surface of tumor cells makes it possible for the body's immunologic defenses to recognize those cells and destroy them. Proponents of the "immunologic surveillance hypothesis" have suggested that tumor cells are actually formed quite often in the body as the result of random mutation, but that these cells are rapidly destroyed by the defense system of normal, healthy individuals. According to this idea, the basis for the development of cancer in the individual could be seen as a failure of the immune system. There is some evidence for this hypothesis. A number of inherited diseases associated with immunologic deficiency are also linked to an increased incidence of cancer. And patients who receive immunosuppressive drugs following organ transplants (for example, kidney transplants) also run a high risk of developing cancer. However, immunologically suppressed patients tend to develop different kinds of cancer with different frequencies from those of individuals in the population at large; so factors other than immunodeficiency must be important in the genesis of cancer and in determining what kind of cancer will develop.

The study of tumor immunology has been intimately connected to the study of immunology in general (see Chapter 7). Both B and T lymphocytes seem to be involved in the immunological response to tumor cells; but it is now clear that the interrelationship of the many different types of T and B lymphocytes, in tumor immunity as well as in other types of immunity, is exceedingly complex. Some types of T lymphocytes may actually inhibit the immunological destruction of tumor cells. As these phenomena become better understood, methods of treatment aimed at boosting tumor immunity will certainly improve.

At present, approaches to improving tumor immunity in cancer have been developed from experimental models and empirical clinical trials. Some methods involve the relatively nonspecific augmentation of the immune response. The agent most widely used for this purpose is the attenuated tubercle bacterium BCG (see Chapter 5); experiments in rodents and some clinical studies have suggested that BCG may exert an antitumor effect in the presence of small numbers of tumor cells. A second approach specifically stimulates immunity against the tumor by developing a response against tumor antigens. There is evidence that these antigens can be used to program T lymphocytes in the laboratory to kill tumor cells; the possibility of returning these programmed lymphocytes to the cancer patient for therapeutic purposes is now being studied. Methods of transferring immunity from a donor to the patient (including the transfer of stimulated lymphocytes) are also being investigated.

Experimental and clinical studies indicate that immunotherapy is ineffective against advanced forms of cancer. On the other hand, immunotherapy may be quite effective experimentally in eradicating microscopic foci of disease. Drug treatment (chemotherapy) is more potent than immunotherapy and is probably more appropriate than immunotherapy for the treatment of advanced cancer. But immunotherapy, while less potent, has greater specificity for tumor cells and thus is less likely to produce adverse side effects in the patient. For these reasons many modern approaches combine chemotherapy and immunotherapy in the treatment of cancer.

The quest for a single effective cancer cure is largely a creation of the popular press. There are actually many approaches that are effective, either singly or in combination, in the treatment of different types of cancer in different stages of development. The techniques that have proved most successful so far have been chemotherapy, surgery, and radiotherapy.

Chemotherapy

Perhaps the most important problem in the drug treatment of cancer is to develop agents that will effectively kill tumor cells while doing as little damage as possible to the healthy cells of the body. For this reason, the discovery of quantitative differences between tumor and healthy cells (often resulting from the study of the molecular biology of tumors) has been very useful in improving the drug treatment of cancer.

Biochemical differences between the cellular metabolism of tumor and normal cells may be exploited in drug therapy. Tumor cells may contain enzymes which differ from those found in normal cells and which may catalyze biochemical reactions at a different rate in tumor than in normal cells. Agents may be developed to inhibit selectively the activity of certain essential enzymes in tumor cells without drastically affecting the enzymes that perform the same function in normal cells. Some tumor cells lose the capacity to synthesize the amino acids asparagine, cysteine, and methionine and may need to be supplied with these if they are to survive. Approaches are being developed to remove these amino acids from the medium in which tumor cells grow (for example, by introducing an enzyme that degrades asparagine); these techniques have already been shown to destroy tumor cells selectively in experimental systems and in man. Some of the newer antibiotics (such as the anthracyclines) attack biochemical and molecular targets inside the cell with substantial specificity and have important antitumor activity both experimentally and clinically. And naturally occurring compounds, like the alkaloid chemicals found in many types of plants, are being studied in order to determine their possible use as antitumor agents.

The methodology for using different chemotherapeutic agents in combination has developed rapidly over the past decade and has already substantially improved the treatment of many types of relatively advanced cancer. Even the most effective chemotherapeutic agent may have no effect on one tumor cell in a million. If such a drug is given when there are a billion tumor cells (out of some 40 trillion cells in the patient's body) a thousand tumor cells may survive, and the cancer will not be eradicated. But if another equally effective drug with a different mechanism of action is given simultaneously, a better opportunity for cure exists, since the thousand cells that were resistant to the first drug should be destroyed by the second. Combination chemotherapy can be designed to minimize the dangerous side effects that may accompany drug doses high enough to be effective in the treatment of cancer. Two different agents which both have the same toxic effects (for example, depression of bone marrow function) could only be used together safely if the dosage of each were decreased to half the dosage used when either drug was given alone. But when two drugs with qualitatively different mechanisms of action and side effects are given, both drugs may be employed at full dosage to achieve an additive effect.

Combination chemotherapeutic programs have already been developed for the treatment of two types of cancer of the lymph tissue, histiocytic lymphoma and disseminated Hodgkin's disease. Even the best drugs when given alone could produce complete remission in no more than 10 percent of patients with these disorders. With combination chemotherapy, complete remission is now achieved in more than 80 percent of all cases; and with appropriate treatment during remission, 30 to 60 percent may be cured. Recently, chemotherapy has been effectively combined with surgery and radiotherapy in cancer treatment.

Surgery and Radiotherapy

Surgery and radiotherapy are the major local forms of treatment for cancer and are capable of curing 35 to 40 percent of all cancer patients (excluding those suffering from skin cancer). These methods are generally curative if the tumor is sufficiently localized. A major drawback is that the removal of tumors by surgery or radiotherapy may often leave behind microscopic numbers of tumor cells, which can then spread and cause a relapse. In circumstances where the risk of relapse is known to be especially high, chemotherapy may be employed immediately following tumor removal. (Chemotherapy actually works best against small or microscopic quantities of tumor cells.) Studies have indicated that such a program of chemotherapy significantly decreases the risk of relapse from osteogenic sarcoma (a type of bone cancer) and breast cancer in certain stages. The maximum follow-up time in these studies was only four years, however; and further follow-up will be necessary to determine whether or not chemotherapy following tumor removal actually increases the likelihood of cure as well as preventing short-term relapse.

Ongoing research is directed at improving the clinical techniques of radiotherapy. Subatomic charged particles are now known to release energy in a much more controllable and localized manner than does conventional electromagnetic radiation. If these particles could be selectively introduced into tumors, it might be possible to damage tumor tissue while leaving the surrounding normal tissues relatively intact. Tumors may also be selectively destroyed through the use of radiosensitizers. Many agents can increase the susceptibility of cellular DNA (and hence of the cell itself) to radiational damage; these agents may incorporate themselves into the DNA of the cell, inhibit enzymes that repair damaged DNA, or may operate by other mechanisms that are less well understood. When these radiosensitizers can be made to concentrate selectively in tumors or to exert a greater effect on tumors than on normal tissue, the procedure of radiotherapy will destroy tumors more effectively with less danger to the patient.

Endocrinology and Cancer

The interaction of the body's hormones with tumor growth is now being studied in the hope of finding new ways to curtail the growth of malignant tumors. As long ago as 1940, Charles B. Huggins demonstrated that certain tumors would only grow in the presence of specific hormones and could be treated by hormone deprivation. Cancer of the prostate and breast may be hormone dependent and may undergo regression following removal of the testes and ovaries respectively. But obviously, such radical surgery has major consequences for the individual; and the uncertain effectiveness of such treatment especially limited its applicability.

It has now become possible to determine accurately which patients will benefit by surgical hormone deprivation. We now know that the action of sex hormones is mediated by specific cellular proteins. It has been shown that estrogen deprivation, entailing removal of the ovaries and often of the adrenal glands, is an effective treatment for breast cancer only when the tumor cells contain specific protein "binders" for estrogen. Since the presence of hormone binders is a clear indication that the patient could benefit from hormone deprivation, the necessary surgical procedures can now be performed selectively on only those patients likely to be benefited by them.

One possible therapeutic alternative to surgical hormone deprivation involves the use of antihormones, that is, substances that interfere with hormone activity. Antihormones are now being identified and used experimentally, and in preliminary clinical trials, to prevent hormones from supporting the growth of tumor cells.

Hormone research has had important implications for the detection as well as the treatment of cancer. It has been known for a long time that certain tumors, including some cancers of the lung and kidney, may infrequently result in syndromes associated with excessive production of the polypeptide hormones (hormones that resemble proteins in molecular structure, but which are much smaller than proteins). It is now possible to measure excessive hormone production directly by radioimmunoassay, a method that uses radioactive antibodies to the substance one wishes to detect (see Chapter 18). Radioimmunoassay can be used to detect elevated hormone levels that are still below the level required to develop associated symptoms. Studies using this technique over the past several years have indicated that several cancers are associated with the excessive release of polypeptide hormones at a subclinical level. No one yet understands this phenomenon, although it seems that the association between cancer and hormone production must eventually prove a source of some insight into the fundamental nature of the disease. But these observations have already provided an effective means of evaluating the presence of a tumor, the extent to which it has grown, and, particularly, the effectiveness of antitumor treatment.

Methods of cancer detection have become an increasingly important subject of research; early detection of cancer is essential if the disease is to be caught when tumors are still small and localized, and when there is the greatest possibility for cure.

Cancer Detection

Several methods for the early diagnosis of cancer have already been put into widespread use, with encouraging results. Probably the best example has been the use of the Papanicolau (Pap) smear (which consists of scraping off and examining cells from the uterine cervix) in the prevention of cervical cancer. It is now generally agreed that the Pap smear has brought about the significant decrease in the death rate from cancer of the cervix that has been observed in the United States. More complex detection techniques have also been developed; these include cellular studies, specialized radiologic techniques (such as mammography and xerography), and endoscopic examination.

Recently, the technology of cancer detection has been greatly advanced by the introduction of computers to radiography. Computerized scanning can now locate tumors as small as one centimeter in the brain and other areas of the body that are hard to examine through conventional radiographic methods. Another development of major importance has been the introduction of radioactive substances that concentrate within or around certain tumors, thus making those tumors easier to detect radiographically. These sophisticated techniques have already proved useful and will certainly play an increasingly important role in cancer detection in the future.

Tumor immunology has also provided new methods for the early detection of malignant tumors. Under certain conditions, antigens may split off from the surface of tumor cells and enter the bloodstream. It may then be possible to detect these antigens with sensitive techniques like radioimmunoassay. At present, tumor cell-surface antigens can only be detected in patients whose cancer has already reached an advanced state; but it is hoped that similar methods may be developed to detect tumors at an early stage, when they are still small and have not yet spread.

As a growing number of effective screening tests for cancer are developed, epidemiologic factors must be considered in their application. It is not practicable, and probably not even desirable, to perform all these diagnostic tests on an unselected population; a better approach would be to administer them only to individuals who have been identified as being at high risk for the development of a certain type of cancer. It is now becoming possible to identify those people who are especially susceptible to different cancers. Epidemiologic (and sometimes genetic) factors that increase the risk of cancer of the breast, lung, and cervix have already been determined, and knowledge of these variables has made it possible to conduct detection surveys more rationally.

Cancer research has been controversial for a variety of political, clinical, and academic reasons. Researchers in this area have debated whether more funds should be allocated to clinical or to basic research, to the study of virology or the identification of chemical carcinogens, to drug research or to tumor immunology. But progress and controversy go hand in hand. These sometimes bitter debates do not arise from the failure of any given approach but rather from the rapid emergence of many new findings in several areas. The controversy in cancer research reflects the speed of progress in many different yet closely interrelated approaches to the problem of cancer.

Genetic Disorders

RICHARD W. ERBE

4

Genetics is a field with applications in virtually all other areas of medicine; it has often been stated that every disease is influenced by genetic factors. Geneticists are concerned with the variation observed between individuals over the entire span of development from conception to old age. Viewed in this perspective, genetic disorders represent extremes of variation of one or more attributes. The point at which genetically caused variation comes to be defined as constituting a disease is sometimes arbitrary; but the presence of a substantial degree of functional impairment usually distinguishes a genetic disorder from the extensive variation that we expect between so-called normal individuals.

Health Burden Imposed by Genetic Disorders

Birth defects, a leading cause of death in infancy, are often genetically caused. Since these serious disorders are manifest so early in life, many more "life years" are lost to genetically caused birth defects than to conditions that are usually seen as more threatening. For instance, it has been estimated that such birth defects claim over four times as many life years as does heart disease, eight times as many as cancer, and ten times as many as stroke. And even when they are not fatal, birth defects may produce chronic disability of physical functions, mental retardation, or both.

It has been estimated that serious genetic defects are present in about 4 percent of newborns. About 40 percent of all infant mortality results from genetic factors, and 20 to 30 percent of all pediatric hospital admissions are related primarily to genetic disorders, with malformations being the commonest cause for hospitalization in North America. Present overall estimates indicate that 12 million Americans have genetically caused birth defects. In addition to substantially decreasing the individual's potential capabilities and contributions, these disorders often necessitate expensive, long-term medical care, which is usually palliative rather than curative.

Genetic disorders may take their toll even earlier, during the period from conception to birth. About 40 percent of conceptions end in spontaneous abortion; somewhat over half of these occur so early that the woman may not be aware she is pregnant. Major chromosomal abnormalities are present in a substantial proportion of all conceptions and are a leading cause of this fetal loss. Undoubtedly many additional spontaneous abortions result from genetic metabolic abnormalities which are not as readily detected as chromosomal changes.

In contrast, other genetic disorders have their most serious consequences later in childhood, in adulthood, or even in middle or old age. The time delay before serious manifestations of these genetic disorders appear and our limited ability to identify major genetic problems before they become clinically apparent may lead us to underestimate the true extent of genetically caused disability. Even today, many physicians and laymen still think of genetic disorders as rare. Until recently almost all genetic disorders were estimated to occur in only 1/100,000 to 1/10,000 of all live births. It is true that many of the more than 2,000 genetic disorders identified so far actually are that rare. But it has now become clear (partly through mass screening programs) that some serious, specific genetic disorders occur in 1/500 or even 1/100 of the general population. And even the rarer types of birth defects represent a substantial health care burden when considered together. Finally, it has long been recognized that certain groups of people distinguishable by geographic origin, race, religion, ethnic background, or other factors run a particularly high risk for some specific genetic disorders which are correlated with (but not caused by) these demographic variables.

There is another reason why the incidence of genetic disorders has only recently been appreciated. The science of genetics has just now progressed to a point where these disorders could be identified, studied, and understood. Although the investigation of inheritance began over a century ago, this work did not begin to find clinical application until the last few decades.

The History of Medical Genetics

The study of human genetics began haltingly, with gaps of many years separating important milestones. Disorders now recognized as genetic have been described since earliest written history. Yet the science of genetics was born when the work of the Austrian monk Gregor Mendel was published in 1865.

Mendel, using sweet peas, deduced the mathematical rules by which hereditary characteristics are passed from generation to generation. To appreciate the magnitude of his accomplishment, one must realize that the functions of the cell nucleus were totally unknown and chromosomes had not yet been recognized, even the word gene did not originate until more than forty years later. Indeed, Mendel's laws, as they are now called, were unappreciated until 1900 when his work was rediscovered and others began to test its general validity in a variety of plants and animals.

By the turn of the century an English physician named Archibald Garrod had begun to make the first major contributions to the study of human genetics. In 1897, through his studies of urinary pigments, he encountered a patient with dark-colored urine and a disease called alkaptonuria, which, according to the theory of the day, resulted from abnormal microbial fermentation within the gut. Garrod's subsequent studies of this patient and others with alkaptonuria led him to reject the popular fermentation theory and to characterize the disorder instead as a "freak" of metabolism. His observation of in-breeding in the parents of many alkaptonuric patients was published in *The Lancet* in 1901 and caught the attention of the geneticist William Bateson, who recognized the precise correspondence to a pattern of inheritance that had been described by Mendel. In 1908 Garrod published a book containing the results of his studies on alkaptonuria and three other diseases (including albinism) which he designated "inborn errors of metabolism." Garrod suggested that in persons with each of these conditions there was a block in some specific metabolic reaction due to the deficiency from birth of a specific enzyme.

As with Mendel, the significance of Garrod's insights was not widely appreciated for several decades. In 1941 studies of mutant strains of yeast with specific requirements for growth led George Beadle and Edward Tatum to formulate the "one gene–one enzyme" hypothesis that metabolic blocks due to the deficiency of a specific enzyme result from alteration of single genes. In 1952 Gerty Cori and Carl Cori produced the first direct evidence that a human inborn error of metabolism, called glycogen storage disease type I, is the consequence of deficient activity of a specific enzyme. (The Coris showed that glycogen, a complex carbo-hydrate, accumulates in large quantities in the liver of affected indi-viduals because of a deficiency of the enzyme necessary to catalyze a step in its breakdown and utilization.) And in 1958 Bert LaDu finally con-firmed biochemically Garrod's prediction of a specific enzyme deficiency in alkaptonuria.

Since the late 1940s new findings in diverse research fields have been brought together to provide a firm scientific basis for an identifiable discipline of human genetics. Many types of hereditary abnormality are now understood. Genetic disorders are inherited in different ways; and some important disorders of the genetic material are not really inherited from the parents. On the basis of their causes genetic disorders can be divided into three basic groups: the chromosome disorders, the Mendelian (or single-gene) disorders, and the multifactorial (or polygenic) dis-orders.

The Chromosome Disorders

Chromosomes are structures within the cell composed of highly coiled deoxyribonucleic acid (DNA) and protein; in their DNA the chromosomes contain all the genetic information for every cell. Although chromosomes were first described in the 1870s, it was not until 1956 that the number of human chromosomes was correctly determined to be 46. Twenty-three like-membered pairs of chromosomes are present in all cells of the body except the sex cells (ova and sperm); one member of each pair is inherited from the mother and one from the father. (Each sex cell contains 23 unpaired chromosomes.) The different types of chromosomes can be identified by size, overall shape, and by specific details present on some chromosomes. In 1959 the first three chromosome disorders were described in rapid succession. The study of two of these disorders led to an understanding of human sex determination. It was discovered that two of the 46 human chromosomes are sex chromosomes that are alike in females but not in males; females have two X chromosomes, and males have an X and a Y chromosome (Figure 4-1).

Chromosome disorders result from deviations in the amount of chromosomal material present. Portions of individual chromosomes may be absent (deletions) or may be detached from their normal locations and attached instead to other chromosomes (translocation); or an extra segment of one chromosome may be present. Entire individual chromo-

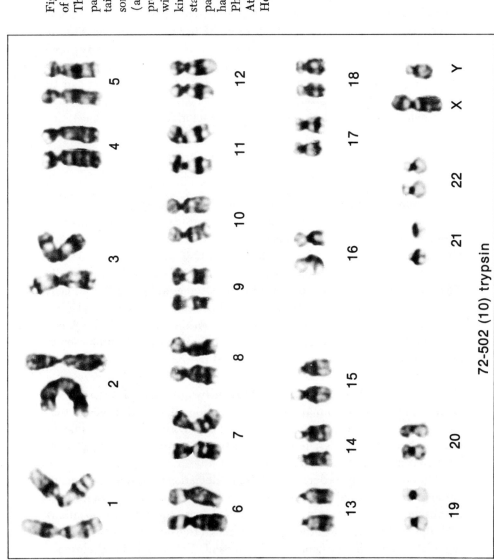

Figure 4–1. The chromosomes of a normal (46,XY) male. This banded karyotype shows a pattern called G banding obtained by exposing the chromosomes to a solution of trypsin (an enzyme that breaks down protein) and then staining them with Leishman stain. (Another kind of staining, Giemsa staining, also gives a G banding pattern in chromosomes that have been exposed to trypsin.) Photograph courtesy of Leonard Atkins, Massachusetts General Hospital, Boston.

72-502 (10) trypsin

somes can also be missing or present in extra numbers. In short, the chromosome disorders can be described as diseases of too much or too little chromosome material, or too many or too few chromosomes.

The causes of the various chromosomal disorders are unknown; but in almost all instances, they are not inherited. In other words, these disorders are not transmitted by a parent who had similar chromosomal abnormalities. Instead, they arise in the children of normal parents through abnormalities in the egg or the sperm at the time of conception. These "sporadic" chromosome disorders are nonetheless classified as genetic because they involve the chromosomes, which are the carriers of genetic material.

Chromosome abnormalities are a major cause of spontaneous abortions, particularly those which occur in the first half of pregnancy. But 5 to 10 percent of fetuses with serious abnormalities may survive gestation and birth. Nearly three quarters of these disorders cannot be detected by physical examination of the infant, but only by chromosome analysis or karyotyping. Studies in which populations of infants have been surveyed by karyotype analysis at birth indicate that about 1/150 of all newborns suffer from major chromosome abnormalities, most of which have a detrimental effect on the child's physical or mental function, or both.

The chromosome disorders can be divided into two major classes: those which involve the sex chromosomes and those which affect some of the other 22 pairs of chromosomes (the autosomes).

Down's syndyrome, a form of severe mental retardation associated with definite physical and chemical abnormalities, is the most common of the autosomal chromosome disorders (see Chapter 10). It is caused by the presence of extra material from the chromosome number 21; either an entire extra chromosome or an extra segment of the chromosome may be responsible. Unfortunately, the precise mechanism by which this extra chromosome material produces these abnormalities remains unknown.

Ninety-five percent of all cases of Down's syndrome result from the presence of an entire extra chromosome number 21, called trisomy 21 Down's syndrome. Of the remaining 5 percent, about 2 percent of the total have so-called mosaic Down's syndrome in which the separation of the chromosomes has been disrupted sometime after the first cell division following fertilization so that some cells have trisomy 21 and others are entirely normal. In general the severity of the resulting abnormalities is proportional to the number of cells which contain the extra chromosomes. The remainder of cases of Down's syndrome, about 3 percent of the total, results from the presence of an extra copy of only a portion of chromosome 21 which has become attached to another chromosome. In about one third of all such cases of translocation Down's syndrome, one parent, usually the mother, will be found to be an unaffected carrier of this translocation in its "balanced" state; that is, she or he has only one normal chromosome 21 in addition to the translocated segment, instead of the two normal chromosomes 21 plus the translocated segment present in the affected child. (The parent thus has a normal amount of chromosome 21 material and is unaffected by the translocation.) It is only when one parent has a balanced translocation of chromosome 21—a circumstance that accounts for only 1 percent of all cases of Down's syndrome—that the defect is actually inherited.

The most frequent of the sex chromosome disorders is Klinefelter's syndrome, which occurs in about 1/1,000 male births. This disorder results from the presence of an extra X chromosome, which gives a 47,XXY chromosome makeup. (Normal females with 46 chromosomes have two X chromosomes and are designated 46,XX, while normal males have one X and one Y chromosome and are designated 46,XY.) Individuals with Klinefelter's syndrome appear to be normal males until puberty, when they develop eunuchoid body proportions with breast enlargement and sparse facial hair. The testes fail to function and produce neither sperm nor adequate amounts of male hormones, so that affected individuals are sterile. Male hormones can be administered to achieve appropriate masculinization but do not correct the sterility nor the complex behavioral abnormalities which are usually present.

Almost as frequent as Klinefelter's syndrome is the occurrence in males of an extra Y chromosome, resulting in a 47,XYY chromosome makeup. The features of this syndrome are still incompletely characterized but it is known that these males are unusually tall, are normally masculinized and fertile, and do not pass on sex chromosome disorders to their sons. (XYY males might be expected to produce sperm with extra chromosomes and thus pass on the abnormality; but unidentified factors apparently select against the production or function of sperm with extra sex chromosomes in these males.) It is likely that XYY individuals have unusual behavior patterns, but the nature, severity, and even the existence of specific XYY behavior abnormalities are still in question. Since the initial observation that XYY individuals were found with unusually high frequency as inmates of institutions for the criminally insane, much misinformation has been widely disseminated in connection with sensational trials of bizarre individuals. Convicted mass murderer Richard Speck, who was widely thought to have a 47,XYY chromosome makeup, was actually known by medical and legal authorities from the outset of the trial to be a chromosomally normal 47,XY male. It now seems clear that the behavioral alterations which may result from the 47,XYY chromosome makeup are complex and cannot be characterized simply as "a tendency to criminal and impulsive behavior"; still, the behavioral correlates of this not uncommon chromosome pattern are important enough to merit further study.

An extra X chromosome (47,XXX), which occurs in about 1/1,100 of female births, is apparently not a cause of abnormality. In contrast, Turner's syndrome, resulting from the absence of one sex chromosome (45,X), results characteristically in short stature, a shield-like chest with widely spaced nipples, cardiovascular malformations, and other changes, all of which are apparent at birth. At puberty, the breasts do not develop and menstrual periods do not occur; although these changes can be induced by the administration of female sex hormones, the sterility associated with Turner's syndrome (resulting from a failure of the ovaries to develop) is irreversible. Behavioral changes are seen beyond those attributable to the hormonal and physical abnormalities of Turner's syndrome. The severity of the impairment produced by the 45,X makeup is suggested by the high frequency with which it results in spontaneous abortion; only 1/64 of 45,X conceptions are liveborn, and only about 1/10,000 of live female births are 45,X. About 40 percent of these individuals show chromosomal mosaicism, with both 46,XX and 45,X cells being present; as with mosaic Down's syndrome, the degree of abnormality is correlated with the proportion of 45,X cells.

One important clue to the mechanism of the chromosome disorders has been the observation that maternal age dramatically increases the risk that a child will be born with trisomy 21 Down's syndrome (see Chapter 10) or with trisomies 18 or 13 (rare conditions in which an extra chromosome number 18 or 13 is present). Children of older mothers run an increased risk of being born with Klinefelter's syndrome (47,XXY) as well. The mechanisms that may underlie this observed correlation are under active investigation.

New insight into the mechanism of chromosome disorders may also come from innovations in the techniques for identifying the different chromosomes and studying their function. The study of chromosomes was revolutionized in 1970 with the introduction of banding techniques that allow the researcher to stain different areas of the individual chromosomes. The bands thus seen are much larger than individual genes; even the smallest band probably contains dozens if not hundreds of genes. But these staining techniques reveal details of chromosomal structure that allow each chromosome to be identified uniquely, make it possible to detect rearrangements of very small segments of chromosomes, and can be used to visualize many variations that are not associated with any apparent abnormality. Banding techniques are a vast improvement over conventional karyotyping, which is often made especially problematic by structural abnormalities that may exist in the chromosomes being studied (Figures 4-1 and 4-2).

The banding techniques have been useful not only clinically but also in research to map the location on human chromosomes of specific genes for enzymes and other proteins. The method, in brief, is as follows. Rela-

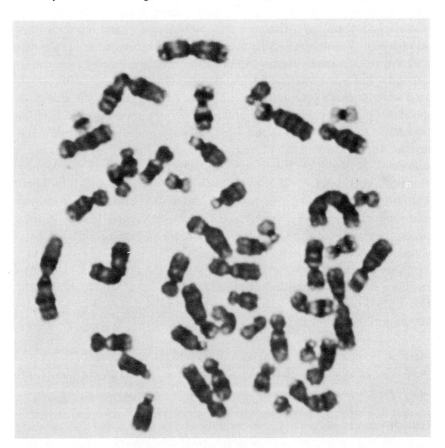

Figure 4–2. The original picture from which Figure 4–1 was taken. Chromosomes from a cell were stained and then photographed at the metaphase stage of cell division to give the picture shown here. The pictures of individual chromosomes were then cut apart from each other and rearranged in pairs to give Figure 4–1. Photograph courtesy of Leonard Atkins, Massachusetts General Hospital, Boston.

tively hardy and unspecialized cells called fibroblasts can be taken from the skin and cultured outside the body in special serum-containing media where they will grow, multiply, and produce many of the enzymes and other proteins present in the human body. Where human fibroblasts are mixed in culture with fibroblasts from the mouse and certain viruses or chemicals are added to promote interaction of the cell membranes, some cells will fuse completely to form hybrid cells that initially contain complete sets on both human and mouse chromosomes. For reasons still incompletely understood, during subsequent divisions of these hybrid cells the human chromosomes are randomly but progressively eliminated. Eventually cells are produced that retain a complete set of mouse chromosomes but only a single human chromosome; the specific human chromosome differs between different hybrid cells and can be identified through banding techniques. The hybrid cell can then be analyzed to determine which specific human enzymes and other proteins it makes; and in this way the genes present on the human chromosome in that cell can be determined. To date about 100 genes have been mapped to specific human chromosomes in this way, and all chromosomes except number 22 have at least one mapped gene on them. This is a major accomplishment which has been carried out just over the last few years.

Mendelian Disorders

The Mendelian or single-gene disorders, which are inherited according to the classic patterns described by Mendel, do not involve abnormalities of whole chromosomes or relatively large portions of chromosomes; instead, they stem from small but important changes in a minute fraction of the DNA that makes up the genes.

Each gene on the 22 pairs of autosomal chromosomes is represented twice in each cell, once on each member of the chromosome pair. Recall that the individual inherits one member of each chromosome pair, and therefore half of his or her genes, from each parent. Studies indicate that about 20 percent of an average person's gene pairs contain different genes from the mother and father; in other words, each individual shows this type of internal variation for at least 20,000 of the 100,000 genes estimated to be present in each cell. One can appreciate intuitively that the degree of variation between two unrelated individuals must be vastly greater. It is thus no mystery that no two persons (except identical twins) are exactly alike genetically.

While a very large proportion of genes vary within and between individuals, a relatively small number of these variant genes result in genetic disorders. Autosomal dominant disorders can be produced by an abnormal gene present on only one member of an autosomal chromosome pair, even if the gene for that same function on the other member of the chromosome pair is normal. In contrast, autosomal recessive disorders occur only when two disease-producing genes are present, one on each member of the chromosome pair. An individual having a recessive gene on one chromosome but not on the other, designated a carrier, can pass the gene on to offspring but does not manifest a genetic disorder (Figure 4-3). (It has been estimated that each of us is a carrier of six to eight

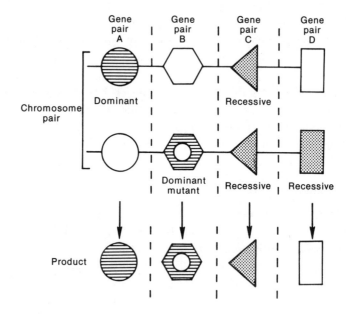

Figure 4–3. The expression of autosomal dominant and recessive traits. In schematic form, this diagram shows how different types of gene pairs determining individual traits are expressed. When one member of the gene pair is dominant, the product of that gene pair—some genetically determined trait— will be entirely determined by the dominant gene. This situation is shown here for gene pairs A and B; in gene pair B, a new type of abnormal trait has developed through the mutation of one gene to a dominant form. Both genes of gene pair C are the same recessive form; this is the only situation in which a completely recessive gene can be expressed. If only one of the genes is recessive, as in gene pair D, the individual is a carrier and does not show the recessive trait. For many genetic disorders, however, the carrier state can be detected using special tests even though the carrier does not manifest the disorder.

recessive genes for disorders which would have been exceedingly serious if we had inherited a like pair of genes.) In the third major Mendelian pattern, X-linked recessive, the sex of the individual is an important factor in the expression of the disorder. Females have two X chromosomes, one inherited from the father and one from the mother. Even if one of these X chromosomes bears an abnormal recessive gene, the other will likely have a normal gene to prevent a deficiency, making that female a carrier who does not experience a genetic disorder herself. Males, however, have only one X chromosome, the other member of the sex chromosome pair being the Y, which has a different (and still almost entirely unknown) genetic makeup. Lacking a second, normal gene, the abnormal X-linked recessive gene on the single X chromosome of the male will be expressed as a genetic disorder.

Many Mendelian disorders which initially appear to form a single disease entity are shown on further study to be divisible into two or more separate disorders associated with distinctly different modes of inheritance, clinical features, biochemical changes, or pathological abnormalities. A publication in 1958 listed 412 Mendelian disorders. Ten years later, Victor A. McKusick had catalogued some 1,545 Mendelian disorders and single gene products; and the 1975 edition of his catalogue contains 2,336 listings. About half of these disorders are well established, and half are probably or possibly separate and specific disease entities. Although this increased recognition has been dramatic, the one or two thousand Mendelian disorders currently recognized constitute abnormalities of a mere 1 or 2 percent of the 100,000 genes probably present in the whole human genetic constitution. Clearly there is still much research to be done in delineating additional Mendelian disorders.

Let us consider briefly a few examples of the vast array of Mendelian or single-gene disorders.

Recent evidence suggests that the most common of the serious autosomal dominant disorders is the group of hyperlipidemias. About 2 percent of the general population has a gene which results in marked increases in blood cholesterol or triglycerides or both. These disorders are particularly important because of their high frequency and because they lead to the premature development of coronary artery disease, which now kills 60 percent of all Americans (see Chapter 12). A detailed study of 176 survivors of heart attack and their relatives led to the identification of three distinct autosomal dominant disorders in which plasma cholesterol or triglyceride is elevated. About 20 percent of the heart attack survivors studied who were below 60 years of age had one of these dominantly inherited disorders. Compared to persons with normal plasma cholesterol and triglyceride levels, white, middle-class males with hyperlipidemia were five to forty times more likely to have a heart attack by middle age, the precise risk factor depending on which of the three disorders was involved. Hyperlipidemia can in many instances be diagnosed in childhood either through testing younger relatives of heart attack patients or by screening in the general population. But the proper course for preventing the serious consequences of these disorders once they have been identified is not yet clear. Furthermore, while it seems likely that a gene produces elevated levels of cholesterol and/or triglyceride which in turn directly damage the blood supply to the heart, the alternative possibility that the gene itself acts by an unknown mechanism to cause both the elevated lipids and the vascular damage simultaneously has not yet been entirely excluded. The frequency and health impact of these inherited disorders indicate that a high priority should be placed on studies directed at answering these questions.

One productive approach, used by Michael Brown, Joseph Goldstein, and associates (and by others), has used fibroblasts cultured from skin specimens obtained from persons with familial hypercholesterolemia (hyperlipidemia in which plasma cholesterol is elevated). These cells synthesize cholesterol and can be used for studies of the regulation of this lipid. In fibroblasts from patients with familial hypercholesterolemia the activity of the enzyme catalyzing the critical first step in the biological synthesis of cholesterol is markedly increased, resulting in a large increase in the rate of cholesterol production. Yet the enzyme itself is not abnormal. Instead, it turns out that cells from these patients are deficient in the cell-surface receptors which normally play a crucial role in regulating the synthesis and breakdown of cholesterol (see Chapter 12). The elevated plasma cholesterol levels in patients with familial hypercholesterolemia thus result from both increased production and decreased degradation of cholesterol. Familial hypercholesterolemia is one of the first autosomal dominant disorders in which a specific defect at the subcellular or molecular level has been identified.

Several genetic cancer syndromes occur among the autosomal dominant disorders. In a disease called familial adenomatous polyposis, which affects about one person in 8,300, a single gene results in the appearance of from several dozen to thousands of glandular outgrowths confined strictly to the colon, or large intestine. Unless treated by removal of the colon, at least 80 percent and probably all individuals with this disorder develop bowel cancer by age 50, with an average age of appearance of 39 years; this contrasts markedly with bowel cancer in the general population, which occurs at an average age of about 60 years. In this genetic syndrome, the cancer usually develops at several separate locations in the colon simultaneously. Such early onset and multiple foci of origin are characteristic of genetic cancers, the molecular basis for which is entirely unknown. Another autosomal dominant cancer syndrome is retinoblastoma, a disease that produces one or more malignant tumors in the eyes of children under the age of five; these tumors may even be present when the child is born.

Huntington's disease, also known as Huntington's chorea, is a rare but very serious autosomal dominant disorder. Because the clinical manifestations of this disease do not begin until an average age of about 40 years, many persons who develop Huntington's disease have already had children; and those children will have a 50 percent chance of developing the disease. Once an individual who has inherited the gene for Huntington's chorea begins to have symptoms, the course is usually one of progressive neurologic and intellectual deterioration over the course of three to five more years; no effective therapy is presently available.

Despite extensive research efforts, primary molecular defects still remain to be identified in nearly all of the one thousand known autosomal dominant disorders. As a result we are not only ignorant of the causal mechanism in these disorders but also, in most instances, have no laboratory tests available for establishing precise diagnoses and are forced instead to rely on clinical findings which are often equivocal. Prenatal diagnosis (with the option of selective abortion) is also impossible for virtually all these disorders.

More than 900 disorders are inherited in the autosomal recessive pattern in which two unaffected, carrier parents give birth to one or more affected children. Since each parent has a 50 percent chance of passing on the gene, the risk of the disorder on each pregnancy is 25 percent; autosomal recessive disorders occur only when the child inherits a gene for that disorder from both parents.

The most frequent serious autosomal recessive disorders in the United States are sickle cell anemia and cystic fibrosis. About 1,200 children with each of these diseases are born each year, and both generally suffer chronic disability and a shortened life span. Although similar in their impact, the two disorders otherwise differ greatly.

Sickle cell anemia may affect as many as 25,000 Americans. In the United States, this disease occurs almost entirely in blacks where the frequency is 1/625 at birth. Almost every vital organ can be damaged in this disorder and life expectancy is substantially reduced; it is estimated that only 50 percent of affected individuals survive beyond the age of 20. Carriers have one gene for this disorder and one normal gene, a condition referred to as sickle cell trait. Contrary to earlier claims, sickle cell trait is medically benign and results in no physical limitation, although it does carry with it the risk that, if the spouse also has sickle cell trait, a child may have sickle cell anemia. The carriers with sickle cell trait (8 percent of American blacks) are about 50 times more numerous than people with sickle cell anemia.

The study of sickle cell anemia has included many of the milestones of research in human biochemical genetics. The clinical features of the illness as well as the sickle-shaped distortions of the red blood cells from which the disease name derives were clearly described in 1910. In 1949 Linus Pauling and colleagues observed that hemoglobin (the oxygen-carrying protein of red blood cells) that came from patients with sickle cell anemia migrated more rapidly than normal hemoglobin when placed in an electrical field (a laboratory procedure called electrophoresis). In 1957 Vernon Ingram demonstrated that the faster electrophoretic migration rate of sickle hemoglobin resulted from a change in one of the 146 amino acid building blocks of the hemoglobin molecule. One specific amino acid had been substituted for another because of a change in the gene coding for hemoglobin. Through Ingram's work, sickle cell anemia became the first genetic disorder in which the precise nature of the genetic defect was identified on a molecular level. Four years later, Marshall Nirenberg and Heinrich Matthai made the first of a series of observations that led to an understanding of the genetic code, the set of rules by which the makeup of genes determines the specific makeup of proteins. Subsequently over 100 variant hemoglobins resulting from specific mutations have been identified. (Only a few of these mutant hemoglobins produce serious disease.) Hemoglobin is now the most extensively characterized human protein molecule from a biochemical and genetic point of view.

Despite the progress in laboratory research on sickle cell anemia, no cure has been developed, and there is at present no fully effective and satisfactory therapy. Over the past several years, mass screening and genetic counseling programs have been established; the aim is to inform couples where both have sickle cell trait of the risk that their children will have sickle cell anemia before the birth of the first affected child. The results of recent research may soon make possible the prenatal diagnosis of sickle cell anemia early in the course of pregnancy, thus offering carrier couples a means of having children without the risk that they will be born with this disease.

Cystic fibrosis is the most common serious recessively inherited disorder in the white population of the United States, occurring with a frequency of about one in 2,000 births. Knowledge of the clinical and pathologic aspects of this disorder has increased substantially since the original description of the disease in 1936. The disease affects nearly every organ and tissue in the body. In about 10 percent of patients the diagnosis can be made at birth; most instances of cystic fibrosis, however, go unrecognized until some time during childhood when either the failure of normal absorption in the gastrointestinal tract (with accompanying failure to thrive) or recurrent pulmonary problems bring the child to medical attention. At present the most accurate and useful diagnostic test is the so-called sweat test, which involves the analysis of the concentration of minerals, particularly sodium, in sweat collected from the skin. While cystic fibrosis was previously considered to be uniformly fatal in infancy and childhood, improvements in therapy have resulted in a steady increase in life expectancy; the average age of survival was 15 years in 1970 and is probably now somewhat higher. However, cystic fibrosis remains a very serious disease that produces much suffering and chronic disability among children. Despite considerable research effort the primary molecular defect in cystic fibrosis has eluded identification, although it has been suggested, by analogy with other recessively inherited disorders, that the primary defect should reside in a single mutant enzyme or other protein.

Without knowledge of the basic defect and even of a specific diagnostic marker, it is not possible to cure the disorder or treat the abnormalities effectively, nor is it possible to identify the carriers (about 1/20 of the white population) prior to the birth of an affected child. It is not yet possible to diagnose this disorder prenatally. Thus prevention of cystic fibrosis is very limited, consisting solely of informing couples who have already had an affected child of the risk that subsequent children will also have the disease. An understanding of the basic defect in cystic fibrosis remains an exceedingly important goal, but the best and most productive route to that goal is by no means clear.

Tay-Sachs disease is an autosomal recessive disorder in which the affected child appears normal at birth, shows abnormalities of the nervous system at about age one year, and subsequently follows a steady and relentless course of neurologic deterioration leading to death at about age four. About 50 children with this disorder are born each year in the United States. The disorder and the gene occur primarily among Jews of Eastern European origin, among whom the frequency of the carrier state is about 1/30 as contrasted with about 1/300 in the general population. The deficiency of a specific enzyme activity has been identified as the basis of this inborn error of metabolism. Simple laboratory tests have been developed for specific identification of carriers and those with Tay-Sachs disease; these tests are currently in widespread use both for prospective screening, prior to the birth of the first affected child, and for prenatal diagnosis in couples where both are carriers (see Chapter 10). Like all other such programs in medical genetics, these screening and counseling programs are interim measures that make it possible to prevent the birth of children with serious genetic disorders until effective therapy or until a cure is developed.

The X-linked recessive disorders are generally carried by females and expressed in males. Perhaps the best known of the 171 described X-linked disorders are hemophilia A, commonly referred to simply as hemophilia (despite the fact that it is but one of several hemophilia syndromes), and Duchenne's muscular dystrophy, usually known simply as muscular dystrophy (although 10 distinct muscular dystrophy syndromes have been recognized). Both these disorders are quite rare; hemophilia affects about 1/6,500 of all males and Duchenne's muscular dystrophy about one male in 10,000. Yet both can produce severe and prolonged suffering.

Hemophiliacs in different families may experience mild, moderate, or severe hemophilia. Those with severe hemophilia have little activity of a clot-promoting blood protein designated as Factor VIII (see Chapter 15). As a result, they usually experience severe hemorrhages into the skin, within joint spaces such as the knee (leading eventually to loss of joint function), or from almost any site, including the nose, mouth, and gastrointestinal tract. The disorder can be quite successfully treated by administering Factor VIII derived from blood of a normal individual once abnormal bleeding has begun but before it has become severe. The hemophiliac has a great demand for Factor VIII; the treatment of hemophilia A, as a rare genetic disorder, has been estimated by the National Heart and Lung Institute to account for about 25 percent of the total blood and blood products collected in the United States. If Factor VIII were to be administered at regular intervals such as twice weekly to prevent abnormal bleeding from even beginning, such therapy for hemophilia would require more blood than we presently collect for all purposes. It is likely that this problem will eventually be solved by the development of a synthetic Factor VIII, but the possibility of this being accomplished in the near future seems slight.

In Duchenne's muscular dystrophy, the affected males appear normal at birth but develop muscle weakness during childhood; a wheelchair is required by the teens and the victim invariably dies with end-stage muscle wasting by the early twenties. Recent studies have suggested abnormalities of protein synthesis in muscle cells which may help to identify female carriers of this disorder. Other studies of red blood cells from patients and carriers have shown decreased membrane deformability, a phenomenon which may also prove to be a useful marker in diagnosis. However, the specific primary defect remains a mystery, and therapy aimed at slowing the progress of the disease is still ineffective.

Neither for severe hemophilia A nor Duchenne's muscular dystrophy is it now possible to make the specific diagnosis prenatally with a pregnant known carrier of the disorder. One option that does exist is amniocentesis for determination of fetal sex, with abortion of males (which have a 50:50 chance of being affected with the disease) to ensure that no affected males are born. However, couples at risk have seldom elected this option.

The most frequent X-linked recessive disorder in the United States and the commonest inherited enzyme abnormality yet identified is glucose-6-phosphate dehydrogenase (G-6-PD) deficiency. This disorder affects some 100 million males worldwide; about twice as many females are carriers. G-6-PD is an enzyme widely distributed in the body. When it is deficient, the red blood cells become particularly susceptible to a number of ordinarily harmless drugs and other chemicals and, upon exposure, rupture to an extent that can be severe and even fatal. In most types of G-6-PD deficiency, the emphasis is entirely on the identification of susceptible individuals and avoidance of the provocative agents. To date over 85 genetically determined variant forms of this enzyme have been identified, only a few of which are associated with disease. G-6-PD is thus the most extensively characterized enzyme in human biochemical genetics.

The Multifactorial Disorders

The multifactorial (or polygenic) disorders are less strictly genetic than the chromosome or Mendelian disorders. While multifactorial genetic factors increase the risk of developing certain diseases, environmental influences play a central role in determining who will actually manifest the multifactorial disorder. In polygenic disorders, several genes that each exert a small deleterious effect act in combination with one another and with environmental factors to produce observable abnormalities. Some of these disorders are present at birth, such as defects in the structure of heart chambers or valves, congenital dislocation of the hip, and cleft lip (alone or with cleft palate). Others, such as most instances of high blood pressure, arteriosclerotic heart disease and gout, are not evident until adulthood.

Collectively the multifactorial disorders affect a very large number of people. Their management generally falls into the domain of the nongeneticist; in many instances they can be quite effectively treated by nongenetic means. Surgeons repair cleft lip, congenital heart disease, and other types of malformations, endocrinologists treat diabetes with insulin and by regulating the diet, and hypertension can be treated with a variety of drugs. Genetic counseling is particularly ineffective in dealing with polygenic disorders because of their low recurrence risk. The chance that one of these disorders will recur in a child born to parents who have already had one affected child, or in any given child of a parent with one of these disorders, is usually only about 5 percent. Most couples contemplating pregnancy perceive such odds as being quite favorable and generally state that this risk is too small to constitute a reason for limiting family size.

In one group of the multifactorial disorders, however, recent developments suggest that a much more active approach to prevention should be taken. These are the so-called defects of neural tube closure, representing defective development of the brain and spinal cord and their membranous and bony coverings. Early in embryonic development the tissues destined to become the brain and spinal cord form first by migration of cells up and around to produce a tube-like structure which finally closes along its outermost surface. Defective closure occurs for unknown reasons and with widely varying degrees of severity. In anencephaly, the most severe form, the fetus has literally no brain or skull formation above the level of the ears, and the floor of the skull is open to the outside through a large cranial defect. The anencephalic fetus survives gestation because the functions it lacks are largely supplied by the mother but dies at or shortly following birth. The spinal defect meningomyelocele (see Chapter 10) consists of an opening in the bony spinal column at the base of the spine through which protrude the meninges, or fibrous coverings, and the spinal cord or nerves. This abnormality usually entails paralysis of the lower extremities as well as loss of bowel and bladder control and, in males, loss of sexual function. Prenatal detection of the most severe of these disorders has become possible through two means. One is the detection of abnormally high levels of a substance called alpha-fetoprotein in the amniotic fluid, where the protein leaks through the abnormal opening in the skull or the spinal cord. Through early amniocentesis and testing of the amniotic fluid sample thus obtained it is possible to detect accurately all instances of anencephaly and the 90 percent of fetuses with meningomyelocele in which the defect is open to the amniotic fluid (and in which the spinal abnormality is the most severe).

The second major development in prenatal detection of neural tube defects has been ultrasonography. This technique uses reflected sound waves to form an image of the intrauterine fetal structures in much the same way that sonar allows the visualization of underwater objects (see Chapter 18). When expertly done, ultrasonography can be used to detect the prominent skull defect indicative of anencephaly as well as several other major malformations. (Ultrasonography also allows accurate detection of twin pregnancies, which can if unidentified confound the results of many tests.)

A major limitation of attempts to prevent the birth of children with severe neural tube defects has been the fact that not all pregnancies are monitored by amniocentesis, nor is it clear which pregnancies should be so monitored. Since there is a 1/20 risk of recurrence in the children of couples who have already had a child with one of these serious disorders, children of these couples are at much greater risk than the general population, where the frequency of these disorders is ten times less. Yet monitoring for recurrence will still miss the vast majority (about 19/20) of neural tube defects, which occur in families with no prior history of such a disorder.

Very recent research findings have suggested new, more practicable techniques for detecting neural tube abnormalities. In many but not all pregnancies where the fetus has a severe closure defect the level of alpha-fetoprotein is abnormally high not only in the amniotic fluid but also in the mother's serum early in pregnancy. Thus a simple blood test can be used to screen all pregnant women, and if the alpha-fetoprotein level is clearly elevated, amniocentesis can be performed. The maternal serum tests are not foolproof; but until such time as all pregnancies are monitored by amniocentesis, the screening procedures which use maternal serum merit further investigation and refinement.

Prospects for Therapy and Prevention

Presently available treatments of various genetic disorders range from the very effective to the totally ineffective. In all instances, treatment is directed at modifying the environment or the outward expression of abnormal genes. We have no means at present for directly manipulating a person's genes in a controlled manner. Interest in such techniques of genetic engineering has risen in the past few years, particularly since the possibility has been recognized of delivering genes to cells by means of certain animal viruses. But while most would agree that the only true cures of genetic diseases must involve replacement of the deleterious genes by normal genes, opinion is divided regarding both the promises and the perils of such gene manipulation and the likelihood that such techniques will be introduced in the near future.

Currently available therapies involve altering the biochemical as well as the physical aspects of the environment. We can modify the diet to prevent the abnormal production in the body of toxic substances from food; in phenylketonuria (PKU), a diet low in the amino acid phenylalanine during the first years of life prevents the severe mental retardation which occurs with an ordinary diet (see Chapter 10). An inactive or missing biological substance can be replaced with a normal one from an unaffected individual; for example, blood fractions enriched in Factor VIII activity can be given to a male with hemophilia A. In several disorders, most of which are inborn errors of metabolism, administration of very large amounts of certain nontoxic vitamins ameliorates the effects of deficient enzyme activity. And several research groups are now systematically investigating the factors involved in making enzyme replacement therapy successful.

Just as genetic disorders involve many different areas, so we can expect new treatments to emerge from research in various clinical and basic science disciplines. A remarkable example of the clinical application of basic research has been the development of procedures for prevention of Rh disease of the newborn (see Chapter 15). A recent study has estimated that the entire amount of money used to support Rh disease research from 1930 through the successful development of a preventive vaccine in 1966 is equivalent to the present cost of lifetime care for only six children irreparably brain damaged by the disease.

But for many serious genetic disorders that lack a cure and even an effective treatment, attention has focused on preventing the birth of affected individuals through genetic counseling. The aim of genetic counseling is to provide information to couples and individuals at risk for having children with serious genetic diseases so that they can make childbearing plans which they feel are best. This information includes an estimate of the risk that the disorder in question will occur, an evaluation of the types of impairment that the disorder may cause, and an outline of the reproductive alternatives available. Depending on the disorder in question, the reproductive alternatives may include taking chances and having as many children as desired despite the risk; limiting family size or foregoing childbearing altogether and perhaps adopting children; artificial insemination where genetically appropriate; and prenatal diagnosis, for those disorders where this is now possible. Genetic counseling usually requires discussion of the emotional significance of a genetic risk or disorder and giving the counselee enough background information about human biology and genetics to understand what is said and to participate in a meaningful dialogue. Increasingly, various aspects of genetic counseling are being delegated to specially trained nonmedical personnel who function as part of a team.

The ability to diagnose serious genetic disorders in the fetus early in pregnancy has been one of the most important advances in medical genetic care (see Chapter 18). A four-year, nationwide collaborative study conducted by the National Institute of Child Health and Human Development has found that amniocentesis and prenatal diagnosis are safe to the mother and fetus and can accurately detect the presence of serious fetal disorders. However, it is eminently clear from this study and others that only a small fraction of the pregnancies known to be at risk for a serious genetic disorder are actually monitored by early amniocentesis. As a result, these disorders are prevented much less often than they could be.

Another factor reducing preventability relates to the difference between occurrence and recurrence risk. Although the mathematical details are somewhat complex, modification of plans for childbearing after the birth of the first affected child will have only a limited effect on the frequency of the disorder; most genetic disorders are seen in the first, and usually the only, affected child in the family. Methods for decreasing the first occurrence of affected children in families can substantially reduce the frequency of serious genetic disorders, while even very effective measures directed at preventing recurrence in children born after the first affected child can reduce the overall frequency of the disorder very little.

The recognized importance of preventing the birth of the first affected child and the increasing availability of methods of carrier detection have stimulated the development of mass screening and genetic counseling programs in the past two years. These programs aim to identify couples where both individuals are carriers and to inform them of the risks, the potential burden of the disorder, and the reproductive alternatives prior to the birth of the first affected child. Efforts to prevent sickle cell anemia and Tay-Sachs disease have received the most widespread attention. In particular, the federally funded sickle cell screening program launched in 1972 has produced much controversy; some have questioned specific details of program design, while many have raised fundamental issues relating to screening, selective abortion of fetuses with genetic disorders, and genetics and health care in general. Ethical issues in human genetics have been widely discussed; despite their importance, they will be reviewed only briefly here.

Concern has been expressed about the potential for childbearing plans to be misdirected by geneticists who through ignorance or malice seek inappropriate ends. For example, some aspects of the more active mass screening and genetic counseling programs have caused some observers to recall—with understandable dismay—the unfortunate practices which appeared in earlier years under the banner of eugenics. But these early, misguided policies were generally aimed at changing very complex human attributes including intelligence, physical appearance, and personality characteristics. The chromosome, Mendelian, and multifactorial disorders that are the focus of modern medical genetics are simple by comparison, and their nature is much better understood. And while there is no single agreed-upon value system in medical genetics, most geneticists seem to believe that decisions regarding childbearing are those of the couples alone, that information in genetic counseling should be as objective as possible and free of judgments regarding right and wrong choices, and that the geneticist should serve the best interests of the couple and future child rather than a notion about what is good for society. In order to protect the rights of the childbearing couple, most geneticists have felt that complete confidentiality is essential and that there should be no intrusion through legislation or other governmental action. In fact, fears of possible political involvement have led most screening and counseling programs to dissociate themselves from government as much as possible.

Unfortunately, there is still much potential for misunderstanding because the general public's comprehension of medical genetics and human biology is woefully deficient. For example, carriers of autosomal recessive disorders may be unnecessarily stigmatized. The coincidental high frequency of certain genetic disorders in particular racial and ethnic groups may also be misinterpreted.

Like the giving of information, the decision to withhold information also raises ethical issues. For example, imagine that a geneticist detects a carrier state for a serious disorder in an individual consulting him and that this carrier state implies that children of the patient's relatives might also be at high risk for the disorder; yet the patient refuses to transmit this information to his relatives. Given that privacy and confidentiality must be respected, what is the obligation of this geneticist? And is a physician who believes that abortion is wrong under any circumstances entitled not to discuss the options of prenatal diagnosis and selective abortion with a couple whose future offspring are at risk for a serious genetic disorder?

The ongoing discussion of these and many other ethical issues relevant to medical genetics is not likely to yield definitive answers; but such debates have already resulted in raising the consciousness level of medical geneticists and have made it increasingly clear that those practicing medicine in this special field need very special sensitivities.

Future Directions

Recent advances in many clinical and basic science fields have resulted in a remarkable momentum in medical genetics. A number of predictions can be made on the basis of current trends. Although the surgical correction of malformations is already highly refined, the list of inborn errors of metabolism which can be treated effectively will probably increase steadily. Those disorders which produce irreparable damage early in gestation despite the link to the maternal circulation will clearly be the most difficult to treat. Our ability to make specific diagnoses both prenatally and postnatally will continue to improve as additional biochemical markers are identified, as more genes are mapped on specific chromosomes, and as methods are devised for deriving more and more information from cultured skin fibroblasts, small samples of blood, and amniotic fluid and cells.

The central challenge in genetics today is to decipher the organization of the human genetic material. We already know that the genetic code for protein synthesis is essentially the same in all life forms that have been studied; and there has been much recent progress made in understanding the physical chemistry of chromosomes and their function at the molecular level. Yet a remarkable void exists in the area of genetic regulation. If human genes contain regulatory mutations of the types so well characterized in microorganisms, where are they and what is their nature? What makes particular mutations dominant or recessive? What turns genes on and off during development and makes them more or less active during metabolic regulation? The answers will not come solely from the study of the genetics of microorganisms. In microorganisms, for example, the structural genes which encode functionally related proteins are often immediately adjacent to one another on the chromosome and are all under the control of a nearby regulatory gene. But closely related functions in people seem to be controlled quite separately; even the different subunits of one protein structure may be located on completely different chromosomes.

The insights that will unravel the mysteries of human genetic organization could come at any time and from almost any related research area. If the progress that has been made over the past several decades is any indication, the field is ripe for such a major advance.

Bacterial Infections

LOUIS WEINSTEIN
MICHAEL J. BARZA

5

Although some infections had been known for many years to be communicable, it was not until the development of the science of microbiology that a firm scientific basis for the study and treatment of infectious disease was established. The first microbes recognized as causes of disease were fungi (1836) and protozoa (1865). The first bacterium proved to be a cause of an infectious process was *Bacillus anthracis*, the agent responsible for anthrax. Robert Koch established the microbial etiology of this disease in 1876 and also formulated four criteria (Koch's postulates) that are still used to establish the specific relation of a microscopic organism to the disease it causes. During the latter part of the nineteenth century, methods were developed for isolating and growing the organisms responsible for cholera, typhoid, diphtheria, pneumococcal pneumonia, tetanus, and staphylococcal, meningococcal, and gonococcal infections. The first half of the twentieth century saw many more species of bacteria identified.

Since the time of these early investigations, many years of laboratory studies and clinical experience have made it eminently clear that infection is a varied and complicated biological phenomenon. Some organisms very readily invade the body and cause disease, while others can produce illness only in unusual circumstances. In certain diseases (like pneumonia and meningitis), bacteria and other infectious agents produce their effects by eliciting local inflammatory reactions that damage tissues, blood vessels, and organs. Some infectious processes cause disease at least partially through an allergic reaction; tuberculosis and the late com-

65

plications of streptococcal infection (rheumatic fever and kidney damage) are examples of such allergic disorders. Other diseases—including tetanus, botulism, diphtheria, and cholera—are not due directly to the invasive activity of bacteria but result instead from the action of bacterial toxins released into the tissues or bloodstream. In these cases, the infectious process itself may be trivial; it is the intoxication that is responsible for illness and even death.

The mechanisms of bacterial intoxication and ways to prevent it remain objects of intensive study. Bacterial exotoxins (substances excreted by bacteria) are firmly fixed to tissue almost immediately after contact and, once fixed, cannot be neutralized even by huge concentrations of antitoxin. Scientists are now trying to develop methods for inactivating bacterial toxins with chemical substances other than specific antitoxins. Endotoxin, a toxic substance produced and retained within the bacterial cell and released when this breaks up, produces circulatory abnormalities, fever, and other characteristics of severe infection. These effects of endotoxin are well known, but the exact role the toxin plays in the pathogenesis of infectious disease remains unclear.

Although the infectious process may not be completely understood for some time, striking progress has been made in the treatment of bacterial infections for decades. The first breakthrough came in 1936 with the clinical introduction of the sulfonamides, chemical compounds that were used effectively to treat many kinds of infectious diseases. But the sulfonamides were soon made obsolete by penicillin and the other antibiotics that were shortly developed. The antibiotics—substances naturally produced by microorganisms (such as molds and bacteria) that can kill dangerous bacteria—completely revolutionized the treatment of infectious disease.

The Golden Era of Chemotherapy

Alexander Fleming's discovery in 1928 of penicillin offers a particularly striking example of the unanticipated benefits of basic research. Fleming, a microbiologist, was examining the production of pigment by staphylococci. By chance, some of his bacterial cultures were contaminated by a mold, *Penicillium*. When Fleming examined these cultures he noted that there were no staphylococci in the areas of the culture where the mold had grown. Ten years later, this basic observation began to be exploited. In 1941 chemists, microbiologists, and clinical investigators finally purified penicillin, the active substance made by *Penicillium,* and subsequently produced it in sufficient quantities for use in the treatment of human infections. This achievement opened the "golden era of chemotherapy."

The proven curative activity of penicillin stimulated the search for other effective antibiotics. Following Fleming's serendipitous discovery, substances thought to be effective antibiotics were systematically sought for in organisms present in soil. Over the past 35 years, basic scientists in diverse fields (such as microbiology, chemistry, and pharmacology) have discovered more than 40 effective antimicrobial agents. These drugs differ, even within a given class or group, in the specific organisms against which they are active, in their behavior in the body (excretion, metabolism, penetration into various tissues), and in the unwanted effects or reactions they may produce.

The effectiveness of the antibiotics as curative agents is readily apparent when one compares the death rates from some of the common infections in the preantibiotic era with present rates (Table 5-1). A very common kind of pneumonia caused by the pneumococcus was reported as being fatal in 20 to 85 percent of all cases in the 1941 edition of an authoritative textbook on medicine. The 1963 edition of this same book states that the risk of death from this disease, in cases treated with an antibiotic, is only about 5 percent. Prior to 1945 infection of the heart valves (subacute bacterial endocarditis) almost always proved fatal. Proper antibiotic treatment lasting about one month has now reduced the death rate for this disease to about 5 percent. The outlook for uncompli-

Table 5–1. Effects of antibiotics on death rates of several common infections

Disease	Percent deaths	
	No antibiotics	Antibiotic therapy
Pneumonia (pneumococcal)	20–85	About 5
Subacute bacterial endocarditis	99+	5
Meningitis (*H. influenzae*)	100	2–3
Meningitis (pneumococcal)	100	8–10
Meningitis (meningococcal)	20–90	1–5
Typhoid fever	8–10	1–2

Source: L. Weinstein, "Antibiotics: Curative Drugs," in Samuel Proger, M.D., ed., *The Medicated Society* (New York: Macmillan Co., 1968). Copyright © 1968 by Tufts–New England Medical Center.

cated recovery in three common forms of meningitis has also been strikingly altered by treatment with these drugs. And the chance of death from typhoid fever, a disease still very common in many of the developing areas of the world, has been reduced by the use of the antibiotic chloramphenicol.

Antibiotics have also proven highly effective in decreasing the complications and duration of nonfatal illness. Penicillin treatment has converted three infections caused by the streptococcus—"strep sore throat," scarlet fever, and the skin disease erysipelas—from prolonged, uncomfortable, and potentially dangerous experiences to mild diseases of short duration and benign outcome. Most infections of the lungs, except those caused by true viruses, are cured by antibiotics. Boils and more life-threatening infections due to the staphylococcus respond remarkably well to antibiotic treatment. And infections of the kidneys and bladder can be readily suppressed in the acute stage by moderate doses of any of several drugs given for ten to twelve days. (Chronic disease of this type is more difficult to cure but can be controlled by treatment over an extended period.)

The impact of the antibiotics on the veneral diseases has been tremendous. Before penicillin was available, eradication of syphilis involved one or sometimes two years of weekly injections of an arsenic compound. This long period of treatment discouraged many patients; some dropped out before they were rid of the disease and not only endangered their own survival but also constituted a menace to the public health. Today, one daily injection of a special preparation of penicillin can cure all cases of syphilis within two weeks. (Tetracycline is an adequate substitute in patients sensitive to penicillin.) The effects of antibiotics in gonorrhea are just as impressive.

In addition to their effectiveness in curing established infections, antibiotics can sometimes prevent epidemic outbreaks of disease. Many communities contain clinically healthy carriers who harbor the organism responsible for diphtheria and spread the disease to others; now, about two weeks of treatment with erythromycin eliminates the dangerous carrier state. Carriers of salmonella bacteria, which cause food poisoning, can also be given antibiotics to prevent them from spreading disease. And a developing epidemic of dysentery may be halted abruptly by giving an antibiotic that can kill the responsible bacteria (shigellae) to healthy people who have come into contact with it.

Finally, antibiotics have enabled many persons with readily curable infections to be treated at home and be spared the extended periods of hospitalization once required. (The availability of therapeutic drugs has brought about especially dramatic changes in the treatment of tuberculosis.) Each year antibiotic therapy represents a huge financial savings in terms of the costs of hospital care for the millions of Americans who suffer from certain infectious diseases. In addition, rapid cure allows people to return to work much earlier than they could before chemotherapy was available. Other nonmedical benefits of antibiotic treatment include reduction of the social disruption that may result from the removal of one of the parents from the home to the hospital and avoidance of the psychological trauma incident to hospitalization (especially in young children).

But antibiotics are not panaceas. The decades since their introduction to medicine have shown these powerful antimicrobial agents to be totally ineffective in certain clinical situations. Worse, it is now only too clear that the indiscriminate use of antibiotics can itself lead to the initiation or spread of disease.

The Limitations of Antibiotic Therapy

The initial enthusiasm that greeted the advent of antibiotics was soon dampened by recognition of a problem of major clinical importance: the development of bacterial resistance to these drugs. Shortly after penicillin was introduced it became evident that staphylococci were becoming resistant to this agent. Certain strains of staphylococcus can produce a substance (penicillinase) that destroys the antibiotic. As penicillin came into widespread use, these resistant strains survived; and within ten years or so, about 15 to 30 percent of staphylococci in the community and the majority of those present in hospitals were of the type unaffected by the drug. Infections due to these organisms began to reach epidemic proportions in some instances, until chemists succeeded in developing derivatives of penicillin that were not inactivated by penicillinase. This pattern of events leading to the development of bacterial resistance has characterized the history of virtually all antibiotics after they have come into broad clinical use.

Among the most important contributions of basic scientists to the treatment of bacterial infections has been the elucidation of the mechanisms involved in that pattern. Three factors may make bacteria resistant to antimicrobial drugs. The bacterial wall may lack surface receptors to which the drug can attach. The antibiotic may be unable to penetrate into the interior of the organism. Or the bacteria may produce substances that destroy the activity of the drug. One or another of these mechanisms may come into play through spontaneous mutation of an organism; exposure to the antibiotic then eliminates the sensitive bacterial cells and favors growth of the mutant forms. Resistance may also develop through the transfer of genetic material among members of the same bacterial species, or to organisms of a different species. (This transfer can occur through a form of sexual mating, or a virus can carry genetic material from one bacterium to another.) Recent years have seen a spread of resistance to many antibiotics among staphylococci in Europe, and shigellae (a bacterial cause of dysentery) and salmonellae in Japan, Mexico, and the United States. The worsening problem of bacterial resistance is largely due to the widespread and sometimes indiscriminate use of antibiotics.

The overuse of antibiotics can have other serious consequences besides causing strains of bacteria to become resistant and hard to eradicate. In some instances, antibiotics may actually be toxic and directly harmful to the individual using them.

All antimicrobial agents may produce a variety of reactions ranging in severity from mild to potentially fatal; under certain circumstances, some antibiotics can cause deafness, bone marrow damage, or injury to the kidney or liver. Since many antibiotics act by disrupting the processing of genetic information or the synthesis of protein in cells, some extremely basic and elusive biological processes have been studied in the attempt to understand the effects of these drugs. Basic research has led to the development of techniques for monitoring the concentrations of various antimicrobial agents in the serum in order to avoid excessively high (potentially toxic) or low (ineffective) concentrations.

Penicillin, the first clinically useful antibiotic, has proved over the past thirty years to be one of the safest antimicrobial agents; yet reactions even to this drug do occur in unusual circumstances, especially when penicillin is given in massive doses to patients with decreased kidney function or brain disease. Allergic reactions, which may be produced by all types of penicillins, range from mild skin rashes to high fever, from difficulty in breathing to sudden death. Basic studies of the mechanisms involved in these reactions have identified certain metabolic products of the antibiotic that are responsible for both the relatively mild effects and the life-threatening ones. The presence of these substances can indicate that the user of penicillin may risk such untoward consequences. Studies are in progress to develop safe and useful ways of detecting sensitivity to penicillin by measuring these metabolic products.

Even if antibiotics are not directly toxic to the patient, they may disrupt the bacterial ecology of the individual; and this action, too, can lead to serious medical problems. All animals, including man, normally harbor large populations of a variety of microorganisms in various sites of the body including the upper respiratory tract, intestine, genitals, and skin. The huge number of bacteria, fungi, and viruses that inhabit the intestinal tract cause no difficulty as long as their normal relationships to each other are not disturbed. A delicate system of checks and balances operates in the intestine; the microorganisms that live there compete for food, and some species of these organisms synthesize metabolic products that inhibit or suppress the growth of others. Antibiotic treatment may eliminate certain members of the microbial population and disrupt the protective balance, allowing the bacteria that have not been affected by the drug to overgrow. As a result, disease may occur in the intestine or at any other site if invasion of the bloodstream occurs. Infection may also develop if organisms normally present in the upper respiratory or genital tracts accidentally escape and lodge in other sites.

When one considers that people are uninterruptedly exposed to a huge number of diverse microorganisms in the internal and external environment, it is remarkable that infections do not kill babies shortly after they are born and that older children and adults are not constantly infected. Actively functioning defense mechanisms, some present from birth and others developed during life, are essential to the individual's survival. Some of the most important defense mechanisms are special cells (phagocytes) in the blood and tissues that can ingest and kill bacteria with which they come into contact; the development of antibodies; and cell-mediated immunity, a response to some types of infection, notably tuberculosis, carried out by highly active cells (type T lymphocytes) that kill bacteria and other infectious agents (see Chapter 7).

When these vital defenses malfunction, antimicrobial therapy becomes ineffective and the individual is left dangerously susceptible to infection. This problem is especially serious in hospitalized patients with Hodgkin's disease or cancers (like leukemia) that damage the body's defenses and in individuals treated with immunosuppressive drugs that decrease or completely abolish the activity of normal mechanisms of defense. These people run a high risk of being infected by their own bacteria. In addition, the hospital environment is swarming with microorganisms that normally colonize areas on the skin of hospitalized patients shortly after their admission; these organisms are harmless to people with adequate defenses but can lead to disease and even death in those whose defense mechanisms are not fully operative. Routine surveillance cultures of the nose, throat, skin, and stool of patients with inadequate immunological defenses are now carried out in many hospitals to detect infection before it becomes a serious problem. There is also an increasing trend to systematic, hospital-wide surveillance programs aimed at anticipating and preventing epidemic outbreaks of disease, monitoring the development of resistance in the bacteria found in the hospital, and detecting contamination of sterile devices (such as respirators) used in patient care. The effectiveness of such monitoring programs has not yet been accurately determined and is currently being investigated.

In spite of these measures, however, infection is a worsening medical problem. Organisms that were once considered harmless are now becoming increasingly common causes of infection; fungal and protozoal disease, for example, is now almost commonplace. Many of these infections are called "opportunistic" because they involve organisms with very little intrinsic invasive potential and generally attack individuals whose defenses have been altered. Such individuals are increasing in number for four reasons: the longer life span of patients with leukemia and other forms of cancer, the use of potent immunosuppressive drugs to control those disorders, the increasing frequency of organ transplants (which also require immunosuppressive therapy), and the surgical implantation of artificial devices like heart valves, grafts, and various shunts. The origins of opportunistic infection are still very unclear; for example, no one knows exactly why artificial devices implanted within the body are so prone to bacterial colonization, or why those bacteria are so difficult to eradicate even when highly effective antimicrobial agents are administered. The techniques of molecular biology and epidemiology will have to be used in the study and eventual solution of this problem.

Much recent work has been aimed at finding direct ways to improve the immunological defenses of patients with conditions that make them especially susceptible to infection. Because phagocytes (special cells that ingest and destroy bacteria) play a critical role in defending against microbial invasion, one possible way to boost immunological defenses could be the transfusion of phagocytes from normal donors. (This approach has already been shown to be feasible and beneficial in a number of instances.) Infection with certain innocuous types of bacteria may actually protect the individual from some serious bacterial and viral infections and may even increase his resistance to some kinds of cancer. This phenomenon has long been observed in animals; but the mechanisms involved are still poorly understood, and this type of therapy cannot yet be widely applied to human disease. (However, there is some evidence from human studies that inoculation of the bacterium known as BCG may destroy some types of cancer, or at least keep them from spreading.) Certain chemicals and an organism, *Corynebacterium parvum*, that appear to stimulate immunological mechanisms are also under investigation. If these approaches prove to be clinically practical, physicians will have at their command effective methods that complement the action of antibiotics. These methods could vastly improve the treatment of infections in patients with inadequate immunological defenses.

Immunization can effectively prevent patients with inadequate defenses from developing serious infections; for example, burned patients can be immunized against pseudomonads (bacteria responsible for various types of pus-forming infection) by a vaccine made from these organisms. Active immunization, a procedure designed to stimulate the body's own defenses, involves the repeated injection of dead bacteria or their toxins; if the process is successful, specific protective antibodies to the injected organism will develop. In passive immunization, the individual is injected with serum containing antibodies obtained from animals (horses, rabbits) or human donors who have been hyperimmunized to a specific organism or bacterial toxin.

The most widespread application of immunization techniques has been their use in the prevention of infectious disease in immunologically normal people.

Preventive Vaccination

The introduction by Edward Jenner in 1796 of vaccination against smallpox was the earliest and most successful approach to the prevention of an infectious disease; but the principles underlying this procedure were not appreciated until Pasteur, almost a century later, successfully used killed or attenuated (weakened) organisms to immunize against cholera, anthrax, and rabies. Today, immunization is most commonly practiced in the United States against the bacterial diseases of diphtheria, tetanus, and whooping cough. Protection against tetanus and diphtheria by injection of altered bacterial toxin is almost 100 percent effective when properly performed.

An effective vaccine against pneumococcus (the commonest cause of bacterial pneumonia) was first developed and used, in limited fashion, in the late 1930s. When it became apparent in the early 1940s that the sulfonamides, penicillin, and other antibiotics were highly active in curing pneumococcal pneumonia, the vaccine was abandoned in favor of drug treatment. But in the late 1950s physicians began to recognize that this type of pneumonia was still sometimes fatal in older persons, despite therapy with penicillin and other potent antibiotics. Consequently, interest has revived in preventing pneumococcal pneumonia in selected older populations through vaccines containing antigens from the types of pneumococcus that most often cause this disease.

Meningococcal meningitis can also be prevented by immunization. The vaccine against meningococcus was made possible by elegant studies of the biochemical nature of the organism; a single molecular substance isolated from the bacterium has proved to stimulate the production of high levels of protective antibodies against two types of the meningococcus. The vaccine has already proved its usefulness in preventing the spread of meningococcal infection in this country and in Brazil. Efforts are now underway to develop an effective vaccine against *Hemophilus influenzae,* a common cause of meningitis in children under three years of age.

Diarrheal disease due to bacteria is a serious disorder very common in many of the developing areas of the world (see Chapter 16). The approaches now being employed to develop against a vaccine shigella (one type of bacterium that can cause diarrhea) illustrate the importance of basic research. Mutants of shigella have been developed that require the antibiotic streptomycin for growth. When large numbers of these bacteria are given orally in the absence of streptomycin, they don't grow and thus produce no disease; but the mutant bacteria do induce the production of antibodies. Since these antibodies are also effective against normal shigella, they increase the individual's resistance to this bacterial cause of diarrhea. Genetic hybrids of shigella and *Escherichia coli,* an essentially harmless inhabitant of the intestine, also appear to protect people against infection without producing disease. Finally, basic researchers are attempting to modify the toxin produced by the cholera bacterium in the hope of producing an effective immunizing agent (see Chapter 16).

The Future of Bacterial Research

One of the most important current goals in bacteriology is simply to improve the basic experimental methods for growing and studying bacteria. Hospitals and clinics throughout the world still employ essentially the same techniques that were developed fifty years ago. Cultures of various body fluids, surfaces, and tissues are taken and placed on media that favor bacterial growth; the resultant "colonies" of organisms are then studied to determine their biological characteristics and their susceptibility to different kinds of antibiotics. Unlike the methods employed in chemistry and hematology, those used in clinical microbiology are not largely automated; as a result they are costly and subject to error. They are also time-consuming. Most bacteria require at least 24 hours to produce sufficient growth for study, and some organisms may have to be incubated from one to four weeks.

In the past decade, researchers have begun to develop new, faster techniques for measuring bacterial growth. These methods are based on the measurement of biological and physical processes that occur in different phases of the bacterial life cycle. The growth medium can be analyzed at different times for the presence of metabolic products (like carbon dioxide) and adenosine triphosphate (ATP, a substance produced by all living cells). The acidity of the medium can serve as a sensitive indicator of bacterial growth. And the density of microorganisms growing in a liquid can be determined by measuring transmission of a light through the liquid. All these new techniques are still in early stages of development and have yet to be made economically, technically, and clinically practical. But some of these methods should be perfected, and others developed, as our understanding of the life cycle of bacteria improves.

As techniques of bacteriological research become more sophisticated, researchers are turning increasingly to the study of microorganisms that previously were difficult or impossible to investigate. Special attention has recently been given to the so-called anaerobic bacteria. While many microbes thrive in both aerobic (oxygen-rich) and anaerobic (oxygen-poor) environments, anaerobic bateria are exquisitely sensitive to oxygen and will multiply only in the absence of the gas. Anaerobic bacteria are very important members of the microbial population of the human body; they are ten times more common than aerobic bacteria in the mouth and vagina, and a thousand times more common in the intestine. Anaerobic bacteria also outnumber aerobic ones on the skin by a factor of ten. The mechanisms involved in permitting survival of anaerobic bacteria on the skin, which is constantly exposed to oxygen, are not yet clear. It has been suggested that these organisms are protected against the lethal effects of this gas by living in crevices of the skin, that other microorganisms may alter the chemical environment in ways that allow anaerobes to survive, or that the lipids of the skin are protective. This problem requires the application of further basic research for its solution.

The role of anaerobic bacteria in disease has been recognized for a long time; the anaerobic clostridia, for example, are known to cause tetanus, gas gangrene, and botulism. But the specific mechanisms involved in the production of disease by these bacteria have remained poorly understood. It has simply been very difficult to study these organisms; since oxygen fills our environment, special techniques have had to be devised to study the bacteria that cannot live in the presence of this gas. During the past few years, new, sensitive techniques have been developed for detecting the presence of some anaerobic bacteria in human infections. Gas chromatography can now be used to measure the metabolic products of these bacteria in pus and other infected material; different bacteria can be identified by the presence of these metabolic products. As the anaerobic bacteria have been increasingly well characterized, the mechanisms by which they cause infection have also been investigated, with some unusual results.

As with intestinal bacteria, the ability of anaerobic bacteria to cause disease is markedly affected by the presence of other microorganisms. Intestinal bacteria may be innocuous until the use of antibiotics upsets the intestinal ecology; when the microorganisms that normally compete with it are killed off, one type of bacterium may take over to a dangerous extent. Just the opposite kind of interaction is frequently seen with anaerobes. Many anaerobic bacteria are virtually harmless by themselves, but in the presence of certain other bacteria they may markedly increase their capacity to invade tissue and produce serious disease. This phenomenon of synergy is still poorly understood, but clearly has great implications for the study and prevention of human disease. At least some of the synergistic interactions of bacteria seem to stem from the ability of one organism to effect chemical changes in the tissue that allow the anaerobic bacteria to grow. The metabolism, cell wall structure, chemistry, and pathogenicity of anaerobic bacteria are now being studied intensively in an attempt to understand how synergistic interactions take place.

Much recent research has focused on the problem of shock, a life-threatening complication of bacterial and other infections (see Chapter 24). This syndrome, which basically consists of a failure of the circulation to nourish and maintain normal function, now seems to be determined by many different factors. The nature of the primary injury, the patient's age, the presence of other diseases (such as diabetes, alcoholism, or heart disease), and the variety of effects produced by chemical substances released by the body's tissues during shock, all determine the character and intensity of the clinical picture. The purpose of ongoing investigations into the basic nature of the process is to develop techniques to identify quickly the biological mechanisms that are malfunctioning and to provide drugs or other forms of treatment to interrupt the vicious cycle of circulatory collapse. Devices for measuring the acidity, oxygen content, and blood flow of critical tissues are now becoming available. Studies now in progress may provide information that will permit physicians to reverse the circulatory abnormalities that can prove fatal in patients who develop shock in the course of an infection. A major priority of research in this area is the development of specific agents to treat shock, since use of the wrong type of treatment may actually worsen the condition. The drugs now available for restoring the badly disturbed circulatory functions to normal are relatively blunt tools. Even when treated with potent antibiotics, nearly half of the patients who develop shock die from this disorder.

In general, the limitations of antibiotic therapy are still too little appreciated. Death occurs frequently in individuals with leukemia and other diseases who develop infections despite therapy with powerful antimicrobial agents. In patients with structural abnormalities of the urinary tract or chronic bronchitis, recurrences and relapses of infections are very common; these often fail to respond to the use of antibiotics. Such infections represent difficult therapeutic challenges even though the bacteria that produce them are often very susceptible to antimicrobial drugs. Basic scientists are now addressing many questions stemming from this problem. Why do patients succumb to infections despite therapy with effective antibiotics? How may the nature of the infecting organism and its susceptibility to antibiotics be recognized more promptly? What is the role of the immunological defenses in the cure of bacterial infections (and how may these be bolstered)? These questions impinge in a fundamental way on the biologic response of patients to infection and are being intensively explored.

Research into the bacterial infections has come full circle. During the early part of this century, biologists interested in the control of infection focused their attention primarily on the cells that normally protect the body against invasion by bacteria and other organisms. With the advent of chemotherapy and the rapid development of a large number of drugs capable of curing infections, interest in the basic aspects of the body's defenses waned. Now, however, the inadequacy of antibiotic therapy in certain cases has become clear; and research is focusing increasingly on identifying the factors involved not only in the pathogenesis but also in the clinical expression of infection. Much has already been learned about the mechanisms by which phagocytes kill bacteria, antibodies interact with bacteria, and cellular immunity comes into play. But much more basic research is needed before the understanding of these complex processes will be advanced enough to be translated into methods for the effective clinical management of infectious disease.

Viral Infections

LOUIS WEINSTEIN
TE-WEN CHANG

6

The fight against viral diseases has seen some of the great successes of modern medicine. Smallpox, once a major cause of death and disability, has virtually disappeared from the globe; and yellow fever, too, is now almost unknown. Closer to home are the modern American experiences with poliomyelitis and measles. A few decades ago these two diseases infected thousands of children and adults in this country, often with crippling or fatal results. Today, effective vaccines have all but eradicated polio and have reduced the number of measles cases.

But many viral diseases are still common. As measles and polio have been disappearing, other childhood diseases—rubella (German measles), chicken pox, and the mumps—have remained prevalent. Members of the group of herpes viruses surround us. One of these viruses is the agent responsible for infectious mononucleosis, which often appears in localized epidemics in colleges and universities; and two other herpes viruses, closely related to each other, give rise to infections of the mouth and upper respiratory tract (often with a cold sore on the lips) and to a type of genital infection that is now second in incidence only to acute gonorrhea among the venereal diseases. Even more prevalent is viral infection of the upper respiratory tract, which we experience as the common cold; about four fifths of all viral disease involves this area, and it has been estimated that every American experiences an average of five episodes of respiratory infection per year. In addition to being highly contagious, this type of disease can sometimes have serious consequences; the possible complications of upper respiratory infection include pneumonia, meningitis, and infections of the middle ear.

In spite of advances that have been made, viruses are still responsible for a larger proportion of human illness—and of animal and plant diseases —than any other type of microorganism. They are transmitted more readily than other pathogenic microbes and are the cause of the great majority of epidemics and pandemics of disease that have struck large areas of the world periodically. Such outbreaks of viral disease can affect substantial portions of the population; bacterial infections (like salmonellosis) may involve large numbers of people when they become epidemic, but epidemics of viral diseases generally affect even more. Clearly, the study and control of viruses are essential to the improvement of human health.

The Development of Virology

The term virus is derived from the Latin word for poison, or slime. It was originally applied to the noxious stench emanating from swamps that was thought to cause a variety of diseases in the centuries before microbes were discovered and specifically linked to illness. But it was not until almost the end of the nineteenth century that a true virus was established as a cause of disease.

The nature of viruses made them impossible to detect for many years, even after bacteria had been discovered and studied. Not only are viruses too small to be seen with a light microscope, they also cannot be detected through their biological activity, except as it occurs in conjunction with other organisms. In fact, viruses show no traces of biological activity by themselves. Unlike bacteria, they are not living agents, in the strictest sense. Viruses are very simple pieces of organic material, composed only of nucleic acid, either DNA or RNA, enclosed in a coat of protein made up of simple structural units. (Some viruses also contain carbohydrates and lipids.) They are parasites that require human, animal, or plant cells for growth. The virus replicates by attaching to a cell and injecting its nucleic acid; once inside the cell, the DNA or RNA which contains the virus's genetic information takes over the cell's biological machinery, and the cell begins to manufacture viral proteins rather than its own (Figure 6-1).

While viruses may invade any organ or tissue of the body to produce localized inflammatory reactions and cellular destruction, each different type of virus has a tendency to restrict its attack to specific tissues in the body. This phenomenon is known as tropism. The agent of poliomyelitis, for example, invades primarily nervous tissue; that of measles, the

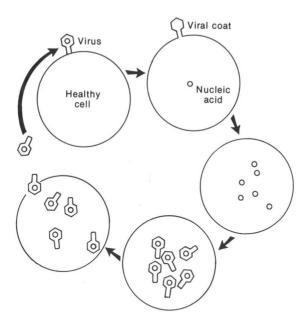

Figure 6–1. The process of viral infection. The virus attaches to a cell's surface and injects its nucleic acid into the cell. The nucleic acid multiplies and then orders the cell to make many copies of complete viruses. Finally, the newly made viruses burst out of the cell, killing it in the process, and spread to infect other cells. Although other kinds of cycles of viral infection and replication also occur, this is the most general model. In this drawing, the size of the virus and its nucleic acid relative to the size of the cell has been magnified by several orders of magnitude for illustrative purposes.

respiratory tract and skin; the agents of hepatitis, the liver; and influenza, the upper respiratory tract. (Most bacteria, in contrast, can produce disease almost anywhere in the body, although they may be more likely to invade some sites than others.) In general, viral infections are self-limited and do not produce permanent damage; but acute attacks of some viruses, such as those that cause poliomyelitis and encephalitis, may have permanent crippling results. The long-range damage caused by such infections may be due to the direct action of the virus or to the development of allergic reactions to tissues that have been altered by viral activity.

Viruses may also have serious effects that are not immediately apparent but that become evident months or years after the acute stage of the infection is over. This phenomenon of "slow virus infection" was first described in 1954 by the Icelandic veterinarian B. Sigurdsson, who correctly attributed three types of sheep disease to slow viruses. In the past two decades, slow viruses that may cause human disease have been studied extensively. Most of the slow viruses we now know of cause prolonged infection and eventual degeneration of the nervous system. (These are discussed extensively in Chapter 11.) Recent evidence suggests that even multiple sclerosis may result from a slow virus infection. But not all slow viruses affect the nervous system. Warts are caused by a specific virus and may persist for years once they develop. German measles acquired by babies *in utero* persists in them for months to years after birth; similarly, infectious hepatitis may be featured by persistent and chronic activity, with long persistence of the virus in the blood. Although chicken pox develops acutely, the virus that produces it (varicella) usually becomes latent in cells and persists for very prolonged periods or even for life. Certain triggering events (still largely unknown) may cause varicella to leave the cells where it is sequestered and migrate to the skin, where it causes shingles, an acute skin inflammation.

Early virologists were ignorant of the different ways that viral infections could develop. Even the basic process of the viral infection of cells has become understood only recently, since the introduction of the modern biochemical technology required for its study.

Early researchers could only show the activity of a virus by a process of elimination. If it could be shown that disease was caused by a preparation that did not contain any known pathogenic agents (such as bacteria), then the illness could be ascribed to a virus—although no one knew exactly what viruses were or how they worked. In 1892 a Russian botanist, D. Iwanowski, became the first to demonstrate that an agent capable of passing through a filter that held back bacteria produced disease. He noted that a filtered extract of ground-up diseased tobacco leaves reproduced the original disorder when applied to healthy leaves of the plant. Although the results of this experiment were clear-cut and reproducible, questions were raised as to whether it was a virus that had been transmitted or whether the changes in the plant were due to toxic particles of organic material. But one year later, the first virus involved in an animal disease—foot and mouth disease in cattle—was discovered and its prime role in this infection proved.

The first viral agent proven to be a cause of human illness was found by Walter Reed and James Carroll at the turn of the century. This was the agent of yellow fever, an infection that was responsible for a large number of deaths among the personnel engaged in the construction of the Panama Canal. Yellow fever, which is carried by mosquitoes, was the first viral infection shown to be caused by the bite of an insect. (We now know of 250 viruses that are transmitted by insects, usually mosquitoes and ticks.) This understanding of the spread of yellow fever—together with the earlier demonstration that malaria was carried by mosquitoes— lent some credence to the old concept that disease came from the swamps, since swamps are the areas in which mosquitoes breed and multiply.

The characterization of viruses and their role in human disease progressed slowly for many years, in spite of the exciting prospects that virology offered. One of the most difficult problems facing early virologists was the paucity of methods useful in the recovery and cultivation of viruses. Mice were used extensively as experimental animals in attempts to isolate viruses from various infected fluids and tissues. However, one of the difficulties associated with the use of these rodents was the fact that they carried latent viruses. Material suspected of containing a virus could be injected into the mouse experimentally, but even if death followed, this did not prove that the material itself had proved fatal. It was known that the trauma of injection, especially into the brain, might activate a latent virus; and it might be this latent virus that produced the lethal effect observed. Despite these limitations, mice and a variety of other animals were used in attempts to recover viruses from infected tissues and fluids. In 1909, for example, K. Landsteiner and E. Pepper succeeded in transmitting the agent that caused poliomyelitis to Rhesus monkeys, which developed a disease identical with that occurring spontaneously in people.

The chance to eliminate the problem of animal experimentation from virology came with the discovery that viruses can multiply in cultures of tissue grown outside animal or human bodies. This methodological breakthrough opened the way to growing large quantities of pure virus for identification and study. Alexis Carrel demonstrated that the virus reponsible for a tumor in chickens, Rous sarcoma, replicated in tissue culture; and the virus of cowpox was cultivated in testicular cells of rabbits in 1920. But in spite of these preliminary suggestions that some viruses were capable of multiplying in tissue cultures grown outside the body, very little progress was made until much later in the development and use of this method. A major remaining problem was that fluids and tissues obtained from infected persons or animals were often contaminated, even after filtration, with bacteria and other organisms that destroyed the tissue cultures.

The development of antibiotics and other antimicrobial agents was the vital step that made it possible to cultivate many viruses outside the body; these agents were used to inhibit the growth of contaminating microbes that destroyed cells in tissue culture. If antimicrobial agents had not been developed, the field of virology might never have reached the advanced stage of development it presently occupies. The usefulness of antibiotics was demonstrated in 1954 when researchers at the Harvard Medical School succeeded in cultivating the virus responsible for poliomyelitis in cells derived from human foreskin. Their success opened the modern era of virology. It was finally possible, by proper selection of cells and media in which to grow them, to isolate and identify most of the viral agents involved in animal and human diseases. As with a number of other discoveries that have led to dramatic advances in knowledge, it was the development of a new basic method of research—the use of tissue culture —that opened and expanded this important scientific and clinical field.

Once viruses could be grown with relative ease outside the body, new viruses were rapidly discovered. Half a century ago, only about 10 viruses were known; and 20 years ago, only 70. But the method of tissue culture led to the identification of over 300 viruses. Some have been associated with infections that had already been known for many years; others turned out to be the cause of newly described infectious diseases. Viruses have been classified on the basis of their size, the type of nucleic acid they contain, the sites in which they multiply in tissue, the means by which they are transmitted to man, and their shape as revealed by the electron microscope. (They may be rod-shaped, round or oval, icosahedral, helical, hexagonal, square with rounded corners, or even filamentous.)

Virology more than any other field of biology demonstrates the important contributions to clinical medicine and to the definition of fundamental biological processes that may accrue from purely basic scientific research. All the presently available information concerning the classification of viruses and the diseases they are involved in has been the product of years of basic research in virology and molecular biology. Tissue culture, immunological techniques, electron microscopy, and biochemical studies have supplied all the details of viral structure and behavior. These methods have been used to prove the direct relationship of different viruses to specific infections, to develop methods for early and late diagnosis, to study the antiviral effects of drugs and other agents, and to produce safe and effective immunizing preparations, vaccines.

Immunization against Viral Disease

Successful immunization has demonstrated the potential value of preventive medicine. Because there are presently no proven effective means for treating viral infections after they occur, attention has been directed primarily to the development of vaccines that will produce immunity against viral diseases. Thus, the main thrust has been in the direction of prophylaxis rather than therapy and will probably continue to be so until drugs are discovered that are effectively therapeutic.

The impact of the combined efforts of basic scientists, clinicians, and epidemiologists has been reflected in the large number of effective vaccines now available for protection against many viral infections, including influenza, measles, poliomyelitis, mumps, and rubella (German measles). Immunization works by exposing the individual to a harmless form of a virus (the vaccine), so that antibodies to the virus will be developed even though the virus does not cause disease. Widespread immunization requires a method for producing some harmless form of a virus in large quantities. Tissue culture has made it much easier for researchers to produce variants of a virus that may be effective immunizing agents and for clinicians and epidemiologists to carry out careful field trials to determine both the effectiveness and the safety of a proposed vaccine. And once a vaccine has been developed, it can be produced in tissue culture in quantities large enough to make mass immunization possible.

The value of this new technique has been striking. Before modern methods were developed, there were only three viral vaccines of any value: the vaccines for influenza and for yellow fever (both cultivated in chicken eggs) and the vaccine for smallpox (grown on the skin of calves). Vaccines for yellow fever and smallpox are now being produced in tissue cultures and are safer and easier to produce than the old vaccines. Although smallpox immunization had been available since the end of the eighteenth century, the disease remained highly prevalent in the developing areas of the world, where it killed thousands each year until very recently. In the past few years, new methods for mass immunization have been applied to vaccinate huge numbers of people for smallpox, and the disease has been almost totally eradicated. (It now appears that smallpox is no longer present anywhere on earth except in a small area of Ethiopia.) All viral vaccines, except the one for influenza, are now grown in tissue culture.

In addition to developing new ways to grow vaccines, basic scientists have made a major contribution by devising methods to weaken (attenuate) pathogenic viruses so that, although they lose the ability to cause disease, they still stimulate the production of antibodies and thus make effective vaccines.

One method of changing viruses to produce vaccines has been to alter the virus genetically. This approach has been successful in many cases and has been one of the main methods of producing attenuated viruses; and it is likely to find more applications in the future. Two major mechanisms—mutation and recombination—are involved in the induction of genetic variation in viruses.

Mutation consists of a change at one specific point in the nucleic acid that makes up the genetic code of the virus. Mutation may occur spontaneously in many types of virus, although the chance of a given virus experiencing a mutation is only about one in a million. But a number of viruses—like those that cause measles, mumps, rubella, chicken pox, and poliomyelitis—do not mutate spontaneously; they have remained genetically unchanged since they were first identified and characterized. Mutation of these stable viruses may be induced in the laboratory by exposing the virus to chemical or physical agents that produce alterations in nucleic acid.

Recombination involves the exchange of genetic material between two viral agents that are present simultaneously in a cell. This process results in the production of a new strain of virus (the recombinant) that possesses characteristics that are not found together in either of the parent viruses. The new combination of characteristics may result in an attenuated virus.

The field of genetic manipulation of viruses, as well as of bacteria and animal cells, has attracted a great deal of attention in the last few years. Efforts at genetic manipulation have raised considerable controversy because of the danger that such experiments may accidentally result in the production of new organisms that are actually more dangerous to man. But to date, genetic changes have successfully been used to alter viruses so as to make them less, not more, dangerous. Some of the live attentuated viral vaccines now available are the product of spontaneous mutation. Living poliomyelitis vaccine was developed by cultivating strains of the virus in tissue culture repeatedly until attenuated strains capable of producing immunity but not disease appeared. Similar approaches have been used to develop effective vaccines for mumps, German measles, and measles.

The introduction in 1956 of a vaccine for poliomyelitis had rapid and dramatic results; the disease quickly began to disappear (Table 6-1).

Table 6–1. Number of cases of and deaths due to measles and polio, Massachusetts, 1945–55 and 1962–72

Year	Measles		Poliomyelitis[a]	
	Cases	Deaths	Cases	Deaths
1945	7846	10	527	22
1946	38400	14	378	19
1947	12065	12	345	12
1948	37081	118	175	5
1949	26394	12	1782	51
1950	12850	2	518	9
1951	16728	5	288	11
1952	52866	17	548	17
1953	2290	1	635	28
1954	23526	6	1035	18
1955	50619	19	3950	175
TOTAL	280,665	216	10,181	367
1962	26969	0	7	3
1963	4978	0	3	0
1964	7265	1	0	0
1965	19152	4	1	1
1966	853[b]	0	5	0
1967	420	0	2	0
1968	385	0	2	1
1969	262	1	0	0
1970	482	0	2	0
1971	276	0	1	–
1972	1189	–	0	–
TOTAL	62,231	6	23	5

Source: L. Weinstein, "Infectious Disease: Retrospect and Reminiscence," Journal of Infectious Disease 129 (1974), 480–492; reprinted by permission of the University of Chicago Press. Copyright © 1974 by the University of Chicago.

[a] Use of killed poliomyelitis vaccine started on nationwide scale in 1956.

[b] This reflects the wide use of measles vaccine.

This first polio vaccine contained virus that had been killed. Once injected, it produced immunity against infection of the nervous system; but it unfortunately did not appear to prevent wild strains of poliomyelitis from colonizing the intestinal tract and possibly being transmitted to susceptible individuals from there. Today, a live attenuated vaccine, which was developed to solve these problems, has completely replaced the original vaccine in clinical practice. Since there are three antigenically distinct types of poliomyelitis virus, all three must be given, either together or sequentially. Unlike any of the other viral vaccines presently in use, polio vaccine is given by mouth; once swallowed, the virus lives and multiplies in the intestine, where it stimulates antibody production. It is interesting, and fortunate, that this vaccine tends to spread in families; if one person in a family is vaccinated, the virus may spread to all the others in the group and immunize them. Immunization of 75 percent or more of all preschool children also protects most nonimmune adults by reducing the pool of wild virus, present primarily in youngsters, from which the disease is spread. (This phenomenon is known as herd immunity.)

The measles vaccine, also a living attenuated virus, has proven to be highly effective (Table 6-1). Although it is considerably attenuated, the measles vaccine may produce mild measles occasionally; but this can be prevented by giving the vaccine together with a dose of human gamma globulin containing antibody to the virus. More recent preparations, which are less virulent (more attenuated), do not require the administration of globulin. In spite of their possible side effects, live attenuated measles vaccines are more effective than vaccines containing killed virus. Even the live vaccine may fail to produce long-term immunity in some children; some youngsters may develop measles despite previous immunization. This phenomenon suggests the need for booster doses.

Until recently, German measles (rubella) has been a very common viral infection, sometimes occurring in worldwide epidemics. Rubella has posed the greatest threat to the unborn children of pregnant women infected with the virus. Although other viral diseases, including mumps, measles, influenza, and infectious hepatitis, have been thought by some to cause birth defects or death *in utero* in the children of pregnant women they infect. This is much less of a problem than rubella. (It is also possible—although there are no valid supporting data for this—that a number of viral illnesses that are not yet fully characterized may, if severe, lead to premature delivery.) But rubella has been responsible for birth defects more often than any other virus. Table 6-2 illustrates the levels of risk to the fetus exposed to rubella while in the womb. The greatest danger to the unborn child is during the first month or two of pregnancy; after 20 weeks, the danger has practically disappeared. The defects that have been observed in such children have involved the heart, eyes, brain, ears, blood-forming organs, and bones.

Table 6–2. Incidence of congenital malformations and rubella syndrome in infants of mothers with rubella during pregnancy

Country and year		Number of pregnant women	Number of live-born infants	Number of children with major defects	Stage of gestation (weeks) and percent born with defects						
					0–4	5–8	9–12	12–16	17–20	First trimester	Total pregnancies
Worldwide, 1946–61	R	–	1231	96	33	25	9	4	1	20	8
	C	–	–	–	–	–	–	–	–	–	–
Sweden, 1951	R	1140	1121	51	11	11	8	1.4	0.5	10	6.6
	C	712	698	5	–	–	–	–	–	0.7	0.7
United Kingdom, 1951	R	578	547	37	15.6	19.7	13	4.2	2.2	15.6	6.4
	C	5767	5655	128	–	–	–	–	–	2.3	2.3
France, 1953–64	R	48	42	23	100	63	40	–	75	66.6	50
	C	571	551	0	–	–	–	–	–	–	–
Australia, 1957–61	R	145	707	20	60	33	33.4	5.7	–	23.6	10
	C	–	–	–	–	–	–	–	–	–	–

Sources: R. Lundström, "Rubella in Pregnancy," Acta Paediatrica 51 (1962), 9–102; M. M. Manson, W. P. D. Logan, and R. M. Loy, "Rubella and Other Virus Infections During Pregnancy," Ministry of Health Report on Public Health and Medical Subjects, no. 101, pp. 1–110 (London: Her Majesty's Stationery Office, 1960); M. Lamy and M. E. Séror, "La Rubéole de la Femme Enceinte," Archiv für die Gesamte Virusforschung 17 (1965), 377–390; D. Pitt and E. H. Keir, "Results of Rubella in Pregnancy," Medical Journal of Australia 2 (1965), 647–651.

R = Mother had rubella during pregnancy.
C = Mother had no rubella during pregnancy.

Because rubella is a potentially serious threat to the developing fetus, a number of vaccines have been developed for this disease; and a widespread program of immunization has led to a marked decrease in the number of cases reported in the United States during the past decade. But the effectiveness of presently available vaccines in preventing birth defects by immunization of young children alone has been questioned. The authors have found that these vaccines produce only relatively weak immunity and that people immunized against rubella may still contract a clinically inapparent form of the disease if they come into contact with a wild strain of the virus. The effectiveness of the rubella vaccine will probably depend at least partially on the age of the individuals who are immunized. Since the type of herd immunity that occurs when young children are vaccinated against polio does not occur with rubella, inoculation of children cannot be expected to protect adults in the population as well. Because this disease is most dangerous in pregnancy, some have suggested that the vaccine be administered at the time of puberty in girls and immediately after the birth of a child in other women. Prevention of rubella may be facilitated in the near future by a new attenuated rubella vaccine, which can be instilled into the nose; this vaccine now appears to be safe and to afford long-term protection from German measles.

In addition to measles and German measles, the other well-known viral diseases of childhood—chicken pox and mumps—continue to account for much serious illness, some of which has led to permanent damage and even death. In the United States, there were between 140,000 and 180,000 cases of chicken pox each year between 1972 and 1974; the annual number of deaths from this disease over the same time period ranged from 81 to 153. Mumps has been almost as prevalent; there were 60,000 to 120,000 cases of mumps annually between 1968 and 1974, with 12 to 50 patients dying of the disease during each of those years. But researchers continue to develop new ways of fighting the childhood diseases. A mumps vaccine has been developed recently and may reliably prevent this infection.

To be effective, a vaccine must be designed to confer immunity to a very specific infectious agent; a vaccine against one type of virus that can cause a given disease will not protect the individual against other viruses that may have the same clinical effects. As mentioned before, polio vaccines contain attenuated forms of three distinct types of poliomyelitis virus; although all of these viruses cause polio, immunization against one alone will not protect the individual against the other two. A goal of one branch of viral research is the accurate identification of viral agents so that vaccines against them may be developed.

Researchers are now attempting to develop vaccines against hepatitis, and immunization against this disease may become possible within a decade. Two main types of virus, type A and type B, have been known for some time to cause infectious hepatitis. Type A hepatitis is usually transmitted by the fecal-oral route, through various types of food, shellfish, water, and human carriers. Type B hepatitis—which is generally more serious—is usually transmitted in the course of blood transfusion or the use of blood products, or from exposure to contaminated needles and syringes. Studies of the type B virus have demonstrated the importance of basic sciences such as biochemistry and immunology; the nature of a number of proteins present in the virus have been identified immunologically, and it has been suggested that these are associated in specific ways with the infectiousness and severity of the disease.

It now also appears that there may be a third type of hepatitis virus, nonA nonB (some prefer to call it type C). Hepatitis nonA nonB closely resembles hepatitis B; it is also transmitted through blood transfusion. However, the virus that may cause this third type of hepatitis has yet to be identified. If a nonA nonB virus is characterized, it may become possible to develop a vaccine against it as well. (Although these three viruses are responsible for most cases of infectious hepatitis, it should be mentioned that other unrelated viral agents, such as yellow fever virus, may produce a similar type of liver disease.)

Even when a specific and effective vaccine is developed, it may be rendered obsolete by genetic changes in the virus it is designed to protect against. Such spontaneous viral mutation has been a major obstacle to the effective prevention of influenza.

Influenza is so common that we have become accustomed to the epidemics of influenza, resulting from type A or type B strains of this virus, that occur somewhere in the world every year. But influenza is more than an annoyance; it can be a serious, and even lethal, disease. The influenza virus may fatally invade the brain, the lung, or the heart; or invasion of the intestinal tract, with severe abdominal pain, vomiting, and diarrhea, may occur. The potential ferocity of the influenza virus is best illustrated by the worldwide pandemic it caused in 1918, which affected the entire globe (except for a few small islands and Australia). Although the pandemic lasted less than three months, it involved at least 500 million people and caused about 20 million deaths; the number of deaths caused by influenza in this short time matched the fatalities over comparable time periods during the epidemics of yellow fever and bubonic plague that occurred in the seventeenth and eighteenth centuries. When the influenza epidemic was raging at its worst, it killed an average of 175 people a day in Boston, 600 to 700 in New York City, and 1,700 in Philadelphia.

Fortunately, such disastrous loss of life did not occur during three subsequent pandemics. In fact, pandemic influenza in 1957 was not any worse clinically than influenza in 1947, a nonpandemic year. The bacterial complications of influenza that were responsible for most deaths in the 1918 pandemic are no longer life-threatening, thanks to antibiotics and modern medical care. But if the consequences of influenza epidemics are less serious now than they were fifty years ago, the epidemics themselves remain very hard to prevent.

The prevention of influenza epidemics is made unusually difficult by the genetic mutability of some of the viruses that can cause them. Although type B virus remains relatively stable from year to year, strains of type A frequently undergo major or minor genetic changes that alter the proteins of the virus. Since antibodies recognize and attack the virus by recognizing these proteins, it may be impossible for antibodies formed against an earlier strain of influenza virus to combat the new, altered strain. Thus the value of immunization (which relies on the formation of specific antibodies) becomes unpredictable; vaccines prepared for protection against disease during one epidemic may be ineffective in the next. To produce an effective vaccine, it may be necessary to determine the type of virus responsible for each outbreak, isolate it, and grow it in large quantities in time to make it available for use in immunization; but this is often not possible until after an epidemic is already under way. Constant worldwide surveillance by virologists and epidemiologists is needed to detect genetic shifts and drifts (minor and major genetic changes, respectively) as early as possible. In 1976 such surveillance uncovered cases of influenza due to the swine influenza virus, the agent thought to have been responsible for the pandemic of 1918; and the early detection of this virus made it possible to begin plans for national immunization almost immediately. (As this chapter is being written, it is still not possible to predict whether or not the epidemic of 1918 will repeat itself in the immediate future.)

Attempts are also being made to improve the effectiveness of the influenza vaccines that are developed. One area that has been a major focus of research attention has been the development of an effective live influenza vaccine (the vaccines now available use killed influenza virus). Temperature-sensitive mutants (viruses that can survive only at relatively low temperatures) have now been developed and used experimentally. These temperature-sensitive viruses can be introduced into the nose, which is somewhat colder than the rest of the body; here they stimulate antibody production but do not produce disease. The technique of recombination has also been applied to make new types of influenza virus and to develop other strains that will become effective and safe live vaccines.

Immunization is the most powerful tool for combating viral disease that is now available; but it is not the answer to all the problems posed by viral infection. Effective vaccines remain to be found for several serious viral illnesses. And even the best vaccines can only prevent disease from developing; they can do nothing for the person who has already contracted a viral infection. While immunological programs continue, virologists have begun to intensify their search for chemical agents that can be used to prevent or to treat viral disease.

The Search for Antiviral Agents

Unlike the search for drugs to treat bacterial infections, which has been essentially a process of "search and find," the development of antiviral compounds has been, with few exceptions, based directly on knowledge of the dynamics and biochemistry of viral replication. The invasion and replication of viruses in cells involves several sequential steps; drugs that disrupt any of these steps will keep the virus from growing and producing disease. The specific nature of each step is determined by the type of virus, the site of its multiplication within the cell, and the kind of cell with which it becomes associated. Our knowledge of the process of viral infection has been acquired from very basic studies utilizing the techniques of molecular biology. These studies, which have indicated possible approaches to treatment based on interruption of viral replication by drugs that act at specific stages of the process, will surely be essential to the further development of potent antiviral drugs.

Although intensive effort has been directed for many years to the discovery of effective agents for the treatment of established viral infections, little has been accomplished so far. A major obstacle has been the complexity of the biological processes involved in viral invasion and replication in cells. The problems of viral disease are much more complex than those of bacterial disease because viruses multiply within the body's cells; there is a constant danger that agents that injure viruses will also produce irreversible damage to the cells in which they are multiplying. The timing of the viral life cycle also partially accounts for the failure of many drugs to alter the course of viral disease after clinical manifestations have become apparent. Within 12 to 48 hours after the virus has penetrated the cell, the virus has taken over the cellular machinery for its own purposes and has begun to replicate itself. Evidence of infection often does not appear until a week or more has elapsed and is therefore probably not due to the viral activity itself as much as to the resultant damage to invaded cells. Thus, drugs with potent antiviral activity in the laboratory may have little or no effect on the course of viral disease that has already developed because they cannot correct the cellular dysfunction set in motion days or weeks earlier. Their only beneficial activity may be to prevent the spread of virus from infected to uninfected cells, a process that probably goes on during and after clinical manifestations have developed.

Very few effective antiviral agents are currently available. Although many drugs are effective in tissue culture, most have failed to alter the course of infection in experimental animals or man. Some drugs that have proven beneficial when given to people have been limited in their usefulness because their toxicity has made them too dangerous for clinical application. The few chemicals that do appear to hold some therapeutic promise are quite restricted in their activity. Each is effective against only one or two specific viruses. Idoxuridine is of value in the treatment of eye infections due to one type of herpes virus; it is incorporated into the DNA of the virus and increases its susceptibility to breakage. Amantadine prevents the penetration of type A influenza virus into cells and produces a prophylactic effect when given to persons exposed to type A influenza virus, but it is of no value against type B strains. Cytosine and adenine arabinosides act on viruses by inhibiting two enzymes involved in viral replication. The cytosine compound appears to be beneficial when applied locally in eye infections caused by idoxuridine-resistant strains of herpes simplex, but it is not effective in other diseases produced by this virus. Because of its toxicity, it has been suggested that it not be used clinically. Adenine arabinoside is without effect when applied locally in infection due to *Herpesvirus hominis,* but it has promise, when given intravenously, in the management of severe disease caused by this virus. The drug also exerts a beneficial effect on shingles in immunosuppressed but not in immunologically normal patients.

Recent research has begun to turn from synthetic antiviral agents to natural substances that suppress viral activity. Within 12 to 48 hours after intracellular viral multiplication has reached its maximum, it is rapidly brought to a halt by interferon, a substance produced by the infected cells. All cells have the capacity to make this compound, although they do not make it under normal circumstances. Infection by some viruses—and exposure to some other kinds of agents—induces the cell to start making interferon. Different kinds of interferon have been demonstrated under various experimental conditions; they constitute a special class of proteins whose common property is their capacity to inhibit the replication of viruses. (Actually, interferon itself does not inhibit viral multiplication; it stimulates the synthesis of another protein that is the active inhibitory agent.)

Interferon should be an ideal antiviral agent. It is a potent inhibitor of the replication of both DNA- and RNA-containing viruses; it is virtually nontoxic; and it can be given repeatedly without causing the individual to develop antibodies to it. Attempts have therefore been made to use it in the treatment of human viral disease. Interferon is strictly species-specific; when produced by the cells of chickens, mice, or rabbits, for example, it is effective only in the species in which it was made. For it to act in people, it must be made in human cells. The first studies employed interferon obtained from cultures infected with virus; however, the difficulty of producing adequate quantities of interferon by this method limited its application. But it has now been found that human white blood cells and cultures of certain other human cells are rich sources of interferon.

Interferon would seem to hold much clinical promise; but despite the fact that this antiviral agent has been known and studied intensively for the past 18 years, it has not yet found practical therapeutic use. Patients with severe viral infections fail to respond when given interferon intravenously. However, local applications of this substance may prevent the development of disease at the site where it is applied. For example, when sprayed into the nose, interferon has been noted to exert a favorable effect on type B influenza and common colds caused by certain viruses.

The approaches that have been used to develop antiviral agents dramatically illustrate the importance of studies of the molecular biology of viruses. The various antiviral chemicals now being investigated have all been selected for evaluation because of their effects on viruses at the molecular level. And the existence of interferon came to light through very basic studies of the biochemistry of cells and the viruses that infect them. It seems certain that future advances in virology will continue to come from such highly sophisticated studies of the basic processes and mechanisms of viral infection.

The Immune System and Diseases of Inflammation

K. FRANK AUSTEN

7

The immune response is essential to human life; it is the body's principal means of defense against the hostile bacteria and viruses that exist in the environment. For this reason, malfunctions of the immune system can lead to sickness and occasionally to death. When the body's defenses are not functioning fully, the individual becomes much more susceptible to infections of all kinds; it is even likely that the risk of developing cancer may increase when the normal immunological response to malignant cells is deficient. It is easy to understand why such immunological deficiencies should be dangerous. However, disease is often caused by overreactions of the immune system rather than by inadequate reactions. In certain disorders, the body's defenses may mount a full-scale attack against an innocuous bit of foreign material or may even begin to attack the body's own cells, with harmful results. This chapter deals with diseases caused by precisely this type of immunological error.

The response to foreign material in the body is carried out by special types of white blood cells. Many molecules, including viruses and bacterial products, induce the production of circulating antibodies by cells derived from white cells called type B lymphocytes. (Molecules against which antibodies are made are called antigens.) Antibodies are formed so as to attach themselves specifically to the introduced antigen and not to any other type of molecule. Bacteria, toxins produced by bacteria, and some viruses are rendered harmless when bound to antibodies and can easily be digested by other kinds of white cells (the phagocytes) in this form. Molecules on the cell surface of bacteria elicit antibody formation; when antibodies have bound to these antigens, a circulating substance known as complement attaches itself to the antigen-antibody complex, thereby enhancing digestion by phagocytes or rupturing the bacterial wall, with death of the bacterium. Other types of antigens do not induce production of circulating antibodies at all but are attacked directly by white cells known as type T lymphocytes.

To be optimally effective, these types of immune response are often preceded by changes in the circulatory system. Such changes are controlled by specialized cells known as mast cells that are found in connective tissue throughout the body and that are especially concentrated in the skin and in the lining of the respiratory and gastrointestinal tracts. When tissue is injured in infection, the mast cells release various chemicals, including histamine, into the bloodstream. Histamine acts on the circulatory system to increase blood flow and make the venules more permeable to antibodies and complement. These local changes, which result in a state of inflammation, facilitate the destruction of the infectious agent by antibodies, complement, lymphocytes, and phagocytes.

Inflammation itself can become a problem, however. At best, it is a painful process, accompanied by redness, swelling, and heat in the affected tissue. At worst, excessive release of histamine and other chemical mediators in inflammation can strain the circulatory system to the point of collapse. Malfunctions in the inflammatory response are intimately tied to errors in antibody function, which are of two basic types: errors in antigen recognition and errors in antibody response. When antibodies inappropriately identify drugs and pollens as foreign invaders, the cellular damage that follows the resultant immune response may lead to dangerous local inflammation or systemic shock. And even when the right antigens are attacked, an excessive response may damage host tissues. The different types of adverse reaction of the immune system, known collectively as hypersensitivity reactions, are in fact the basis of allergies, arthritis, and several other disorders that are major health problems today.

Allergic Disease

Allergic diseases are the most common example of errors in response in the immune system. In these disorders, basically innocuous antigens trigger an unnecessary immune response, mediated by special kinds of antibodies of the class immunoglobulin E (IgE). Allergic disorders differ in their symptomatology and seriousness, depending largely on what antigen is eliciting the hypersensitivity reaction. Asthma, a recurrent, generally reversible condition of obstructed breathing, is the most serious in terms of medical care required and attendant disability; about 9 million Americans suffer from this disease (but only a portion are clearly allergic). Another 14.5 million have an allergic inflammation of nasal passages or hay fever (allergic rhinitis); about 11.8 million have other types of allergy, including skin problems (such as hives and eczema) and hypersensitivity to foods, drugs, and insect stings. Although usually only damaging or disabling, allergic diseases can be fatal, particularly in the case of asthma; hundreds of cases of sudden death also result annually from anaphylaxis, an acute reaction that can occur minutes after an insect sting or after drug injection. The economic cost of allergic disease is considerable; in 1969, 345 million dollars were spent on physician services and 235 million dollars on drugs used in the management of hay fever and asthma.

It has long been known that hay fever and bronchial asthma frequently occur together in the same individual and that both conditions often run in families. This observation suggests that the tendency to develop an allergic reaction is largely inherited. However, the specific materials which elicit asthma, hay fever, and hives are determined by environmental conditions, both current and past. For example, an individual growing up in Europe, where there is no ragweed, may manifest ragweed hay fever within three to five years after moving to the United States. Interestingly, once an individual develops this type of sensitivity, it can persist even when the affected person has been away from a pollen-generating area for many years. The problem is not limited to pollens; individuals may react allergically to a variety of foods, industrial agents, household molds, materials present in household dust, and animal danders. The same person may react to different allergens at different times in his or her life.

Recent research has clarified the biological and genetic basis of the allergic reaction. It is now known that allergies stem from a genetic tendency, inherited through recessive genes which may control amounts of IgE antibodies as well as the specificity of the material recognized as foreign. IgE antibodies, which are present in relatively small numbers in the bloodstream, affix themselves strongly to mast cells. When an allergen such as pollen enters the body of an allergic individual it reacts with the IgE on the mast cells, causing secretion of the cell's noxious substances. In the skin, the result is hives; in the nose, runniness and stuffiness; in the lung, asthma; and in the stomach and intestines, vomiting and diarrhea.

If the allergen enters the bloodstream, as does insect venom, the mast cells are diffusely involved throughout the body and the individual may suffer shock with or without preceding breathing difficulty. The specific substances that an individual becomes allergic to are determined by the nature of the excessive IgE antibodies; a person with an overabundance of IgE antibodies to pollen will show an allergic reaction only to pollen. This specification of IgE antibodies, and hence of the allergen, appears to be controlled by both environmental and genetic factors.

Treatment of allergies begins with the identification of the allergen so that the patient can avoid it. Detailed investigation of the individual's work, living, and eating habits may be required, along with skin testing with extracts of known, naturally occurring, allergens. (Skin tests for allergy to drugs and chemicals generally give unsatisfactory results.) Test tube techniques for identifying the specific IgE antibody involved are under development and should be helpful in the future. Once the allergen has been determined, avoidance may involve such major disruptions as a job change, a move to a new locale, or severe limitation of diet. Some allergens are virtually unavoidable. In these cases a process known as desensitization or immunotherapy may be used; extracts of the allergen are injected in gradually increasing doses over many months to induce the production of another kind of antibody, IgG, and minimize the reproduction of IgE antibodies. (If many IgG antibodies to the allergen are produced, then these circulating antibodies should bind to the allergen when the individual comes into contact with it, thus preventing IgE from reacting with the allergen.) The efficacy of this approach has been established for prevention of anaphylaxis (severe systemic reaction) to certain types of insect stings and for the treatment of hay fever. When the allergen cannot be detected or when desensitization is not helpful or justified, drugs are used to inhibit or limit the allergic reaction. Antihistamines, adrenaline-like drugs, and caffeine-like drugs are particularly helpful and may obviate the need for desensitization treatment. Drugs like cortisone are also effective, but their side effects limit their systemic use to only the most intractable problems; however, local instillation of such steroids may prove to be a workable effective approach.

Research on many levels is directed toward identifying the normal mode of action of genes which control production of IgE antibodies. Other research is aimed at understanding IgE attachment to mast cells in the hope of finding ways to block this step. Exciting progress has also been made recently in identifying the diverse mast cell products besides histamine which produce allergic symptoms, in the hope of eventually being able to delineate and pharmacologically prevent the biochemical steps in their generation, release, and action.

Systemic Lupus Erythematosus (SLE)

Although the precise factors causing this inflammatory disease remain unknown, most patients with systemic lupus erythematosus (SLE) develop circulating antibodies to components of their own cells, particularly nuclei and deoxyribonucleic acid (DNA). The symptoms of SLE are varied and can be quite serious. The disease may be marked by skin lesions, hair loss, sun sensitivity, arthritis, nephritis (kidney disease), recurrent fevers, anemia, and inflammation of the outer lining of the lung and heart. Less frequently it may involve the central nervous system. Patients with SLE need not develop all these signs but usually have various combinations of them. The disease affects an estimated 500,000 Americans; women, especially those in their twenties and thirties, are afflicted nine times as frequently as men. Each year approximately 50,000 new cases are discovered and 5,000 people die from SLE.

SLE and related disorders may be noted among members of the same family, suggesting that genetic factors play a role in the etiology of this disease. This speculation is supported by the observation of inherited complement deficiencies in patients with SLE and by the high concordance for SLE in identical but not in nonidentical twins. Environmental factors also play a role, however. The disease may be triggered by sun exposure, infections, or the use of certain drugs. The detection of antibodies to certain viruses and of one type of viral antigen in some SLE patients suggests the influence of viral infections. These separate observations lead to the conclusion that the etiology of SLE probably includes many factors, with inherited abnormal immune responses to microorganisms and tissue antigens resulting in tissue damage through the deposition of immune complexes.

Treatment of this disease is still primarily empirical and is aimed at preventing permanent tissue injury by suppressing inflammation. Research on SLE is presently focusing on many areas: the clarification of the role of antibodies to different nuclear antigens and nucleic acids; elucidation of the nature and implications of abnormalities in the components of the complement system; exploration of the possible contributions of viruses, including an attempt to isolate viruses from patients and animals with SLE; determination of the role of genetic factors; and development of new drugs which will be more effective and safer than the presently employed agents.

Rheumatoid Arthritis

Arthritis probably represents the most important public health problem of the diseases of inflammation; it is widespread, serious, and poorly understood. Arthritic disease affects 20 million Americans of all ages; approximately 10 percent of all physician visits in the United States are accounted for by individuals suffering from arthritis and related musculoskeletal disorders. Arthritis is the second leading cause of illness for all age groups, disabling a total of nearly 3.5 million persons, and is the primary cause of limited mobility in individuals over the age of 45. Disability payments to workers crippled by arthritis are approaching one half billion dollars annually and are expected to pass the one billion dollar mark by the end of this decade. The total annual cost of arthritis including medical care was estimated at 9.2 billion dollars in 1972, and there is reason to believe that this cost is increasing at the rate of one billion dollars per year.

The most prevalent and crippling form of arthritis is rheumatoid arthritis, which affects 4 to 5 million Americans. (Unfortunately, there are still very few physicians specializing in this disorder; there are only about 1,500 to 2,000 fully qualified rheumatologists in the United States.) This disease affects approximately three times as many females as it does males, usually beginning in the fourth or fifth decade of life, and appears equally prevalent in all climates and among all races. Rheumatoid arthritis disrupts the tissues involved in joint function. The normal human joint is designed to provide painless motion with stability; the two bony surfaces of the joint are covered with articular cartilage, a pearly white, elastic substance that allows the bony ends to glide over each other with little friction. A capsule surrounding the joint is lined by a tissue called synovium which nourishes the joint and produces synovial fluid to keep the joint lubricated. In rheumatoid arthritis the essential defect is an inflammation of the synovium, called synovitis; over a period of years, this process can permanently cripple the individual by eroding the cartilage and bony structures of the joint (Figure 7-1). Although the synovium is the prime organ affected by rheumatoid arthritis, other organs are commonly involved, including the eyes, blood vessels, bone marrow, and the tissues overlying both the heart and the lungs. Rheumatoid arthritis is actually a generalized illness in which the patient, unlike someone with a sprained ankle, is sick in addition to being stiff; patients experience generalized fatigue and a sense of not being well.

While the cause of this disease is unknown, some progress has been made in the description of the biochemical changes that accompany it.

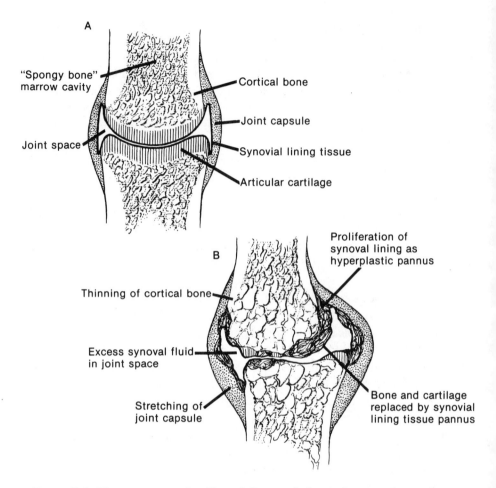

Figure 7–1. The synovium in health and disease. A shows the normal synovium in a joint. B shows the changes that occur with advanced rheumatoid arthritis: inflammation of the synovium is accompanied by an excess of synovial fluid, stretching of the capsule, and erosion of the cartilage and bony structures of the joint. The drawing was based on a sketch by Edward D. Harris, M.D.

Because the inflammatory nature of the disease resembles that of an infectious illness, repeated attempts have been made to isolate an infectious agent from patients with this condition. Such efforts have been unsuccessful, and epidemiological data also suggest that the disease is not infectious, at least not in the usual sense. The basis of the disease process in rheumatoid arthritis seems to involve an antigen-antibody reaction. Patients with rheumatoid arthritis have antibodies called rheumatoid factors mistakenly directed against their own circulating antibody proteins; these substances combine to form antigen-antibody complexes—with circulating antibodies acting as antigens to the rheumatoid factors—which activate complement in the joint fluid. The subsequent interaction of complement proteins generates biologically active byproducts which produce a state of inflammation: blood vessels leak, inflammatory cells enter the site of injury and release their destructive enzymes, and certain cell types die. The recognition that local antibody production, formation of immune complexes, and activation of the complement system occur in rheumatoid arthritis implies that the local joint injury seen in this disease is a form of hypersensitivity. Furthermore, the synovium lining of the joint not only produces antibodies from B lymphocytes but also is rich in T cells, suggesting a form of what is called cellular or delayed-type hypersensitivity. Although this information does not reveal what caused the immune response in the first place, it is sufficient to merit new therapeutic approaches and requires continued investigation.

Although there is presently no treatment which will guarantee a cure, rheumatoid arthritis can be brought into remission in many instances; and when this is not possible, its symptoms can be alleviated. Approximately 10 percent of patients undergo a spontaneous remission, although this is unlikely to occur if the patient has had the disease for more than one year. Certain drugs (gold salts and antimalarial agents) can induce a remission in many patients; but the success of this therapy is unpredictable, and the mechanism of its action is unknown. If a remission takes place before permanent structural damage to the cartilage and bone occurs, the patient will be able to return to full activity and a normal state of health. For patients in whom a remission is not obtained, numerous drugs, such as aspirin, other nonsteroidal anti-inflammatory drugs, or even occasionally corticosteroids, may be used to suppress inflammation. Cartilage, unlike bone, lacks the ability to regenerate or repair itself; once the joint surface has been destroyed, the sole means of correction is to replace it. The rapid development within the last few years of the technique of total joint replacement with metal or plastic prostheses (see Chapter 23) has given orthopedic surgeons the ability to repair structurally destroyed joints; with these techniques, few if any patients with rheumatoid arthritis need be crippled to the point of being bedfast. Joint replacement by itself is not a treatment of choice, however. It is costly, time-consuming, occasionally hazardous, and limited by the fact that it is local therapy and does not alleviate the generalized symptoms of rheumatoid arthritis.

Areas of investigation related to this disease which are likely to be productive in the future include: genetics; virology; research into cartilage synthesis and degradation; and the study of synovial tissue inflammation, the stimulus for its initiation, the mechanisms of its control, and the reasons for its continued activity. These issues are all poorly understood and can best be attacked by fundamental research into the basic mechanisms of tissue inflammation and normal joint physiology and biochemistry.

Juvenile Rheumatoid Arthritis

Juvenile rheumatoid arthritis (JRA) begins in children up to the age of 16 and can continue or recur throughout life. It afflicts approximately 250,000 children in the United States, females three times more frequently than males. It may affect the internal organs as well as the joints; it can threaten mobility, vision, and life itself. Although JRA resembles adult rheumatoid arthritis in some respects, there are many clinical and laboratory features in which these two diseases differ. As with adult rheumatoid arthritis the cause of JRA is unknown. Climate, emotional stress, physical exhaustion, and repeated infections may all exacerbate the disease, but these cannot be considered causative factors. The search for an infectious agent has so far been unrewarding. However, abnormalities of the immunoglobulins and the complement proteins have been implicated in the pathogenesis of this disease. As in adult rheumatoid arthritis, these abnormalities lead to tissue injury within the joints. Studies of the familial incidence of JRA and the frequency of its occurrence in the identical twins of JRA patients do not support the concept that the disease may be simply genetically transmitted; as in SLE, the abnormalities that cause this disease appear to be both environmental and inherited in origin.

The treatment of JRA is difficult and complex. Since there is no known cure for JRA, medical therapy must be directed to the suppression of inflammation. A majority of patients need the combined knowledge, experience, and skills of specialized physicians and allied health professionals to prevent and correct crippling, prevent blindness, and deal with complications such as inflammation of the covering of the heart (pericarditis). Early institution of treatment is essential to prevent irreversible damage. Of primary importance at the present time is the development of a better diagnostic test for JRA; the test for rheumatoid factor used in adults is positive in only 20 percent of patients with juvenile rheumatoid arthritis.

Gout

Unlike rheumatoid arthritis and JRA, the joint inflammation seen in gout has been traced to a definite, correctable abnormality: an excess of sodium urate in the bloodstream. Everyone has some sodium urate in the blood, since uric acid is one of the products of the utilization of food in the body; but in people with hyperuricemia, or gout, the levels are high enough to cause the precipitation of urate crystals in the cartilage of the joints or in the joint fluid. This abnormality results in attacks of acutely painful and often disabling arthritis. The urate is deposited not only in the soft tissue around joints in chronic gouty arthritis but also at various pressure points such as the tips of the fingers, elbows, knees, and bottoms of the feet; even more dangerous are urate deposits in the kidney, causing destruction of renal tissue often accompanied by infection, hypertension, renal failure, and kidney stones. The complications of hyperuricemia can occur singly or in various combinations; they may simply constitute a painful nuisance or may lead to severe disability and premature death. These complications usually emerge in the late forties, with an earlier onset being associated with higher degrees of urate elevation; asymptomatic hyperuricemia is not uncommon and occurs in as many as two thirds of those whose urate levels are considered elevated.

In the past decade research has revealed much about the pathways of urate metabolism and the role of specific enzymes in those pathways. In addition, the production of inflammation by urate crystals in acute gouty arthritis has been studied. Apparently the electric charge on the crystals, which are engulfed by white blood cells, prompts these cells to release substances which attract other white cells; the result is acute inflammation.

The factors that initially lead to high uric acid levels are varied and are being actively investigated. Primary hyperuricemia (gout stemming from basic defects in the way the body uses and processes food) may be caused by an enzymatic defect. The most severe example of this is the Lesch-Nyhan syndrome; this disorder appears in children and is characterized by severe mental retardation, abnormal body movements, and self-mutilation, as well as by the complications found in all types of gout. In most cases of primary gout, however, no specific enzymatic defect has yet been identified. In cases of secondary hyperuricemia, abnormalities arising from other diseases raise the level of uric acid in individuals whose uric acid level had previously been normal. Kidney failure, for example, lowers the excretion of uric acid and raises its level in the bloodstream. In the treatment of leukemia, large numbers of blood cells may be destroyed over a short period of time; this releases the building blocks of urate into the bloodstream, resulting in an elevation in the blood urate level. Today, the most common cause of secondary hyperuricemia and gout is the use of diuretic drugs designed to control high blood pressure or to decrease the retention of fluid in the body; many of these drugs also interfere with the excretion of uric acid by the kidney. The use of these medications is increasing the frequency of hyperuricemia in the population.

The emergence of new therapeutic drugs has markedly improved the outlook for most patients with gout. The development of the drug allopurinol, which decreases urate formation, has made it possible to reduce levels of serum urate to normal in patients with gout and has facilitated prevention of the complications of hyperuricemia. Unfortunately, it has been ineffective in treating the mental retardation and self-mutilatory behavior of children with Lesch-Nyhan syndrome. A number of therapeutic agents—colchicine, indomethacin (a nonsteroidal anti-inflammatory agent), and corticosteroids—are useful in the management of attacks of acute gouty arthritis, although the mechanism of their action unfortunately remains unclear.

Since gout is one of the few forms of acute arthritis related to a defined abnormality, further clarification of the sequence of events in gouty inflammation could be fairly rapid. It should also be possible to discover how hyperuricemia affects the kidney and why arteriolar nephrosclerosis (hardening of the kidney blood vessels) and hypertension so often develop. Such knowledge could profoundly influence the preventive medicine employed in this and related circumstances.

Ankylosing Spondylitis

Recent research has also played an important role in characterizing the disease ankylosing spondylitis, a type of spinal arthritis (once thought to be a variant of rheumatoid arthritis) that affects an estimated 2.5 million Americans. Ankylosing spondylitis is now known to be distinguished from rheumatoid arthritis by the lack of rheumatoid factors in this disorder, by its preponderance in males, and by strong evidence for its heritability. Studies of the blood cells of patients with ankylosing spondylitis have revealed that 95 percent of individuals suffering from this disease have a special kind of antigen called W27 on the surface of their white cells. Since the disorder is apparently inherited, relatives of people with ankylosing spondylitis can now be tested for the presence of W27 on their white cells; this test can be used to detect the disease in its early stages, when the individual may merely experience an unexplained pain in the lower back. (If the disease is allowed to continue unchecked, the patient may eventually experience severe stooped posture, or heart, lung, or eye problems.) It is also interesting that the W27 "marker" has been found in very high frequency in other forms of arthritis, including Reiter's syndrome, and psoriasis and gastrointestinal disorders associated with arthritis. Research on these disorders has been greatly facilitated by the discovery of this genetic marker.

Future Research

Many aspects of the etiology and treatment of these inflammatory disorders remain to be clarified. Vasculitis, a group of disorders stemming from inflammation of the blood vessels, is still very poorly understood and can at present only be treated with potent anti-inflammatory immunosuppressive drugs which have adverse side effects for the patient. The genetic factors regulating the production of IgE antibodies in allergy, as well as the hereditary aspects of SLE and gout, remain to be clarified. Other specific areas such as the study of articular cartilage physiology are also in need of further research. Also on a basic level, the process of inflammation itself needs much further study before it can be understood and controlled. The same is true for proliferative processes such as occur in the synovial tissue (joint lining) in rheumatoid arthritis, adult and juvenile. Several diverse mast cell products important in the allergic reaction have recently been identified and are being structurally defined. One type of white bood cell, the eosinophil, has recently been observed to contain the enzymes which inactivate many of the substances produced by mast cells. There has been great progress in defining the proteins and inflammatory by-products of activation of the complement system; indeed, an alternative nonimmunologically initiated pathway to activation has recently been rediscovered. As the biochemistry of inflammation is better understood, it should become possible to develop pharmacologic agents to prevent excessive inflammation without disabling the initial immune response.

Biomedical Approaches
to Behavioral Disorders

PART THREE

The Biological Bases of Mental Illness

SEYMOUR S. KETY

8

Although schizophrenia, manic depression, and other forms of mental illness are not major causes of death like cancer or heart disease, they rank with these among our most serious national health problems. More than 10 million Americans will experience one or more episodes of serious mental illness before they reach old age. The care of the mentally ill, inadequate as it often is, accounts for a major share of the budget of each of the fifty states; the national total is well over five billion dollars annually. Less easily calculated is the human cost to those affected and their families.

Human disease in general is multifactorial; its origins are not found exclusively in the innate biological processes of the body or in environmental influences but on the continuing interaction between them. In the case of mental and behavioral disturbances especially, these influences would include the important psychological and social components of life experience which act together with biological and physical factors to determine mental health and illness.

Biomedical research has been effective in the past in determining the biological bases of several serious forms of mental illness and making their prevention possible. General paresis virtually disappeared as a cause of insanity in America once its syphilitic origin was established; similarly, pellagrous psychosis ceased to be a public health problem when it was found to be caused by a correctable dietary deficiency of nicotinic acid. But schizophrenia and manic-depressive illnesses have remained with us, and their seriousness is matched only by our ignorance regarding them.

We do not yet know their causes or understand the processes through which they develop, and thus we do not know how to prevent them. Their treatment, although it has improved dramatically through the use of recently discovered drugs, still leaves much to be desired. Over the past two decades, however, substantial research has indicated that these serious mental illnesses do have biochemical origins; and powerful new techniques and concepts have been developed which make the search for these causes more promising then it has ever been before.

Early Biological Approaches

The idea of a biological basis for insanity is not new. The Hippocratic physicians of ancient Greece argued against the then popular belief that insanity had supernatural causes: "And by the same organ [the brain] we become mad and delirious and fears and terrors assail us . . . All these things we endure from the brain, when it is not healthy but is more hot, more cold, more moist, or more dry than natural, or when it suffers any other preternatural and unusual affliction."

The modern biochemical approach to mental illness can be traced to Johann Thudichum, a physician and biochemist who hypothesized nearly a century ago that many forms of insanity were the result of toxic substances fermented within the body, just as the psychosis of alcohol was caused by a toxic substance fermented outside. He received a research grant from the Privy Council in England that enabled him to spend ten years examining this hypothesis. Significantly, Thudichum did not go to mental hospitals to examine the urine and blood of patients; instead he went to the slaughterhouse, obtained cattle brain, and began to study its normal chemical composition. It is very fortunate for us that he did, because in so doing he laid the foundations of modern neurochemistry, which is the essential basis for studying the abnormal chemistry of the brain. If Thudichum had been less wise and courageous, or if the Parliament had been more insistent that he do "relevant" research, what contribution could he have made with the little knowledge that existed at that time? He would have frittered away the public funds and wasted ten years of his life in a premature and futile search. By following the course he did, Thudichum was able to identify a large number of substances in the normal brain which were later found to play a role in a variety of neurological disorders.

Fifty years ago, biochemistry began to trace the complex processes of metabolism by which foodstuffs and oxygen are utilized and energy made available. This understanding was eventually applied to the brain, the brain's dependence on glucose was discovered and the oxygen utilized in various mental functions was measured. Many clinical states of mental abnormality were found to be associated with diminished oxygen consumption in the brain; these included senile psychosis, diabetic and other forms of coma, and a larg variety of conditions in which there are clear primary metabolic interferences with the energy utilization of the brain. These findings raised the hopes that other forms of mental illness might also have their roots in a simple deficiency of energy supply. Research soon showed, however, that a schizophrenic's brain uses exactly the same amount of oxygen as does the brain of a normal individual. Oxygen usage was also found to be unaffected in normal sleep, LSD psychosis, and the performance of mental arithmetic. The study of these four states led to a very important insight: the brain is qualitatively different from most other organs in the body. While the heart, the muscles, and the kidney show a work output which has something to do with their energy utilization, the output of the brain cannot be measured in such simple terms. The brain uses the same amount of energy whether the individual is talking nonsense or speaking brilliant prose; it takes just as much oxygen to think an irrational thought as it does to think a rational one. It soon became clear that what mattered in mental functioning was not so much the supply of power to the brain as the way in which that energy was utilized later on.

Once the major psychoses were not found to be explained as energy deficiencies, a number of other biochemical hypotheses were proposed. One hypothesis developed 20 years ago was that adrenaline was changed chemically in the blood of schizophrenics to a substance called adrenochrome, thought at one time to be hallucinogenic. This hypothesis encouraged Julius Axelrod to elucidate the normal pathways of the metabolism of adrenaline and related substances in the body and brain. His fundamental contributions here provided an important base for much of current research. When the metabolism of adrenaline in schizophrenics was examined, however, no evidence for adrenochrome formation could be found. Other chemical theories of schizophrenia abounded; the disease was ascribed by some to the presence of particular psychotogenic proteins in the blood, described by some as "taraxein," by others as "S-protein." These claims were not confirmed. In retrospect, the difficulty with the theories proposed at that time is quite obvious. These heroic efforts were simply premature. They were attempting to bridge the great gap between existing biochemical knowledge and mental illness in one span, before the foundations had been laid. The numerous "break-throughs," which turned out to be illusory, led many to believe that biology was not applicable to the field of mental illness and that those disorders were primarily psychological and social problems.

In the absence of credible biochemical findings pertinent to schizo-phrenia and manic-depressive illness, observations suggesting hereditary nature of these disorders became crucial. Clear evidence that these ill-nesses had important genetic bases would justify a continued search for biochemical causes, since genetic factors can express themselves only through biochemical processes.

The Genetics of Schizophrenia and Manic-Depressive Illness

The evidence for the operation of genetic factors in the major mental illnesses was compelling but not conclusive, since other than genetic fac-tors could account for the observations that were available. Psychiatrists had known for a long time (and every epidemiologic study has confirmed that observation) that these illnesses run in families. There is an approxi-mately 10 percent risk for the occurrence of schizophrenia in the parents, siblings, and children of schizophrenic patients, and manic-depressive illness shows a comparable familial tendency. Although this is compatible with genetic transmission, it is by no means proof. Wealth and poverty run in families but are not genetically transmitted; and the familial occur-rence of pellagra once fostered a belief in the genetic nature of what we now know to be primarily a nutritional disorder. Members of a family share not only their genetic endowment but also their environment, and either or both of these factors may be responsible for familial disorders. In addition, the study of the familial occurrence of mental illness poses some special difficulties. First, there is the problem of ascertainment and selective bias. If there are more people with serious mental illness than are known to psychiatrists, then it stands to reason that a family with two cases has a greater chance of being discovered than a family with only one. There is, therefore, a built-in bias in favor of finding familial forms of mental illness. A second problem is the obvious subjective bias in-volved in diagnosis. Schizophrenia is not a disorder diagnosed by blood tests or X-ray findings but a collection of subjectively evaluated symp-toms. A diagnosis of schizophrenia represents an opinion on the part of psychiatrists that a patient has enough of these symptoms to be con-sidered schizophrenic. And although subjective evaluation can be very sensitive, it is also easily influenced by preconceived notions and irrele-vant information.

For many years, the best evidence for the importance of genetic factors in mental illness came from studies of the twins of schizophrenic and manic-depressive individuals. These studies have generally shown a high incidence of schizophrenia among the identical twins of schizophrenics and a low incidence among their fraternal twins; similar results have been obtained for the manic-depressive psychoses. These findings are compatible with genetic theories, since identical twins share all their genetic endowment while fraternal twins are no closer genetically than are ordinary siblings. Recent twin studies have been able to avoid ascertainment and subjective bias and still find the same results. But because these studies could not control environmental factors they did not provide conclusive evidence for genetic transmission. Identical twins share more of their environment than do fraternal twins. They usually live together and sleep together, their parents parade them in the same perambulator and dress them alike, they have the same friends and experiences. Unless one could randomize their environment one could not be sure to what extent the shared psychosis in identical twins was due to ego identification, mimicry, or other environmental factors they shared in addition to their genetics. There were loopholes in the genetic evidence large enough that whole schools of psychiatry could march through them, denying that mental illness had any genetic or biological basis.

Over the past 15 years, however, a new approach has been used which appears to have succeeded in separating genetic from environmental factors in the transmission of schizophrenia. This consists in the study of adopted individuals, who share their genetic endowment with their biological relatives but share their environment with their adoptive relatives. In the several studies which have been completed to date the results are quite consistent. Schizophrenia continues to run in families, but now its high prevalence is restricted to the biological relatives of schizophrenic adoptees, with whom they share some genes but few, if any, environmental factors. The adoptive relatives of schizophrenics, who reared them and shared their environment, show no more tendency to schizophrenia than does the population at large.

This is stronger evidence than that previously available but is not conclusive, because adoptees are not separated at the time of conception. They share nine months of *in utero* environment and a minimum of a few days of infancy with their biological mothers; in these interactions it is not impossible that nongenetic influences might be acquired that could produce schizophrenia years later. But even that possibility can be ruled out. The biological parents of adopted individuals are usually young and fertile; they have many other children, often with different partners. This is especially true for the biological fathers so that the adoptees have a large number of paternal half-siblings who did not have the same mother and shared none of the environment—*in utero,* neonatal or postnatal—with the adoptee. When the half-siblings of schizophrenic adoptees and of normal control adoptees were examined for schizophrenia (by procedures designed to protect against subjective and ascertainment bias), the results were striking. Schizophrenia was significantly concentrated in the paternal half-siblings of the schizophrenic adoptees while the half-siblings of the controls had the low prevalence found in the general population. This constitutes the most definitive evidence to date for the operation of genetic factors in the transmission of schizophrenia.

Studies using adopted populations have not yet been completed for manic and depressive illness. However, there have been two reports recently that manic-depressive illness occurs in certain families in association with traits (such as color blindness and a specific blood group) known to be controlled by genes on the X chromosome. Although this association does not occur in all families with these disorders, where it does occur it suggests an X-linked genetic transmission.

Taken together, these studies force one to the conclusion that genetic factors play a crucial etiological role in the majority of patients with typical schizophrenia and in many with manic-depressive illness. But this is not the only evidence that justifies a continued and augmented search for the biological substrates of mental illness.

Chemical Synapses and Psychopharmacology

While the nature/nurture controversy was going on, those equipped to study the fundamental processes of the brain had not been idle. The past twenty-five years saw a dramatic growth in the neurosciences and an unprecedented development of knowledge regarding the brain and behavior. One of the breakthroughs that occurred, with special pertinence to psychiatry, was the recognition and demonstration of chemical transmission at the synapse, the highly specialized junction between nerve cells through which information is carried.

Previously, the brain had been thought of as a highly complex electrical computer. While the ultimate energy source for this computer was known to be biochemical, involving the utilization of oxygen and glucose, it was widely believed that the "wiring" of the computer itself was electrical rather than chemical in nature. The discovery of chemical synapses changed this picture radically. It now became evident that the brain was different from any machine which had ever been devised by man; it was a computer in which the billions of switches were not electrical but chemical switches which could be affected by biochemical processes. Since sensory processing, perception, the storage and retrieval of information, thought, feeling, and behavior all depend upon the operation of these chemical switches, this discovery finally indicated the sites at which chemical substances, metabolic products, hormones, and drugs could modify these crucial aspects of mental state and behavior. If there are biochemical disturbances in mental illness, they could be expected to have effects at the synapses; and drugs which ameliorate these illnesses should exert their influence there as well (Figure 8-1).

Although there may be hundreds of billions of synapses in the human brain, they are organized in a marvelously systematic way along certain pathways that are being mapped by neuroanatomists. Scientists have identified several types of neurotransmitters (chemical substances responsible for the transmission of signals between synapses) and have found these different substances to be associated with different pathways, functions, and behavioral states. The catecholamine transmitters adrenaline, noradrenaline, and dopamine were first identified in the adrenal gland and in the peripheral sympathetic nervous system; they are now known to be important neurotransmitters in the brain, where they appear to be involved in emotional states such as arousal, rage, fear, pleasure, motivation, and exhilaration. Serotonin, first discovered in the blood and the intestine, has also been identified in the brain, where it seems to play a crucial role in sleep and wakefulness, in certain types of sexual activity, and perhaps in modulating, damping, and balancing a wide range of synaptic activity that we are only beginning to understand. Acetylcholine, which is known to be the transmitter between nerve and muscle and is therefore crucial to every voluntary movement, has also been found to be involved in a very large proportion of brain synapses. There are neurotransmitters such as gamma-aminobutyric acid, and certain other amino acids and polypeptides, which have been discovered more recently; and undoubtedly many more remain to be found. Fundamental knowledge of the synapse and chemical neurotransmission has important implications for the understanding and treatment of nervous and mental disease and represents an area of unusual promise for the future.

While noradrenaline and serotonin were being identified in the brain, several drugs were discovered quite independently, and almost accidentally, to exert important effects on mood. The first of these was reserpine, which was known to be useful in the treatment of hyperten-

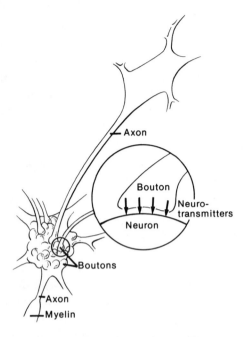

Figure 8–1. The transmission of nerve impulses at the synapse. Although nerve impulses are themselves electrical, the transmission of nerve impulses across most synapses occurs chemically. As shown in this simplified drawing, long fibers called axons extend from each neuron to carry electrical impulses to other neurons. Each axon is coated along most of its length with a material called myelin that increases the efficiency of the electrical impulse. At the end of each axon is a small knob, or bouton, that almost touches the neuron to which nerve impulses are sent. (For the sake of the clarity of the drawing, only a few of the axons connected to these boutons have been shown.) The gap between the bouton and the neuron, shown enlarged many times in the insert, is the synapse. A nerve impulse traveling down the axon causes the bouton to release special chemicals known as neurotransmitters; when these transmitters cross the synapse to reach the next neuron, they initiate an electrical impulse in that neuron, and the nerve impulse is effectively transmitted.

sion. In a small percentage of patients, reserpine produced a state of depression very much like that known to psychiatrists. At the same time, scientists at the National Heart Institute made the important discovery that reserpine caused a decrease in levels of serotonin and noradrenaline in the brain.

A few years later a new drug, iproniazid, was shown to be highly effective in the treatment of tuberculosis. When it was found to cause emotional excitement in some patients, it was supplanted by other drugs equally effective and without such side effects. But this strange side effect of iproniazid, while a hazard in the treatment of tuberculosis, became the basis for an effective treatment of depression. Iproniazid was discovered to block the enzyme monoamine oxidase, which is responsible for inactivating serotonin and the catecholamines. Thus, iproniazid enhanced the effect of these transmitters, an action opposite to that of reserpine. A number of other drugs were developed which were also monoamine oxidase inhibitors and effective in the treatment of depression. Even more effective were the tricyclic antidepressants, including the drugs imipramine and amitriptyline, which enhance the synaptic actions of noradrenaline and serotonin by another mechanism than monoamine oxidase inhibition. Electroshock therapy is effective in the treatment of patients with some kinds of severe depression; and it is interesting that administering similar shocks to experimental animals also increases the levels of noradrenaline and serotonin in their brains.

The foregoing observations suggest that clinical depression may be the result of an inadequacy of noradrenaline or serotonin (or both) at particular synapses in the brain, and similarly, that mania, the obverse of depression, may represent an overactivity of these synapses. The testing of this hypothesis has engaged a number of research groups. Certain types of depression and mania have been found to be associated with a decrease or an increase respectively of a particular breakdown product of noradrenaline in the urine; this substance appears to be derived largely from noradrenaline in the brain. Others examining the cerebrospinal fluid have found evidence of a decrease in serotonin metabolism in the brain of patients suffering from manic or depressive psychosis. A very effective agent in the treatment of mania and the prevention of manic-depressive illness is lithium, a relatively simple ion closely related to sodium (which plays a crucial role in synaptic function); lithium appears to increase the synaptic levels of serotonin. Clearly there is much work which can be done to pursue these interesting leads.

In 1950 a drug was developed which was found to be more effective than any previous treatment in the relief of the major symptoms of schizophrenia. This action was discovered in an interesting and unexpected manner. Pharmacologists had been developing and studying drugs which blocked the action of histamine, an endogenous substance which appears to play an important role in many forms of allergy. One of these drugs also blocked the activity of the sympathetic nervous system. Henri Laborit, a French anesthesiologist, had been looking for a drug which had such properties for use in the prevention of surgical shock, reasoning that both histamine and sympathetic overactivity might contribute to shock in surgical operations. He used this drug in preoperative medication and, because he was a careful observer, he noted that it produced in his patients an unexpected sedation. This sedation was different from that which was known to occur with the barbiturates; Laborit described it as a "euphoric quietude." He felt that such an effect might be helpful in the treatment of disturbed patients and suggested this to some psychiatrists. The drug used by Laborit was the immediate forerunner of chlorpromazine, which revolutionized the treatment of schizophrenia.

Chlorpromazine was immediately seized upon and used throughout the civilized world because it was different from any previous treatment for schizophrenia. While this new drug quieted schizophrenics, it didn't act like a tranquilizer; its action was much more specific. Not only would it quiet a disturbed and aggressive schizophrenic patient, it would also attenuate his hallucinations and delusions and sometimes reduce his apathy. No sedative ever discovered had all those beneficial effects. Here at last was a substance which appeared to be acting almost specifically upon the behavioral and cognitive features that characterized schizophrenia.

In addition to its therapeutic effects in schizophrenia, however, chlorpromazine had an important side effect; it produced in some patients the facial and motor disturbances which are seen in Parkinson's disease. Modifications of chlorpromazine were developed in an effort to preserve the therapeutic benefit while avoiding this drawback, but, with very few exceptions, all the effective agents found also had this side effect. In addition to chlorpromazine and its derivatives (known collectively as phenothiazines), an entirely new chemical class of drugs appeared, the butyrophenones, which were also effective in the treatment of schizophrenia but suffered as well from the tendency to produce symptoms of Parkinsonism. It appeared that the side effect was intimately related to the therapeutic action, but for ten years no explanation of either was possible. That explanation had to wait for a whole area of basic neurobiological research to develop, centered on the study of specific biochemical pathways in the brain.

In 1960 a new technique was employed in Sweden for identifying certain neurotransmitters within the brain by means of their characteristic fluorescence under appropriate conditions. That technique was quickly applied by neuroanatomists and used to trace circuits within the brain which utilized these transmitters. A neurologic pathway which was known to be damaged in patients with true Parkinson's disease was found to use dopamine as a transmitter. This led to the hypothesis and the ultimate demonstration that a partial destruction of the dopamine-synthesizing nerve cells was the basis for Parkinson's disease. Efforts to replenish the lost dopamine by administration of its precursor L-dopa were successful, leading to marked improvement in the patients; this represented one of the major contributions of fundamental research to the treatment of neurologic illness in recent years.

These remarkable findings also had an important impact on psychiatry. It was suggested first by Arvid Carlsson that the antipsychotic drugs might act by blocking the effects of dopamine in the brain, since this would explain their tendency to produce the symptoms of Parkinson's disease. On the basis of his studies and more recent observations in dopamine synapses in the brain and on the components of such synapses studied in the laboratory, it is now clear that Carlsson's insight was correct. A major action of both the phenothiazine and the butyrophenone drugs is to block the dopamine synapses within the brain.

The drug amphetamine also affects dopamine synapses; but amphetamine exaggerates the effects of dopamine rather than diminishing them. Clinically, too, amphetamine can be considered the direct opposite of the antipsychotic drugs. In animals it produces stereotyped movements of various kinds and aimless pacing, behavior patterns also seen in schizophrenia. When it is abused by human subjects it produces a psychosis which is often indistinguishable from schizophrenia and the same drugs which are effective in the treatment of schizophrenia are also specific in terminating an amphetamine psychosis. Amphetamine is also known to exacerbate the psychosis of schizophrenic individuals.

The overall picture is very clear: drugs which enhance dopamine activity in the brain tend to produce or aggravate schizophrenic symptoms, while those which diminish dopamine activity are capable of relieving those symptoms.

These findings do not necessarily indicate that schizophrenia is caused by an overactivity of dopamine synapses. One hypothesis does hold that the disorder is due to an excess of dopamine, stemming perhaps from a deficiency in the enzyme responsible for converting dopamine to noradrenaline; but there are several other possibilities. Dopamine-containing neurons interact with many other neurotransmitters and neurohormones in the brain. For example, dopamine inhibits the release of the hormone prolactin from the pituitary gland; the phenothiazines, by blocking the effects of dopamine, have been shown to raise levels of prolactin throughout the bloodstream and in the cerebrospinal fluid. The activity of dopamine pathways is also affected by neural circuits that use acetylcholine, serotonin and gamma-aminobutyric acid, and it could be these substances that are more directly related to schizophrenic symptoms. But whatever the reasons for the therapeutic effects of the antipsychotic drugs, it is clear that continued and expanded research on dopamine and other neurotransmitters, their distribution and synaptic activity, and on the interrelationship of these neurotransmitters to behavior at very basic as well as clinical levels cannot help but contribute to our understanding of these illnesses. And with this understanding will certainly come more specific treatments and prevention of illnesses.

Other chemical substances besides the catecholamines have also been implicated in schizophrenia, though the evidence for their role in the disease is much less clear. Several drugs such as mescaline, LSD, and dimethyltryptamine (DMT) are capable of inducing hallucinations and some of the other symptoms of schizophrenia and have, to some, suggested hypotheses about the nature of schizophrenia itself. Mescaline and dimethyltryptamine chemically resemble substances normally present in the body but modified by the addition of methyl (CH_3) groups. Shortly after the elucidation of biological transmethylation, by which such groups are added to particular molecules, it was suggested that this normal process might be disturbed in schizophrenia so that abnormal methylated compounds with hallucinogenic properties might accumulate in the brain. This hypothesis received some support from the finding that the amino acid methionine, which can serve as a donor of methyl groups, tends to exacerbate psychotic symptoms in schizophrenic patients. More recently, several groups of researchers have detected an enzyme in the lung and brain of animals and man which is capable of methylating substances normally present in the brain, such as tryptamine, thus converting them to hallucinogenic substances like dimethyltryptamine. In some laboratories, such methylated compounds have been found in the body fluids of schizophrenic patients. These findings, if confirmed, would suggest a link between schizophrenia and the presence of metabolically synthesized dimethyltryptamine or another hallucinogen.

In addition to inactivating serotonin and the catecholamines in the normal brain, monoamine oxidase has the ability to destroy many other amines, including dimethyltryptamine. It is possible that the methylating enzyme present in the normal brain is constantly producing hallucinogenic products that are normally detoxified by monamine oxidase; if monoamine oxidase were deficient in schizophrenics these hallucinogens could accumulate. Recently, several research groups have found that the blood platelets of schizophrenics are indeed low in this enzyme. Especially interesting was the finding that relatives of schizophrenics, especially identical twins, showed this enzyme deficiency, although they may not have been schizophrenic themselves. Clearly, this has potential relevance to the genetic factors that may predispose an individual to developing schizophrenia. At present, however, some laboratories have failed to confirm these findings in platelets and no one has demonstrated a deficiency of monoamine oxidase in the brain.

Whether or not methylated hallucinogenic amines accumulate in schizophrenia is still a matter of controversy. But, the finding that all of us have the capability of forming hallucinogenic substances in our bodies and brains is a striking observation that must be further explored.

Today, the number of new techniques waiting to be applied to the problems of mental illness is legion. There are the techniques that identify and localize specific neurotransmitters and enzymes by means of induced fluorescence. There are procedures employing radioactive tracers that permit one to map the circuits of the brain. Cell culture techniques have made possible the identification of genetic metabolic errors in a substantial number of medical and neurological illnesses. There are sophisticated genetic studies that permit the localization of these defects to particular chromosomes. A number of hitherto obscure medical and neurologic illnesses have been found to result from slow virus infection; and recent advances in virology may uncover similar causes for the mental illnesses as well. Neurobiology and neuropharmacology supply powerful tools for the study of the synapse, which has already led to an elucidation of drug action and to the development of safer and more effective drugs. There are chemical analytic techniques, such as the mass spectrograph, which makes possible the discovery and quantification of infinitesimal amounts of abnormal chemical substances in various body fluids. Rigorous and quantifiable behavioral techniques clarify the relationships of the biological mechanisms to behavior, bringing them to bear upon a wide variety of mental processes such as cognition, learning, motivation, and mood.

A new generation of neuroscientists has been trained, skilled in fundamental research and highly motivated to apply these techniques in unraveling the mysteries of the brain. The time has never been more propitious for progress toward an understanding of the serious disturbances of the human mind.

Alcohol and Drug Abuse

JACK H. MENDELSON
NANCY K. MELLO

9

The discovery and development of substances to provide relief from suffering and distress and to produce feelings of well-being has been one of man's enduring quests. Alcohol is the oldest, most generally available and probably most widely used substance that produces desirable changes in feeling states. The *use* of alcohol for recreation and in ritual ceremonies dates from the earliest agrarian civilizations. The legendary givers of wine, Osiris and Dionysus, were worshiped by the ancient Egyptians and Greeks; and the process of distillation was developed as early as 800 A.D. The *abuse* of alcohol also extends back to antiquity, and the earliest records of human history contain documents which attempt to distinguish between use and abuse.

Biblical records give us a relatively recent example of concern with alcohol abuse in the Old Testament story of Noah's drunkenness. A sculptural depiction of this story, attributed to an unknown artist from fourteenth-century Pisa, dramatically illustrates both the medical and the social concomitants of alcohol abuse (Figure 9-1). According to the Old Testament, Noah was discovered in an intoxicated state by his son Ham, who reported his father's naked stupor to his two brothers. The two brothers covered their father to conceal his "shame" and did not gaze upon his predicament directly. The sculpture shows one son holding a drape covering Noah, and it is clear that both sons are looking away from the embarrassing spectacle. When Noah awoke, he was aware that two of his sons did not voluntarily observe his transgression, but he cursed and eventually drove away the son (Ham) who both witnessed and reported

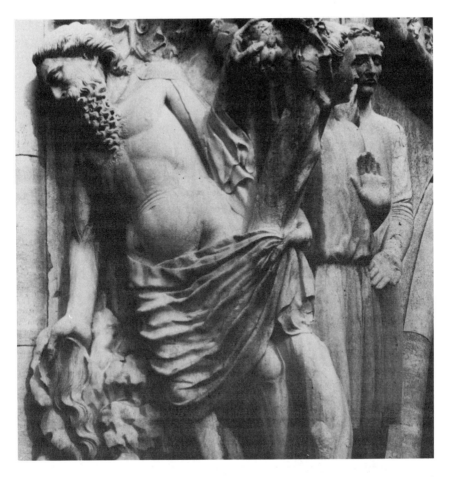

Figure 9–1. A sculpture depicting the drunkenness of Noah and the reaction of his sons. This statue is located on the corner of the Doge's Palace in Venice and is by an unknown fourteenth-century sculptor from Pisa. Photograph courtesy of Jack H. Mendelson.

his state of intoxication. This biblical account anticipates a now common attitude of society toward alcohol abuse; most societies have tended to regard alcohol abuse as shameful and have usually tried to cover up or look away from the problem. This sculpture of the drunkenness of Noah conveys far more than moral or social commentary, however; it is clear that the sculptor selected a model for Noah who had the medical stigmata of chronic alcohol abuse. The distended abdomen and engorged veins of the upper torso and neck are suggestive of advanced liver disease, a condition commonly observed in chronic alcohol abusers. Noah's thin and wasted legs are a typical sign of the peripheral nerve and muscle diseases occurring in alcoholics with poor diet. The relationship of alcohol abuse to disease and disability has long been recognized and is well documented in the medical archives of virtually all societies that have encountered abuse problems.

Although occasional festival drinking has usually been accepted, many groups throughout history have tried to prevent and control the abuse of alcohol. Temperance tracts have been found in the ancient writings of Greece and Rome, India, Japan, China, and Egypt. Contemporary societies have varied in the type of beverage alcohol prohibited and in the fervor with which temperance attitudes have been translated into legislation.

National prohibition continued in the United States from 1920 to 1933; the failure of this attempt to control alcohol use and abuse has been amply documented. Currently, it is estimated that alcohol abuse problems may affect as many as 9 million Americans, including an estimated 5 million alcohol addicts and their families. Because of the severe social stigma associated with alcoholism, precise estimates of prevalence have been impossible to obtain. However, the lack of accurate figures in no way diminishes the fact that the toll of alcohol abuse in economic costs and human suffering is immense. There has been an unfortunate tendency in this country to deny and underestimate the scope of the alcohol problem and its consequences. Reactions to opiate abuse in this country have been less sporadic, and more intense.

Widespread opiate use has existed in the Far East for many centuries; until recently, opium was the major recreational drug of the Chinese people. The ambivalent attitudes of Chinese society toward opium use probably paralleled Western conflicts over alcohol use. China and Britain fought the Opium Wars in 1839 over the issue of opium trade. Britain prevailed and continued to sell the drug (in exchange for silver which was used to purchase Chinese tea). Then as now, it was difficult to determine who in fact consumed these vast quantities of opiates. Opiate use and abuse seem to have occurred at all levels of Chinese society; the opium pipe could be a simple bamboo device for use by any poor person, or could be an elaborate instrument, fashioned with jade, for the nobility.

In Western societies, opium has been used in medicine since the middle ages. As chemistry advanced, crude opium was refined to morphine and later to heroin. Importation of crude opium into this country progressively increased from 1840 to a maximum in 1896 and then declined. Laudanum, a tincture of opium, enjoyed the social acceptance now accorded aspirin until the beginning of this century. Opium for smoking was freely imported into the United States until 1909. The transition from the drug's unrestricted medicinal and recreational use to its prohibition as a feared and vilified drug of abuse has been detailed by David Musto in a historical account entitled *The American Disease*. As this title indicates, opiate abuse in the United States is not a new problem. The consumption of opium on a per capita basis was probably greater in the mid-1800s than during the heroin "epidemic" of the late 1960s; the frequent use of morphine as an analgesic during the American Civil War, the immigration of Chinese laborers to help build the western railroads, and the unregulated use of opium contained in patent medicines may all have contributed to this use pattern. Yet recognition of the many problems associated with opiate addiction proceeded slowly. Finally in 1920, responding in part to the efforts of zealous reformers and to international political considerations, the Supreme Court declared opiate addiction without sufficient medical cause to be illegal.

Current estimates of the prevalence of drug abuse are limited in their accuracy by the same considerations that affect estimates of the incidence of alcoholism. According to a recent estimate, there may be about 500,000 heroin addicts in the United States. The prevalence of barbiturate addiction is unknown. Barbiturates are thought to be a second drug of abuse for heroin and alcohol addicts as well as a common drug of choice for youthful abusers of many drugs; some studies have estimated that 20 to 35 percent of narcotic addicts use barbiturates regularly. While the prevalence of addiction to amphetamines is unknown, it has been variously estimated that between 3 and 4 percent of the population occasionally use these drugs. All these estimates are complicated by the fact that patterns of drug use are not static but are in a constant state of flux.

The medical, social, and economic consequences of alcohol and drug addiction are legion. Treatment and prevention of abuse is especially difficult because these disorders have no single identifiable cause; the initiation and perpetuation of alcohol and drug abuse appear to be related to many interacting psychological, biological, and social factors. The phenomenology of alcohol and drug abuse and their medical consequences is still in an early descriptive phase. In this chapter we will describe some of the questions that have been asked and some current answers, and will explore prospects for future research.

The Nature of the Problem

One recurring question has been central: are problems related to alcohol and drug abuse actually medical disorders, and can their solution be approached by traditional biomedical research methods? Controversy has raged between those who view alcohol and drug abuse in a moral, social, or legal context, and those who consider such problems within the framework of biology and psychology. E. M. Jellinek, whose major work in alcoholism began over three decades ago, was the first to formulate a model which included alcohol-related problems within the traditional framework of human disease processes. Through clinical observations of the development and progression of drinking problems, Jellinek was able to construct a series of typologies of alcohol-related disorders, ranked by severity. This research was basically phenomenological and involved detailed and unbiased observation and recording of human disease processes. The disease model of alcoholism and drug abuse that has evolved from such clinical observations is not very different from the model that has been applied to infectious disease, heart disorders, and even cancer. All these diseases require an agent, such as bacteria or a virus, to produce the disorder. However, although the *agent* is necessary, it is not sufficient to produce the disease. Two other variables must also have certain characteristics for the individual to become sick: the person who is exposed, the *host*, must be susceptible to the agent, and *environmental conditions* must favor the development of the illness. In alcohol and drug abuse disorders there is no mystery about the identity of the agent; alcoholic beverages in their numerous forms and a variety of other drugs are agents, necessary but not sufficient factors for an abuse problem to exist. It has often been said that alcohol problems exist in man and not in wine, beer, or liquor bottles. This may be a time-worn cliché, but it does highlight the importance of host susceptibility and environmental determinants. In the course of examining more specific questions concerning alcohol and drug abuse, we will emphasize the interactions of host, agent, and environment, and the ways in which research relating to each has been carried out.

Causation

Attempts to find one ultimate cause of any human illness are usually destined to fail; since disease occurs as a consequence of a complex interaction between several factors, it is obvious that single-causation notions must prove to be inaccurate and misleading. Nevertheless, many single-causation theories of alcohol and drug abuse have been proposed. Roger Williams, a gifted biochemist and expert in nutrition who made major contributions to biological science in the 1930s, argued that biochemical individuality and nutritional disorders were the basis for alcohol problems. Geneticists have argued that alcoholism is inherited. Psychodynamic theorists have attributed alcoholism to certain personality characteristics, such as dependency, immaturity, hostility, and depression. Selden Bacon, a prominent sociologist, felt that both biological and psychological theories of the causation of alcoholism were inaccurate and that social and environmental causes were most important. Moralists have argued for weakness of character, moral deficiencies, and unrestrained hedonism as the primary causative factors; while William James suggested that alcohol has an enormous sway over mankind because of its ability to affect the mystical properties of human thought processes. Probably all were in error and all were, in part, correct, for each was examining a different side of the host-agent-environment triangle. However, by subscribing to a single-factor theory of causation, each tended to overlook the critical interrelationships of the several variables affecting alcohol and drug abuse.

At the present time most investigators agree that no single biological factor can explain alcohol addiction. Those who have argued that some specific nutritional or biochemical abnormality is the basis for alcohol abuse have not confirmed their hypotheses in controlled research studies. It is true that the alcohol addict may have certain vitamin and nutritional deficiencies, but these disorders are caused by factors associated with heavy drinking, such as poor diet; they are not themselves a cause of heavy drinking. Some decades ago it was suggested that alcohol addicts might suffer from a basic abnormality in the way in which they metabolize carbohydrates, glucose in particular, which might be corrected by their high levels of alcohol consumption. It is true that alcohol intake can affect glucose metabolism; conversely, glucose metabolism can affect the manner in which alcohol is broken down in the body. But no specific problem of carbohydrate metabolism has been demonstrated to be alleviated by alcohol abuse.

Some researchers have hypothesized that heroin addicts may have an innate biological need for opiates, which could result in opiate addiction. This was the basis for one argument advanced to support the development of methadone maintenance therapy programs; methadone, it was contended, would meet this innate biological need, making heroin use unnecessary. But it is now known that methadone is effective in the treatment of heroin addiction, not because it satisfies some metabolic hunger, but because it reduces an individual's ability to achieve a change in emotional state when heroin is used. (This effect is known as the development of cross-tolerance to heroin.)

Some recent evidence suggests the possibility that a genetic component may be associated with the genesis of alcohol problems. Clearly the separation of familial learning variables from genetic factors is a very difficult methodological problem. Studies in Denmark, conducted by Donald Goodwin and co-workers, accomplished this by studying men who had been separated in infancy from biological parents who had been hospitalized for alcoholism; this group had a significantly higher incidence of drinking problems than did matched adoptee controls. In another study, adoptees showed a greater tendency to develop alcohol problems if the biological parent was alcoholic than if the adopted parent was an alcoholic.

Attempts to explain alcohol or drug abuse on the basis of specific constellations of behavioral and personality characteristics have been less successful. Individuals with wide variations in personality, background, and life style have been found to abuse alcohol, drugs, or both. Moreover, people from enormously different social, economic, ethnic, racial, and cultural backgrounds may abuse both ethanol and drugs. Large sample surveys have not isolated reliable sociological predictors of the development of problem drinking; however, some common general characteristics of problem drinkers have been recognized. The largest proportion of alcoholics appear to be persons of lower socioeconomic status living in urban areas; many are unmarried males, under 25, and often report disrupted childhood and a transition from rural to city living. Long-term developmental studies suggest that the same childhood patterns (early school problems, delinquency, drug use, and broken homes) predict drinking problems for ghetto-reared blacks and whites. American Indian and Eskimo populations have also been shown to be at high risk for the development of alcoholism. The correlation between societal alienation and use of alcohol is not straightforward; however, abstainers as well as heavy drinkers have been described as more discontented and more alienated from society than persons who use alcohol in moderation.

It is apparent that there will be no early resolution of the issues involved in the "causes" of alcohol and drug abuse. Research is becoming increasingly directed toward the factors that maintain the abuse pattern once it is initiated, in the hope that the modification of these maintenance factors may eventually permit effective interruption of such patterns.

Natural History

Much work has gone into the investigation of the "natural history" of alcohol and drug addiction; researchers have studied the sequences of events in the lives of individuals that lead up to and accompany the abuse of alcohol and drugs. Knowledge of the factors that influence the transition from normal use to abuse of these substances has been gradually improving, thanks to more careful data acquisition and to the utilization of research techniques adopted from such exact sciences as clinical pharmacology.

Studies of the development of tolerance and physical dependence in alcohol and drug abusers represent an important advance in our understanding of the natural history of these conditions. Tolerance occurs when an individual has to use increasing amounts of a substance in order to produce the same change in feeling state or behavior. Common experience has taught many individuals that reaching the feeling of vitality and relaxation originally produced by one martini may require two or even three drinks after several years of drinking experience. In addition to developing tolerance, the alcohol abuser may actually become physically addicted to ethanol. Hippocrates was the first to point out that tremor and shaking of the hands were associated with the abuse of wine; but many centuries elapsed before it was recognized that these physical disorders were caused not by the *use* of alcohol, but by the *cessation* of alcohol consumption. Excellent descriptions of the alcohol abstinence syndrome were provided by English physicians; the term delirium tremens (DT's) was coined by Thomas Sutton in the early 1800s. Since that time, physicians have debated the cause of this curious syndrome, speculating that alcohol might produce direct toxic effects in the body and particularly in the brain. But the study of the abstinence syndrome is still in its infancy. For example, it was not until the mid-1950s that the careful clinical observations of Maurice Victor and Raymond Adams, carried out at the Boston City Hospital, conclusively established that the alcohol abstinence syndrome was caused specifically by cessation of alcohol use and was not due to toxic or nutritional factors. The study of physical dependence on alcohol has been complicated by the fact that such an addiction generally evolves over a long period of time; whereas physical dependence upon heroin can occur readily within a matter of weeks or months, alcohol addiction usually develops slowly over a number of years. It is now known that no specific pattern of drinking or drug abuse necessarily predicts whether or not an individual will develop physical dependence. For example, although consumption of alcohol during the early hours of the day probably indicates that an individual has developed significant tolerance, it does not necessarily mean that he is on the road to alcohol addiction. (However, the need to consume alcohol upon awakening usually indicates that an individual has developed physical dependence upon alcohol and requires a drink in order to suppress early morning tremor and other incipient withdrawal symptoms.)

Some investigators have proposed that the use of one substance may lead to use and abuse of other substances. For example, they have emphasized the fact that marihuana use often is antecedent to opiate use. But the apparent conclusion that marihuana "causes" subsequent abuse of other drugs is not warranted. Recent studies on the relationship between substance availability and likelihood of multiple drug use and abuse suggests that certain people may simply be likely to use several different types of drugs; hence an individual prone to using marihuana at one stage in life might also be likely to use opiates at a later stage.

There is considerable evidence that an individual's alcohol and drug abuse problems may change, through time, with or without specific preventive or therapeutic interventions. Spontaneous remission can occur in drug and alcohol abuse disorders as in many other conditions. However, despite this possibility, disability and even death are often the terminal consequences of prolonged alcohol and drug abuse. Alcohol addicts are at much greater risk for violent death through highway fatalities, suicide, and homicide than are nonaddicts. Studies carried out in the emergency room of the Massachusetts General Hospital have shown that a very high proportion of individuals who sustain accidents in the home have alcohol-related problems. Drug abusers are constantly in danger of overdose because of unknown variations in drug potency and drug tolerance; and if they obtain drugs through criminal activities, the risk of violent injury or death is high.

Research into the natural history of alcohol and drug abuse has prompted further study of the behavioral and biological factors underlying these problems.

Biological Processes

The study of the biological aspects of alcohol and drug abuse, while concerned with the possible causes of these conditions, has focused primarily on the effects of alcohol and drug usage on body structure and function. Certain diseases of the liver are known to be associated with alcohol abuse; forms of gastrointestinal disease such as chronic inflammation of the lining of the stomach (gastritis) and a serious disease of the pancreas (pancreatitis) are also commonly observed in alcohol abusers. The effects of alcohol on the liver have been documented for centuries, yet the way in which alcohol abuse produces diseases of this organ, particularly cirrhosis, has remained a mystery. The recent development of an animal model for alcohol-induced liver disease has raised hopes of understanding this type of illness. Charles Lieber and Emanuel Rubin have recently reported that they can produce in baboons a full spectrum of liver disease caused specifically by alcohol and not by nutritional or other toxic factors. These investigators offered the baboons a special liquid diet which provided adequate calories and nutrients but also contained ethyl alcohol in amounts proportional to those that might be consumed by human alcohol abusers. The baboons chose to consume copious amounts of alcohol over several years (in contrast to most subhuman primates, who assiduously avoid drinking even small concentrations of ethanol). Rubin and Lieber demonstrated that such consistent high alcohol intake by the baboon produced liver disease similar to that which develops in people over the same time span. This model makes possible the development of animal studies to determine exactly what metabolic, genetic, and molecular processes underlie alcohol-induced liver disease. The importance of this research cannot be overstated; liver disease is widespread in the United States, with cirrhosis of the liver ranking as the third leading cause of death among young and middle-aged males in New York City.

Clarification of the possible role of alcohol in heart disease and cancer has been difficult. One of the major confounding factors is that individuals who abuse alcohol often are heavy smokers. Hence, it has been difficult to separate the effects of heavy smoking from those of heavy alcohol intake, particularly in studies of cancer of the head and neck and premature coronary artery disease. There is some evidence, however, that alcohol may directly damage muscle tissue, including the heart muscle, particularly when heavy drinking is accompanied by a poor diet.

During recent years, an increasing number of patients admitted to mental hospitals with diffuse disease of the brain (organic brain disorders) have been found to have lifelong histories of heavy alcohol intake and alcohol abuse. Many of these patients also have histories of poor diet, and it is not known if alcohol itself damages the brain, or if alcohol in combination with lack of nutritional and vitamin intake is responsible for these disorders. It is known that poor nutrition, when combined with excessive alcohol intake, commonly leads to diseases of the major large nerves which control motor and sensory function in the arms and legs. Some investigators have speculated that even small amounts of alcohol may damage brain cells, on the basis of biochemical studies carried out in the test tube; but direct toxicity of ethanol to the central nervous system has not yet been demonstrated.

Disability and death associated with drug abuse, and particularly heroin abuse, are not usually due to cumulative toxic effects of these drugs on body organs and tissues. More commonly, death may occur from accidental or purposeful drug overdose. However, drug abuse can have many indirect adverse consequences on body function. Infectious diseases such as hepatitis are common to addicts who self-administer heroin intravenously and do not use sterile needles or syringes. And, as with alcoholics, poor nutrition and marginal health habits often are fore-runners of debilitating illness in heroin addicts.

Both alcohol and opiates have complex effects on sexual desire and function. Shakespeare wrote in *Macbeth* that drinking alcohol to excess "provokes [sexual] desire, but it takes away the performance" in males. The biological mechanisms underlying this well-known phenomenon are being explored in studies of alcohol effects on hormones secreted from the pituitary and the testes, which are important regulators of sexual behavior and function. Our laboratory has shown that alcohol intake suppresses testosterone levels in human adult males; very small quantities of this hormone are present when blood alcohol levels are at their highest. This reduction of testosterone is caused by changes in liver chemistry associated with the breakdown of alcohol by that organ. Lowered testosterone levels signal a crucial brain area, the hypothalamus, to stimulate the pituitary to increase its production of luteinizing hormone; this is the body's normal response, since luteinizing hormone stimulates secretion of testosterone. Some investigators believe that this increased release of luteinizing hormone may increase sexual desire during alcohol intoxication, while simultaneously decreased testosterone levels may result in diminished male sexual performance. Narcotic abuse may also produce striking changes in sexual behavior. Heroin addicts report that both sexual drive and performance are diminished, and our laboratory has found that both testosterone and luteinizing hormone levels are very low during peak effects of opiate-like drugs. But the mechanism of hormone suppression produced by narcotics is different from that of alcohol. The major effects of narcotics on male hormone regulation appear to be at the level of the brain; in contrast, alcohol-induced changes seem to involve processes in more peripheral parts of the body.

Behavioral Factors

Most of the basic processes of human behavior remain a mystery, and our knowledge of the ways in which drugs affect behavior is still in an early descriptive phase.

The use of alcohol presents a paradox: while individuals generally drink to reach a state of euphoria, it is well established that changes in behavior and mood following alcohol intake are not always favorable, particularly for those who abuse the substance. Over one half of all arrests made in the United States during the past year were for alcohol-related aggression or disruptive behavior. More than half of all highway accidents and fatalities, and most homicides and suicides, have also been found to be closely associated with alcohol abuse. Carefully conducted studies with alcoholics have helped explain this discrepancy between the observed effects of alcohol and the reasons given for its use. When alcohol addicts are asked to predict how they will feel when intoxicated, they often answer that they will be more calm, less depressed, have enhanced feelings of self-esteem, have less fear about initiating sexual advances, and, in general, achieve a state of well-being. Such effects are not unlike those anticipated by ordinary individuals enjoying a cocktail party. Observation of alcoholics during actual alcohol intoxication indicates that, in contrast to their expectations, many actually become anxious, morose, depressed, angry, and generally dysphoric, not euphoric. But when these individuals regain sobriety, they often recall their anticipated feeling states and experiences rather than the actual behavior and feelings experienced during intoxication.

Why does this strange forgetfulness occur in problem drinkers? Reports in the clinical literature as well as from anecdotal sources indicate that many alcohol addicts experience a profound loss of memory, termed a "blackout." Blackouts during periods of heavy drinking may involve loss of memory lasting anywhere from a few minutes to several days. The mechanism by which alcohol contributes to the blackout phenomenon is unknown. Suggestions that alcohol may disrupt "short-term" memory have not been supported in either clinical or animal studies. (The short-term phase of the memory process is the stage in which information is initially processed by the brain and is temporarily stored there.) Studies of alcohol effects on long-term memory storage processes have been difficult to carry out for numerous technical reasons. It is clear that if we are to understand some of the paradoxical and at times bizarre concomitants of problem drinking we must gain more information about how memory is registered and stored in the central nervous system.

The manner in which opiate drugs both alter mood and produce analgesis (the loss of sensibility to pain) is poorly understood. The subjective nature of pain and mood perception makes the analysis of these phenomena extremely complicated. It appears that opiates change an individual's reaction to pain as well as reducing the sensation of pain per se; in other words, although pain may still be present, the perception of pain becomes less disturbing. Perhaps this dissociative effect is true not only for pain associated with physical stimuli but also for emotional pain and discomfort. One of the most common medical uses of morphine-like drugs is as preoperative medication. Prior to surgery, patients may not be in any specific physical discomfort or distress but are understandably anxious and frightened; and morphine-like drugs reduce such anxiety and fear. As with alcohol, however, the effect of the opiates on mood and behavior changes drastically as the user becomes addicted. Recent studies from our laboratory reveal that heroin use initially produces feelings of elation and reduction of guilt, anxiety, and tension, but that chronic heroin use is associated with dysphoria, irritability, negativism, and hostility. Heroin addicts also report increased concern with bodily functions as opiate intoxication continues. In heroin addiction, as in alcohol addiction, the positive effects of initial use are not sustained.

Since alcohol and heroin addicts apparently do not use these substances to attain a consistent state of euphoria, what do they find rewarding in prolonged drinking and drug use? Perhaps they are not using these substances for pleasure but to avoid those discomforts associated with the cessation of use. There is some evidence that alcohol addicts continue to drink in a purposeful manner in order to avoid experiencing withdrawal effects; some may even taper their drinking through time in order to prevent the abstinence syndrome. However, behavioral studies indicate that the attempt to avoid the abstinence syndrome is not a major reason for perpetuation of drinking. Similar findings apply to the continued use of heroin by heroin addicts. Although addicts may become physically dependent upon heroin, they often voluntarily stop intravenous heroin use even though they recognize that the discomfort of withdrawal will shortly follow. In fact, purposeful cessation of heroin use is a common stratagem to reverse a developed tolerance, reduce the drug dose needed to produce a significant effect, and lower the cost of the habit. Such behavior refutes the common notion that drug users gradually lose control over their use of drugs as they develop physical dependence on them. Recent advances in the behavioral sciences have made it possible to study the behavioral causes and effects of alcohol and drug use more exactly. Ingenious research has been carried out with experimental animals, primarily subhuman primates, in order to examine the processes associated with sustained self-administration of alcohol and drugs; these studies have used methods for the experimental analysis of behavior developed by B. F. Skinner and his associates. Behavioral scientists have also examined group processes, such as decision making and risk taking, in settings where drugs and alcohol are consumed. Their studies have shown that certain types of behavior appear to be specifically evoked by certain substances. For example, aggression very frequently accompanies alcohol use, not only in social settings, but also in experimental research ward studies where subjects are permitted to consume as much alcohol as they like. In contrast, studies where subjects smoke large amounts of marihuana under controlled conditions show that very little, if any, aggression occurs with heavy marihuana use. These differences in observed behavior cannot be explained by differences in the background, personality, education, or culture of the alcohol and marihuana users. It appears likely that these two drugs actually have different pharmacological effects on behavior associated with aggression. Studies of group behavior processes are a microcosm for exploring the social and societal determinants of alcohol and drug abuse, and many new interesting developments have occurred in this area of research.

Sociocultural Factors

Are new, disturbing social problems leading to increased abuse of alcohol and drugs in contemporary American society? It is often very tempting to explain any form of deviance as a consequence of social problems or social change. However, there is no real evidence that abuse of intoxicating substances is greater in our society than in societies with completely different cultures and problems. For example, heroin use is common in Hong Kong, amphetamines are abused in Japan, and alcohol abuse is a major problem in the Soviet Union. Within the United States, overall use of alcohol seems to be relatively constant over time, although individual use varies greatly. Donald Cahalan and co-workers studied American drinking practices in two large-scale surveys which were separated by a three-year interval. Within that brief period, 15 percent of the individuals studied moved into *or* out of the "heavy" drinking group; yet the total size of the heavy drinking group did not change much. (The fact that a large number of heavy drinkers were able to decrease their alcohol consumption is encouraging and demonstrates that heavy drinking does not inevitably lead to chronic alcoholism.)

For obvious reasons, no comparable large-scale survey of opiate use has been conducted in the general American population. However, Lee Robins and her associates have been able to examine changes in patterns of opiate abuse in a sample of Vietnam veterans. It was found that heroin abuse in Vietnam did not necessarily continue once the individual returned to his home community; a two-year follow-up study showed that only 1 percent of those addicted to narcotics in Vietnam continued to use narcotics at home. But many of these former heroin users and addicts began to abuse alcohol following their return to the United States. It appears that substance availability may be the key determinant of substance abuse in these cases; because heroin is much more difficult and expensive to obtain in the United States than in Vietnam, the user and abuser switches to the more readily available compound, alcohol, on his return home.

Robins and her associates have recently concluded a series of very important studies concerning the interaction of social determinants and the epidemiology of alcohol and drug abuse. Their studies of the urban ghetto have found an increasing risk for the development of alcohol-related problems among black women. This risk is significantly greater than exists for white women, although alcohol abuse among white women also appears to be increasing. Paradoxically, the increase in alcohol-related problems among black women appears to be associated with a number of positive changes in life style and behavior. While the exact meaning of this finding is unclear, it demonstrates that social progress as well as social problems may be a causative factor in substance-abuse behavior.

Prospects for the Future

In comparison to most other areas of biomedical research, the study of drug and alcohol abuse has just begun.

Although research into the biological, behavioral, and social aspects of drug abuse is in some respects a more recent endeavor than alcohol-related research, it is more advanced and better supported. One reason is that much contemporary research on drug abuse is solidly based upon work carried out by pharmacologists and other biological scientists during the past four decades. Drugs of the morphine type were always of interest to the anesthesiologist and clinical pharmacologist concerned with problems related to the treatment of pain. Thus a well-trained, sophisticated group of laboratory and clinical investigators established quality standards for research on drug use that were later applied to the study of drug abuse.

Prospects for future advances in alcohol-related research, in contrast, appear rather gloomy. Little investment in time or resources has been made in clinical or laboratory studies of the nature of alcohol abuse. Most private and federal funding has been invested in programs of intervention or treatment, in spite of the fact that the most objective studies carried out to date indicate that no highly effective form of treatment exists for alcohol-related problems. A plethora of techniques and programs, including self-help groups, various forms of psychotherapy, and institutionalization, have been proclaimed as the way to deal with the alcohol problem; yet none of these methods proves to be uniquely efficacious when examined carefully and dispassionately.

More basic research on alcohol abuse is necessary before better treatment programs can be designed. Established priorities of the federal agencies which support alcohol-related research have relegated research funding to a very low level in favor of massive spending for treatment programs of questionable efficacy. Although it is unreasonable to criticize strongly any humane effort to assist people when they are ill, the lack of support for basic research into alcohol abuse is itself a disservice to humanity. By analogy, if a decision had been made during the last polio epidemic to use all available funds to build iron lungs (which indeed can save a polio victim's life), a vaccine for immunization against polio might never have been developed.

Many disciplines can make important contributions to the better understanding of the cause, natural history, and possible treatment of alcohol and drug abuse problems. But each discipline can only contribute at its own current level of development. Advances in basic biochemistry and molecular biology will be needed before we can understand how alcohol acts on nerve cells and brain function. Better techniques in the fields of epidemiology and sociology are essential to improving the study of the prevalence of alcohol and drug abuse. And significant improvements in clinical medicine and psychiatry will be necessary to the evaluation of different treatment programs. It is only through basic research in these fields that we will gain the essential tools, techniques, and models to further our knowledge of alcohol and drug abuse problems. Although it is very probable that some individuals will always abuse alcohol, drugs, and substances yet undiscovered, it is also possible that scientists may, with ingenuity, determine who is most at risk for alcohol and drug abuse and devise ways to intervene effectively to reduce suffering and disability.

Mental Retardation

HUGO W. MOSER 10

It is estimated that there are 6 million mentally retarded people in the United States, and that each year 3.5 billion dollars are expended for their care. The degree of handicap associated with this condition shows a very wide range. It includes, at one extreme, the young person who may be identified as retarded because of unsatisfactory school performance and a low IQ score, but who, after the school years are over, becomes self-supporting, forms a stable marriage, and is no longer considered deviant; and at the other extreme, people who have such serious learning handicaps, with or without added physical defects, that they require life-long care and supervision. Depending upon circumstances, mental retardation may be mainly an educational, a social, or a medical issue; not infrequently, all three components are involved. In recent years a great deal has been learned about each of these three aspects of the problem. There is now every indication that the incidence of mental retardation can be reduced, and that those who are retarded can achieve greater growth and self-fulfillment than had previously been considered possible. In spite of these advances, however, the unknown far exceeds what we do know, and there is a great need for research both at the basic and at the applied level. At least as important is the improvement of care-delivery systems and community attitudes, so that the mentally retarded may indeed enjoy the considerable achievements of which so many of them are capable.

Definition of Mental Retardation

The current manual of the American Association on Mental Deficiency states that "Mental retardation refers to significantly subaverage general intellectual functioning existing concurrently with deficits in adaptive behavior, and manifested during the developmental period." This definition, which upon first reading appears so bland and self-evident, attempts to resolve important and long-standing controversies. The key element is that the term mental retardation is not applied unless subaverage intellectual function (usually ascertained on the basis of IQ score) is associated with deficits in adaptive behavior. To those who have not worked in this field, the precise significance of the term mental retardation may seem an academic point. However, there is abundant evidence that the very designation of an individual as mentally retarded, as the term is now used, may itself be handicapping. Simon Olshansky, who has made outstanding contributions to the habilitation of the retarded, has observed: "To schools the category of mental retardation is a way of classifying some students with learning problems; to the person so labeled the categorization is an attack from which recovery is rarely complete." It is, therefore, important that the term (if its use is to be continued at all) be applied as precisely as possible, and that concurrent steps be taken to change public attitudes and legislative provisions which disadvantage the person labeled mentally retarded.

As is generally known, the average IQ, or intelligence quotient, is set at 100. The standard deviation (depending upon the test used) varies between 12 and 17 points. Intellectual function is considered to be significantly subaverage if performance is more than two standard deviations below the mean. This includes approximately 2.3 percent of the population, and, depending upon the test and its standard deviation, comprises those individuals whose IQ score is somewhere below 67 or 69. The current definition of mental retardation attempts to give due weight to the IQ score but to eliminate the tyranny it had begun to assume. The IQ test was originally designed as a predictor of school performance, and its validity in this respect is well established. Performances in a great variety of IQ tests correlate with each other, suggesting that they do measure some significant common factor. They also correlate significantly with eventual occupational status and other criteria of success in our society. Clearly, these relationships may have a circular quality, since high performance on tests enhances the opportunity for entry into a desired profession, and so on. It would be counterproductive not to utilize quantitative test instruments which have been validated in so many respects; however, great care must be taken not to overestimate their significance.

The Two-Group Approach

E. O. Lewis, E. Zigler, and others have subdivided the mentally retarded into two groups. It would in many ways be preferable if the two groups had separate, distinctive names. However, the dismal array of names that have previously been used in this field (idiot, cretin, moron, imbecile, feeble-minded, mentally defective, and even mentally retarded) makes any attempt to coin new ones appear foolhardly. The main points of difference between the two groups are summarized in Table 10-1.

Group I (the "physiological" group) accounts for the majority of people who are customarily called mentally retarded. Their degree of handicap is milder and appears to be influenced to a great extent by environmental factors. Group II ("pathological") is smaller, more easily and consistently recognized, and in most instances is associated with demonstrable structural or functional abnormalities.

It should be emphasized that the two-group approach is an over-simplification. Actually, hundreds of distinct causes of mental retardation are known. Some people who are only mildly retarded owe their disability to relatively mild organic pathology. Detailed analysis indicates, in fact, that in virtually every instance mental retardation is influenced by both genetic and environmental factors. With present methods of clinical analysis, it may be difficult to know whether a mentally retarded individ-

Table 10–1. Two groups of mentally retarded

Characteristic	Group I	Group II
Names	Physiological Subcultural Culturofamilial Familial	Organic Pathological
Estimated incidence	20–30 per 1,000	3 per 1,000
Most frequent IQ score	50–70	Less than 50
Most common age of ascertainment	During school years	Preschool
Apparent change of prevalence with age	Apparently diminishes after school years	No change
Demonstrable brain abnormality	No	Yes
Relationship to socio-economic status	More common among socioeconomically deprived or disrupted families	None or slight

ual belongs to Group I or II. Nevertheless, the two-group approach is useful in that it increases awareness of the existence of both socially influenced and organically determined handicaps and because, as will be pointed out later, it has important implications in the design of preventive and therapeutic programs.

This discussion will first focus on the smaller, pathological group, for which, complex as it is, there is a greater degree of understanding and unanimity of approach. The chapter will close with a review of present thinking and controversy about the physiological group, which involves large and important issues inextricably tied to our whole social system.

Group II—Severe Mental Retardation

The prevalence of severe mental retardation appears to vary only slightly throughout the world. Surveys conducted between 1925 and 1973 in England, Scandinavia, the United States, Australia, and the province of Quebec, indicate a prevalence of between 3 and 4 per thousand population. Most of these surveys list as mentally retarded people who have an IQ of 50 or less; C. C. Crome has found that over 90 percent of people who function at that level have some type of demonstrable pathology. The lowest prevalence was 2.16 per thousand for northern Scotland; the highest, 5.8 per thousand, was reported for rural Sweden. But of primary importance here is the relative degree of constancy in these figures. Conclusions about individual differences between national prevalence rates are probably not warranted, since the surveys are not exactly comparable in respect to methods of case detection and criteria for case inclusion.

Since there are hundreds (and possibly thousands) of separate causes of severe mental retardation, we will focus here on those that are the most common and those which highlight current approaches.

Down's Anomaly

Down's anomaly (or Down's syndrome) is the single most common cause of severe mental retardation. It is present in approximately one of 700 newborn infants; in surveys of severely retarded populations, it is found to account for 15 to 25 percent of all cases. Down's anomaly was first described in 1866, when the English physician John Langdon Down recognized that some mentally retarded people shared certain physical characteristics, such as small stature, epicanthic folds in the eyelids, a small and underdeveloped nose, an enlarged tongue, and a single horizontal crease in the palm of the hand. Other abnormalities may affect nearly every organ of the body. It is important to note that no one individual shows all these malformations and that these abnormalities also occur in the general population, albeit with a much lower incidence. Until a specific chromosome aberration associated with this disease was discovered in 1959, the diagnosis of Down's anomaly depended solely upon this constellation of physical abnormalities, and in borderline situations even experienced clinicians might disagree. Because of a superficial (but not actual) resemblance of the eyelid formation to that in orientals, this grouping of physical features was referred to as mongolism. Use of this term is now discouraged; it is not accurate, it may be offensive to members of the oriental race, and, most important, it has assumed a pejorative overtone for the child and his family. For these reasons the more neutral term Down's anomaly (or Down's syndrome) is preferred.

The second major advance in respect to Down's anomaly, coming nearly a hundred years after its recognition, was based upon the development of convenient techniques for counting the number of human chromosomes and for studying their size, shape, and other characteristics under the light microscope. Soon after this technique was developed, Jerome Lejeune demonstrated that approximately 95 percent of individuals with Down's anomaly had 47 chromosomes in each cell instead of the usual 46. These individuals were shown to have three (instead of the normal two) number 21 chromosomes; this state is referred to as trisomy 21 Down's anomaly. The other 5 percent of individuals with Down's anomaly suffer from slightly different chromosomal abnormalities (see Chapter 4) that also give them an excess of number 21 chromosome material. The demonstration of this chromosomal abnormality makes possible the unequivocal and early diagnosis of this disease in the fetus.

There is no laboratory test which allows identification of those parents who risk having a child with trisomy 21 Down's anomaly (although parents at risk for producing children with rarer types of Down's anomaly can often be identified). But there is clear evidence that the incidence of trisomy 21 Down's anomaly increases sharply with maternal age, for reasons still unknown. For mothers in their early twenties, the risk is 1/3,000; at the age 35, approximately 1/600; and for mothers age 40 or above, the risk is about 1/40. In recognition of this fact, the attempt to determine whether a fetus in an older mother does or does not have Down's anomaly represents the most common indication for amniocentesis and prenatal diagnosis.

The procedure of amniocentesis basically involves the withdrawal of

5 to 10 milliliters of amniotic fluid through a needle inserted into the womb through the abdominal cavity. The procedure is usually performed between the fourteenth and eighteenth weeks of pregnancy. Appropriate studies can then determine the chromosome makeup of the fetus, as well as the activity of certain enzymes relevant to inborn errors of metabolism such as Tay-Sachs disease (see below). While clearly not to be done for frivolous reasons, this procedure, when performed by a skilled obstetrician, entails a low order of risk and discomfort and is very accurate in assessing the chromosomal makeup of the fetus. Amniocentesis is usually carried out in pregnant women over the age of forty, and in the case of the mother, irrespective of age, who has previously had a child with trisomy 21 Down's anomaly. (In approximately 1 percent of these cases the subsequent child is also affected; this risk factor considerably exceeds that for young mothers in general.)

Unfortunately, for reasons which relate to ethical, social, communication, and financial issues, only a small percentage of at-risk pregnancies are currently monitored. Aubrey Milunsky and Leonard Atkins report that in the United States in 1973, prenatal studies of pregnancies in mothers who were 40 years of age or older detected only 75 fetuses with abnormal chromosomes, whereas it is estimated that women in this age group gave birth to 2,600 children with significant chromosome abnormalities during that year.

The ethical issues associated with prenatal diagnosis will not be discussed here in detail. If prenatal studies indicate that the fetus has Down's anomaly, then the parents must decide, with the advice of religious, legal, and medical counselors, whether or not an abortion is to be done. In most (but not all) instances the families have elected to interrupt the pregnancy. To those concerned with the care of the mentally retarded, our present capacity to diagnose Down's anomaly prenatally has raised ethical issues quite separate from the legal and religious aspects of abortion per se. Many who are not absolutely opposed to this procedure on religious or ethical grounds do favor abortion for fetuses proven to have a fatal disorder such as anencephaly (absence of most of the brain) or Tay-Sachs disease (an irrevocably fatal metabolic disorder). However, the situation is different in respect to Down's anomaly. The implementation of modern child-rearing and training techniques, with emphasis on normalization and home-based care, has demonstrated that many children with Down's anomaly are capable of significant growth and learning, and that they can achieve reasonably full lives and be sources of pleasure and joy to their families.

Perhaps the wisest policy is to take vigorous steps to inform families at risk that prenatal detection of Down's anomaly is feasible and to do everything possible to facilitate the performance of the necessary tests for those families who elect to participate; but the infant with Down's anomaly, once born, must be provided with the same level of medical, social, and educational support services as are all other children.

The history of our knowledge of Down's anomaly provides valuable examples of general research strategies toward mental retardation. The first essential step in the study of this disorder was Langdon Down's recognition, based upon careful observation, that a certain number of retarded people shared specific physical characteristics. It is an obvious but important point that without this initial recognition, nothing else would have been accomplished. At present there are probably several hundred mental retardation syndromes, in which certain physical characteristics are found to be common among different groups of mentally retarded individuals. Such constellations of abnormalities occur in 5 to 6 percent of all severely retarded people; for most of them, our knowledge is still at the level which applied to Down's anomaly between 1866 and 1959. Some of these syndromes are rare, and many others doubtless remain to be recognized. Tentative grouping depends upon careful and often rather tedious observations and measurements. Nevertheless, the proper assignment of these categories is definitely important as a research tool. It often is also valuable in terms of case management, in that it may obviate the need for uncomfortable or expensive tests; and it may be of importance for genetic counseling, since the recurrence risks for some of these syndromes are fairly well established.

The second advance in the study of Down's anomaly, namely the discovery of the characteristic chromosome abnormality, resulted from basic research into the structure of normal human chromosomes followed by applied research to determine if there were unusual features of chromosome structure in people with abnormal physical features. To date, chromosome studies in many of the other mental retardation syndromes have failed to reveal any abnormalities. This does not necessarily mean that these chromosomes are in fact normal but only that the present methods of study are not sufficiently sensitive to detect whatever aberrations do exist.

The way in which the excess 21 chromosome causes mental retardation is still unknown. The anatomical structure of the brain in Down's anomaly as studied with present techniques does not appear to be grossly or consistently disturbed, and no biochemical disorders have been clearly demonstrated to cause the mental retardation. Thus, at this time, the statement that Down's anomaly causes mental retardation rests solely on the consistent statistical association between the two phenomena. This situation reflects the primitiveness of present techniques for the study of brain structure and function.

The Inborn Errors of Metabolism

Of the over one hundred human inborn errors of metabolism which so far have been defined, approximately one half are associated with mental retardation; in all, these account for 3 to 5 percent of severe mental retardation. The inborn errors of metabolism represent very precisely defined abnormalities. Presumably, in each instance, a specific mutation causes a change in one component of a DNA molecule; this in turn causes one amino acid in an enzyme protein to be replaced by another and thus interferes with the function of that enzyme. Because of the extremely small physical size of this defect on the DNA molecule, it cannot be detected by studies of chromosomes under the light microscope. Diagnosis depends upon the demonstration of the deficient function of a specific enzyme, as occurs in Tay-Sachs disease, or the accumulation of a substance whose metabolism is prevented by deficiencies in enzyme function, as in phenylketonuria. Quite remarkable recent advances in basic science and in technology have made it possible to screen for these disorders on a large scale, to treat them when they do occur, and to prevent them through genetic counseling techniques. (Most inborn errors of metabolism are genetically transmitted either through an autosomal recessive or X-linked mode of inheritance.)

In respect to mental retardation, phenylketonuria (or PKU) is the single most important inborn error of metabolism. In the past it accounted for approximately 1 percent of all cases of severe mental retardation. Individuals with this disorder lack the capacity to convert the amino acid phenylalanine to tyrosine, a reaction which is normally catalyzed by the enzyme phenylalanine hydroxylase. Phenylalanine is a component of all proteins; hence, when the person with phenylketonuria eats a regular diet, phenylalanine accumulates in his tissues. As levels of phenylalanine increase, a secondary reaction converts some of it to phenylpyruvic acid (a ketone excreted in the urine after which phenylketonuria is named). For reasons which are not entirely clear, abnormally high tissue levels of phenylalanine cause severe damage to the developing human nervous system (ages 0–4 years) but apparently not thereafter. By changing the diet so that it contains only carefully controlled amounts of phenylalanine, it is possible to maintain normal tissue levels of this amino acid even in individuals with phenylketonuria; if this is done carefully and early enough, the child with phenylketonuria will develop normal intelligence. This impressive therapeutic achievement has provided the impetus for the mass metabolic screening of newborn infants. While these metabolic screening programs always include phenylketonuria, screening for other disorders, such as maple syrup urine disease, galactosemia, and homocystinuria, can be included at relatively little additional cost. (The total cost of these screening programs is approximately two dollars per child.) By 1973 nearly 14 million newborn infants had been tested for phenylketonuria throughout the world, and 1,186 cases of PKU had been discovered. In Massachusetts over 100 phenylketonuric children are under therapy; none are mentally retarded. In fact, since the Massachusetts statewide screening program was begun in 1963, no one has applied for admission to a residential institution for the retarded because of this condition. On the basis of previous experience, ten such admissions per year would have been anticipated. This clearly represents an important humanistic and economical public health advance, since the severely retarded patient with untreated phenylketonuria has a normal life span and nearly always requires life-long institutional care. Therapy for the child with PKU is relatively short-term; dietary treatment can be discontinued, without damage, some time after age four. One important note of caution is necessary, however: dietary control must be resumed when a phenylketonuric woman becomes pregnant. This is due to the fact that abnormally high maternal blood phenylalanine levels can damage the brain development of the fetus. Presumably this can be prevented if a normal blood phenylalanine level is maintained by careful control of the mother's diet. Continued follow-up and communication with the otherwise normal, treated phenylketonuric female thus is clearly essential.

Since phenylketonuria is a treatable disorder, its control focuses on the early identification and therapy of the affected individual. The emphasis is different for Tay-Sachs disease. Tay-Sachs disease is a progressive disorder, transmitted as an autosomal recessive trait, which causes severe mental retardation and leads to the child's death usually by the third or fourth year; in contrast to phenylketonuria, it cannot be treated by any known therapy. It has recently been shown that patients with Tay-Sachs disease lack an enzyme called hexosaminidase A and that unaffected carriers for the disease show half the normal level of this enzyme. Approximately 90 percent of cases of Tay-Sachs disease occur in Jews of Eastern European origin. In this group the disease incidence is approximately 1/3,600 and the carrier rate one in thirty. In several urban areas, hexosaminidase A assays have been offered to all Jewish people in reproductive age. (The hexosaminidase A activity of blood serum can be measured on a mass basis for less than two dollars per test.) If only one of the prospective parents is a Tay-Sachs carrier, then the couple is not at risk, and no further studies are required. If both husband and wife are carriers (the chance of this happening is approximately 1/900), then the recommendation is made that they have no children, or that the pregnancy be monitored by aminocentesis. Statistically, the fetus has one chance in two of being a carrier (clinically normal), one chance in four of being completely normal in respect to hexosaminidase A, and one chance in four of having Tay-Sachs disease. If the latter is the case, interruption of pregnancy is recommended, provided, of course, that this is acceptable to the family on legal, ethical, and religious grounds. It is estimated that screening all Jewish people at risk of producing a child with Tay-Sachs disease would cost approximately 200,000 dollars per year; this represents approximately one third of the purely financial burden of the disease when it does develop.

Tay-Sachs disease is one example of a group of approximately thirty disorders sometimes referred to as lysosomal storage disease. These include Gaucher's disease, Niemann-Pick disease, and Hurler's syndrome (gargoylism), and together account for perhaps 2 to 3 percent of severe mental retardation. In all these disorders there is a diminished capacity to break down certain complex fats or sugars; the substance which cannot be broken down accumulates in a part of the cell called the lysosome, which can be viewed as an intracellular digestive apparatus. The failure of intracellular digestion causes the lysosome to become greatly distended and eventually leads to cell death. Each of the thirty lysosomal disorders is caused by the malfunction of a specific enzyme, which can usually be detected in tests of blood samples and also in the amniotic cells of the fetus. However, most of them lack the clearcut racial predilection of Tay-Sachs disease, and they occur with such relative rarity in the general population that, at present, mass screening of all marriageable adults cannot be justified financially. For most of these disorders, therefore, the screening for carriers is directed toward relatives of known cases. It is estimated that up to 90 percent of Tay-Sachs disease cases and up to half of the cases of the other lysosomal storage diseases could be prevented with the widespread application of these screening techniques.

Mental Retardation Related to Prematurity and to Other Damaging Events Near the Time of Birth

Damage to the nervous system of the infant at or near the time of birth is estimated to cause 10 percent of all cases of severe mental retardation; if the parts of the brain responsible for limb and body movement are injured, cerebral palsy may also result. It is well established that such damage occurs most frequently in premature children. In the past, 33 to 70 percent of infants who weighed less than 1,500 grams (3.3 pounds) at birth were later found to suffer from serious abnormalities, which often included mental retardation; for infants who weighed less than 1,000 grams, the incidence of brain damage was estimated at 80 to 90 percent. One of the truly important recent advances has been the development of the field of neonatology and, with it, the establishment of regional intensive-care units which specialize in the care of premature infants. These nursery units pay the most meticulous attention to the maintenance of proper oxygen levels (too much oxygen leads to blindness), lung ventilation, blood pressure, the control of levels of glucose and other substances in the blood, and provisions for adequate nutrition. Previously the premature infant had often been considered so vulnerable that it was handled as little as possible.

At first, these developments aroused the concern that the ability to achieve the survival of more premature infants might be coupled with a great increase in brain-damaged children. Most fortunately, this fear has been shown to be unfounded. Not only do more premature babies survive, but careful followup studies show that the incidence of brain damage in these children is greatly diminished. In a recent series from London, 68 infants who weighed less than 1,500 grams at birth were reexamined when they were between 2 and 4 years old. Eighty-seven percent were normal, and only 7.5 percent showed signs of damage, as compared to 33 to 70 percent in the past. (The status of the remaining 5 percent in respect to brain function was uncertain.) Similarly, in Sweden, the incidence of low birth weight diplegia (a form of cerebral palsy) has diminished 40 percent, a change which is also attributed to improved neonatal care.

Mental Retardation Due to Infectious Diseases

It is estimated that infectious diseases are the cause of 4 to 9 percent of cases of severe mental retardation. In the first place, certain infectious diseases of the mother are likely to damage the fetus. This is particularly well known in the case of German measles (rubella), where 17 percent of first-trimester and 10 percent of second-trimester infections lead to rubella in the fetus. To prevent German measles in childbearing women it is now recommended that all children be immunized against the disease at one year of age, or in any case prior to beginning school, since immunizations administered during the child-bearing age may affect the fetus. Another important congenital disorder is cytomegalic inclusion disease, which is due to a virus closely related to herpes simplex, and which may be equally widespread. This virus has been known for some time to cause a relatively rare, but serious, disorder of the fetus. Because this virus is found in nearly all human beings at some time in their life, its mere presence does not, of course, establish that it is responsible for damage. However, it has more recently been shown that among certain infants with high blood levels of a certain immune globulin (IgM), approximately 6 percent excreted high levels of cytomegalic virus and showed a significantly above-average incidence of hearing loss and subnormal intelligence. It may thus be possible to pinpoint those infants who suffer brain damage from this or related viruses and to assess how frequently this occurs. Protective vaccines against cytomegalic virus are being tested. The degree to which they will be useful depends upon proof of the vaccine's safety and effectiveness and upon a clearer assessment of how often this virus does cause significant disease.

Viral and bacterial infections in early childhood can also be the cause of mental retardation in later life. Of particular importance here is infection with measles virus, which may cause nervous system damage in one of every thousand cases. Active immunization against measles is available, and its use is strongly recommended. Bacterial meningitis in early childhood may also cause permanent brain damage. The diagnosis of meningitis may be difficult to make in a newborn baby or a young infant and represents a true test and challenge of systems for the delivery of child health services. Once the diagnosis is made, however, antibiotic therapy is highly effective in the treatment of bacterial meningitis. Antibiotic treatment has already reduced greatly the incidence of mental retardation due to congenital syphilis and tuberculous meningitis; it is to be hoped that similar treatment may soon do the same for bacterial meningitis. (For a discussion of other effects of slow viruses on the nervous system, see Chapter 11.)

Mental Retardation Due to Lead Poisoning

There is great current interest in the role of lead poisoning as a cause of mental retardation. While the relatively rare occurrence of full-blown lead poisoning has long been known to be a cause of severe brain damage, there is suggestive evidence that less extreme lead exposure more commonly causes less severe, but significant, behavior abnormalities and learning deficits. Changes of this type have been produced in experimental animals exposed to relatively low lead levels. The main source of lead in people is the ingestion of lead-based paint by children in inner-city slum areas. This represents a particularly pernicious problem, since these are the children who are also most often subject to socio-cultural deprivation, undernutrition and infectious disease. The problem is well understood, and its solution could be achieved by the elimination of lead-based paint and contaminated water; but the implementation of these goals is a point of very great difficulty. Even before the recent financial crisis in New York City, public health officials there pointed out that eliminating this hazard was a nearly impossible task and would necessitate a complete, comprehensive program to improve housing conditions for the poor.

Other Causes of Group II Mental Retardation

Kernicterus, a jaundice of the central part of the brain resulting from Rh incompatibility between mother and fetus in pregnancy, is a long-recognized cause of mental retardation and hearing loss. Fortunately, the incidence of this disorder has been reduced greatly by the prompt performance of exchange transfusions to replace the blood of severely jaundiced infants and occasionally by transfusing a severely affected fetus *in utero*. Of even greater preventive significance are immunization programs for Rh-negative mothers. These programs can prevent the development in the mother of the Rh antibodies which are the cause of the infant's disease (see Chapter 15).

Congenital meningomyelocele, a defect in the closure of the spinal cord or its overlying membranes and bony coverings, is a common and serious form of neurological disability which when severe may also be associated with mental retardation. While early neurosurgical orthopedic and urological intervention can do a great deal to improve prognosis, the large neural tube defects present a serious and continuing burden to the child and family. The condition appears to be inherited as a polygenic trait, determined by the interaction of several genes, in which the risk of recurrence varies between approximately 1 and 5 percent; this represents a degree of risk considerably smaller than is the case for autosomal recessive disorders but 30 to 40 times higher than for the general population. It has recently been shown that 80 to 90 percent of fetuses with significant neural tube defects show elevated levels of alphafetoproteins in the amniotic fluid. It is therefore possible to monitor high-risk pregnancies (those occurring in families in which a neural tube defect has occurred previously) and to identify with considerable accuracy those fetuses which have such a defect. It may be possible in the future to combine such an approach with direct visualization of the fetus (see Chapter 18) or with other procedures which would enable the physician to assess how severe the defect is. Those fetuses in which the defect could be corrected or improved would then be identifiable, and criteria for early surgery, or for abortion, could be developed. Obviously, these new technical developments will lead to new ethical controversies as well.

Group I Culturofamilial or Physiological Mental Retardation

Even though it includes more individuals than the previous group, I have postponed discussion of Group I mental retardation because knowledge about it is limited and it remains very controversial. The field is still plagued by unnecessary controversies about nature versus nurture. An example of an extreme "nature" point of view was that presented in 1866 by Henry H. Goddard, in a paper entitled "The Menace of Mental Deficiency from the Standpoint of Heredity." It was his thesis that the culturofamilial type of mental retardation, as he had studied it in the Kallikak family, was familial and inherited and that such individuals should ideally be prevented from reproducing. While such an opinion appears totally distasteful today, in the early part of this century it was a point of view held by responsible and respected people who were strong advocates for what they considered to be the best interests of the mentally retarded and who did in fact achieve many advances in their care.

It is of course true that the recurrence risk for retardation in future sibs is higher in the culturofamilial group (Group I) than it is for Group II children, where the risk varies with relatively well-understood genetic principles. But the main critique of Goddard's argument is that familial occurrence cannot and must not be equated with heredity. Clearly, the child who is reared in a deprived setting by mentally retarded parents is at a developmental disadvantage. The devastating role of very severe social-environmental deprivation was shown convincingly by R. A. Spitz in 1945. He followed the development of 61 normally developed infants reared in a foundling home which provided adequate physical care, but in which there was a drastic deficiency of personal contact and emotional support during the first year of life. He compared these children with a group in a nursery who were provided with adequate human interaction. The average developmental quotient—a measure of developmental age that is analogous to IQ—fell from a starting level of 131 to 72 among the emotionally deprived foundling-home children, whereas that of the nursery group rose from 97 to 112. Follow-up studies showed that the children deprived during their first year continued to show poor psychomotor development at least until the age of three. The effects were not reversed even when a proper human and training environment was later provided. In spite of apparently adequate physical care, 37 percent of the emotionally deprived children had died by the end of the second year.

Other convincing evidence in support of the influence of environmental factors in respect to culturofamilial retardation is provided by epidemiological studies which Zena Stein and Mervyn Susser conducted in the English city of Salford. These authors identified virtually every mentally retarded individual in this city of 155,000 inhabitants. They demonstrated that in children from families of low social standing, mental retardation with IQ 50–70 in the absence of demonstrable brain disease was the most common form of mental subnormality; but this form was rarely recorded in children from families of high social standing. In other words, the condition was virtually specific to children in particular social categories. These investigators followed the careers of 106 men and women belonging to this group and correlated their eventual success in life with the structure of the family from which they had come. The eventual outcome of the individual's life seemed to depend strongly upon the degree to which his family had remained intact. Of the children who had come from disrupted families, one quarter were admitted to institutions for the retarded by the time they reached early adulthood; this was true for only 3 percent of those who had come from intact families. Similar differences were observed in respect to occupational status as well.

It is only because of the exaggerated claims for the supremacy of either nature or nurture that I restate here the obvious fact that environment and heredity both influence intellectual development and the ability to succeed in life. (The relative degrees of influence are, of course, very difficult to assess.) Recognition of the frequency of Group I mental retardation, of its human and economic cost, and of the fact that it appears to be in some ways environmentally determined has led to massive efforts to identify early those children who are likely to become retarded and to place them in early intervention programs to improve their chances of normal development. Unfortunately, our lack of knowledge and the difficulties of evaluation carry the risk that these efforts may not be successful. A study of signal importance in this respect is the "Milwaukee project," which is being conducted by Rick Heber and other members of the Rehabilitation Research and Training Center in Mental Retardation at the University of Wisconsin. This study has focused on a group of children who are known to have an extremely high risk of culturofamilial mental retardation. These children live in an economically deprived section of the city; it has been shown that if a child lives in this area, and if in addition the IQ of the child's mother is less than 80 (true in 45 percent of all cases), then the child has an 80 percent risk of being mentally retarded. The Milwaukee study is prospective and has involved forty families. Twenty families received very intensive intervention from the time the child was three months old until age 6 years; these families were contrasted with twenty comparable families who did not receive this intensive intervention. In an attempt to ensure that all elements of a training structure and positive intervention program were provided, the program focused on the child's mother as well as on the child. In this way, the intensity and duration of training far exceeded that provided in the usual Head Start programs. Progress evaluations were performed by individuals who were not associated with the intervention program; at the time of the first report, the oldest children were 6 years old. Upon evaluation, the intervention families showed striking gains in respect to psychomotor development. Furthermore, the mean differences in IQ score were 30 points and were particularly striking in respect to language development. While the Milwaukee study is well controlled, and its results are highly impressive, longer follow-up is required before one can be sure that the gains will be maintained. This caution stems from earlier experiences with less intensive Head Start programs. Children in these programs showed impressive gains during their preschool years; but after they entered first grade, differences were no longer demonstrable. As already noted, the Milwaukee study differs from most other programs in that intervention was directed toward both mother and child; the program was designed for maximum constructive impact, which, in terms of family effectiveness, may well be felt even after the formal program is discontinued. If the children's gains are indeed maintained, this finding would have very great practical and theoretical significance.

The Education, Training, and Habilitation of Mentally Retarded Individuals

Most of the advances discussed above aim to treat or prevent brain damage. At the same time, much has been learned in recent years about the education, training, and habilitation of mentally retarded people. Many of these improved training techniques are applicable particularly to the severely retarded, who in the past were often considered incapable of learning even basic skills. These people have benefited greatly from the application of behavior modification principles.

Careful, consistent, and individualized application of techniques for behavior modification can enable people who previously were considered unapproachable to take care of their own basic needs. Once this is achieved, the retarded person can engage in a much wider range of social, recreational, and training activities; in this way he avoids the dehumanizing and degrading side effects of purely custodial care, which separates the person from his known friends and associations and encourages undesirable behavioral traits which then require still greater restriction and incarceration. Seen in this light, the development and the evaluation of ever more effective training methods constitutes a highly significant and important branch of research. Apart from their immediate practical importance, the development of behavioral techniques also makes possible a more reproducible and objective description of a person's behavioral and learning capacities. It is hoped that such endeavors will eventually facilitate the establishment of more precise correlations between the type and location of brain disturbances and their behavioral manifestations. This is an area of research which would not only bring about a better understanding of normal brain function but which, if accomplished, would also undoubtedly help categorize further and eventually relieve the behavioral deficits which represent the main manifestation of mental retardation.

Apart from these specific behavioral techniques, much has been learned in the last two decades about other methods of improving the retarded person's growth and satisfaction with life. Some of these advances represent an unlearning of disadvantageous practices which had been adopted during the previous 75 years. For reasons related in part to inappropriate eugenic ideas, the mentally retarded had long been segregated in large institutions, separated from their normal human ties, stripped of their dignity, and deprived of productive learning experiences. Nonhabilitative institutional care thus compounded initial handicaps, to the extent that these existed. The pernicious effects of these secondary factors are now recognized, and the guiding principle of present-day care is to provide the least restrictive environment appropriate to the person's needs, and a physical and social environment and daily schedule that resemble the normal as closely as possible. The implementation of these approaches requires the design and the evaluation of care-delivery systems to be provided, as much as possible, near the person's home community. Again, these are topics that would benefit from further research. In adition, much applied research is needed to develop and to evaluate habilitative programs for people who have physical or sensory handicaps as well as being mentally retarded.

It is indeed encouraging that the incidence and the degree of disability caused by severe and by mild retardation can be reduced; research has been an important factor in bringing this about. In the prevention of severe mental retardation there are several areas of hope and accomplishment: the reduction of the effects of brain damage at birth through improved perinatal and neonatal care; prevention of brain damage from infectious disease through prompt antibiotic therapy and vaccination programs; the early detection and therapy of inborn errors of metabolism such as phenylketonuria; possible reduction of the incidence of Down's anomaly through genetic counseling and prenatal diagnosis; and reduced incidence of lipidoses through carrier detection and genetic counseling programs. Quantitatively more significant, the recognition of families and of children at risk and the design and evaluation of effective early intervention programs provide the promise of dealing with the very important issues of culturofamilial retardation.

Optimum progress in the field of mental retardation depends upon a multiplicity of approaches and upon the judgment to achieve the appropriate balance between them. Progress in the field has been hampered by narrow, simplistic, and even arrogant formulations which emphasize only a single approach to this broad problem. Examples of this are the nature versus nurture controversies which have already been cited. Other controversies, which have not been dealt with in detail here, center on the extent to which research effort ought to be directed to biological or social aspects, on whether research should be basic or applied, and even more recently, in view of human rights issues, on whether or not research involving retarded human beings ought to be conducted at all.

I believe that future work in the field of mental retardation must employ a multiplicity of correlated approaches. The necessity for basic research in neurobiology is so obvious that it hardly needs emphasis. One example of the primitiveness of our techniques and understanding is the fact that we are still unable to distinguish brain tissue of an individual with Down's anomaly from that of a person with normal intelligence; even more striking, for 30 to 40 percent of the severely retarded we are still unable to find any physiological cause. However, rapid advances are being made in the development of sophisticated techniques for examining the number and structure of brain cells and the connections between them. There is a glimmer of understanding about the forces which determine the migration of nerve cells during fetal life; this is an area of great relevance to mental retardation, since it appears certain that a number of causes of mental retardation are related to disturbances in the ways in which brain cells reach their "addresses" and proceed to connect and relate to other cells. Even though much progress has been made in respect to the inborn errors of metabolism, much more work is required to determine how and why such abnormalities in metabolism derange brain function. This area requires much more research on topics such as chemical transmitter substances and the metabolic process within individual nerve cells, progress which can only be achieved by work in experimental animals. Finally, the field of mental retardation has reaped very great benefits from advances in genetics (see Chapter 4) and will surely continue to do so.

As a person with a background and training in medicine, where the tradition and esteem for research is so firmly established, I have often been surprised by the degree of suspicion and even hostility toward research which exists among highly intelligent and highly motivated professionals and clients in the field of mental retardation. Research workers should examine the reasons for this attitude, evaluate the extent to which it may be justified, and determine what can be done to improve the research image. One of the probable reasons for suspicion toward research is that a great deal of medical research in the field of mental retardation has been directed toward determination of cause and toward prevention and that much less effort has gone into the improvement of care for those who are retarded. It is easy to understand that parents faced with the care of their retarded child are vitally interested in research directed to improving their child's ability to learn and to live in a meaningful and dignified manner. Until recently the United States had lagged behind in these areas, and other countries with fewer resources and less research sophistication had in fact done more to improve the life of their retarded citizens than we had. It has been stated that, in the field of mental retardation, the United States has originated research knowledge and understanding which other countries have applied to help the retarded. It is true that the research worker is not directly responsible for the quality of services offered to our mentally retarded citizens. Nevertheless, for humanistic reasons, and also out of enlightened self-interest, the research worker must join forces with those responsible for service, so that they can together improve the health care, education, and the general life setting of the mentally retarded.

One of the opportunities for resolving these difficult issues is provided by the twelve Centers for Research in Mental Retardation and Related Aspects of Human Development which were established during the Kennedy Administration under Public Law 88–164. The Mental Retardation Research Centers also relate closely to a second set of centers funded under the same law, which are called University Affiliated Facilities for Mental Retardation and which provide interdisciplinary professional training in this field. Together, these two programs provide the opportunity to do basic research of high quality; to apply basic research techniques and knowledge toward the solution of specific problems in the field of mental retardation; to encourage communication and collaborative research between biomedical, behavioral, and social scientists; and to help bridge the personal, cultural, and even geographic barriers which exist between the mentally retarded, their families, and those scientists, service providers, and health-care and social planners who can help them. These efforts, combined with many other programs which are now emerging, should reduce significantly the incidence of mental retardation and allow those who are retarded to lead more meaningful lives.

Neurological
Disorders

NORMAN GESCHWIND

11

Research into neurological disorders did not participate fully in the great flowering of medical investigation that took place in the 1920s. The biochemical advances that revolutionized the understanding and treatment of such diseases as diabetes, disorders of the blood-forming organs, and the diseases of the kidney led to a great expansion of research in departments of internal medicine throughout the United States and abroad. The lag in the study of neurological disorders had many causes. Clinical neurology was poorly developed in many places; indeed, several major medical institutions did not develop departments of neurology until well after the Second World War. Even in the 1920s and 1930s, however, a small number of institutions were making major contributions to the understanding of the nervous system and its disruption in disease. The brain waves seen in the electroencephalogram were first discovered in 1929 by Hans Berger and were rapidly used to distinguish among different kinds of epilepsy by such workers as William Lennox and Frederic and Erna Gibbs. Tracy Jackson Putnam and Houston Merritt developed methods for the experimental study of the treatment of epilepsy in a well-constructed research program which culminated in the development of diphenylhydantoin (still the most widely used of antiepileptic drugs). Abraham Myerson and others pioneered in the study of the biochemical sources of energy for the brain and of the chemical composition of the cerebrospinal fluid, which bathes the surface of the brain and spinal cord and which often shows dramatic changes in many diseases. Increasing anatomical and physiological knowledge led to the development of experimental procedures for controlling various types of disorders of movement and for treating hydrocephalus (expansion of the fluid cavities of the brain due to obstructions to the outflow of cerebrospinal fluid).

The great expansion of research into the nervous system and its diseases has, however, occurred primarily in the last quarter century. In 1939 there was a handful of journals reporting the results of such research; today there are dozens, many of them devoted to highly specific areas of investigation.

Prevalence of Neurological Disease

Despite this enormous expansion of research activity, many laymen are still unaware of the frequent and widespread disability caused by diseases of the nervous system. Neurological diseases rank third as causes of death (after heart disease and cancer). The largest single cause of death among neurological diseases is stroke, of which there are two major types: destruction of brain tissue by blockage of arteries in the brain, and brain damage from bleeding into the brain caused by rupture of blood vessels. At least 200,000 Americans each year die from stroke; many more die of complications resulting from their attack. (Thus, for example, many patients who become paralyzed eventually die as a result of pneumonia.) Neurological deaths form a major component of the mortality from injuries; head injury alone probably accounts for 50,000 deaths each year.

The full cost to society of neurological disease is, however, underestimated even by these impressive mortality figures. Many neurological diseases leave the patient alive but severely disabled; such cases require large numbers of personnel for their care. Mental retardation (see Chapter 10) affects several million Americans and may well be the leading cause of chronic disability in childhood. Muscular dystrophy attacks perhaps 200,000 others, most children. In young adult life multiple sclerosis is probably the most frequent cause of chronic disability, although it is not an important cause of death. Epilepsy, while rarely fatal, seriously affects over a million people. A significant although as yet undetermined fraction of patients in mental hospitals (estimated to be 40 percent by some studies) suffer from chronic abnormalities of behavior stemming from neurological disorders. Stroke leaves over a million patients with chronic crippling impairments, either as the result of paralysis of one side of the body or, when the damage involves the left side of the brain, because of aphasia (disorders in speech, writing, or the comprehension of language). A comparably large number of people are left with permanent impairments after suffering major injury to the brain or spinal cord. Finally, at least 200,000 other patients are chronically disabled by Parkinson's disease, amyotrophic lateral sclerosis, myasthenia gravis, Huntington's chorea, brain tumors, and a host of other disorders.

Disease of the brain is a major cause of disability in the aged. The intellectual decline of many old people, so frequently the most crippling and distressing symptom of aging, tends to be regarded as normal; yet we know that this problem is usually the result of what appears to be a highly specific biochemical disorder of nerve cells in certain portions of the brain. The same disorder may attack people in their forties and fifties, when it goes under the name of Alzheimer's disease. The assumption that senile dementia is normal is probably as incorrect as the medical beliefs of 100 years ago that tuberculosis and body lice were inevitable normal features of the human condition.

In many conditions in which the disease process does not primarily affect the nervous system, disability may result from secondary neurological effects. Thus in many patients with diseases of the kidneys or liver, the changes in the chemical composition of the blood may grossly impair nervous function. Despite the frequency of chronic kidney disease we still do not know what chemical component impairs brain function or how. More specific knowledge might advance greatly our capacity for treating this group of patients.

Fifty years ago there were few clues to determining what types of research might lead to methods for reducing the vast toll of death and chronic disability from neurological disorders. Even today there are many diseases whose causes and possible treatments remain unclear at best. Amyotrophic lateral sclerosis is an example, as is the much more common Alzheimer's disease (and its form in old age, senile dementia). But there are many other disorders, such as multiple sclerosis, for which promising leads do exist. Indeed, despite the vast increase in neurological research in the last 25 years, investigation is now limited by lack of trained personnel and resources rather than by a shortage of justifiable projects.

Neurological research can be divided into two major categories: research into the fundamental causes of disease and research into the nature of functional disabilities and into the means for overcoming them. I shall try to give examples of each of these below.

Basic Causes of Neurological Disease

Many disease processes which may lead to damage to the nervous system affect primarily nonnervous structures. As an example we may consider stroke, or, to use the technical term, cerebrovascular disease. Here the primary site of the disease process is in the blood vessels; arteriosclerosis often leads to the blockage of an artery and a sudden cutting off of the blood supply to a portion of the brain, which dies within minutes. Basic research on arteriosclerosis being carried out by nonneurological scientists should eventually lead to methods for controlling this disorder in the blood vessels of the brain as well as in those of the heart or legs. However, there may well be differences between the blood vessels of the brain and those of other organs; we know, for example, that brain arteries respond quite differently under certain conditions than do the nearby vessels which supply the scalp. Furthermore, certain causes of arteriosclerosis may affect the vessels of the heart and those of the brain differently. Thus diabetes is a major cause of arteriosclerosis in the heart but a much less prominent cause of the same changes in the vessels of the brain, while hypertension (high blood pressure) is a more important cause of arteriosclerosis in the brain than in the heart. Hypertension is in fact the primary cause of arteriosclerosis in the brain and is almost the exclusive cause of cerebral hemorrhage, caused by the rupture of small blood vessels within the brain.

Other areas of research on the causes of neurological disease involve disease processes which are specific to the nervous system. For example, some viruses have a special affinity for specific portions of the nervous system; these will be discussed in greater detail. Certain biochemical abnormalities involve substances found exclusively or predominantly in the nervous system; there is a group of disorders that occur mostly in children, the lipidoses, in which certain lipids (fatty substances) concentrate in certain portions of the brain and derange its functions (see Chapter 10). It is now known that many types of lipidosis are the result of shortages of specific enzymes in the brain which are responsible for the breakdown of lipids under normal conditions. The best known example of this type of disorder is Tay-Sachs, a disease of high frequency confined to infants of Eastern European Jewish background.

Impact of Neurological Research on Other Fields

Research on the nervous system has an impact on medicine that goes far beyond the study of neurological diseases themselves. For example, one of the great advances in the neurological sciences in this century was the discovery by Alan Hodgkin and Andrew Huxley of the mechanism by which electrical activity passes down a nerve fiber. They demonstrated that the voltage difference between the inside and outside of a nerve fiber at rest is the result of the different concentrations of potassium ions (which carry a positive charge) on the two sides. When the nerve is stimulated, an electrical current is observed; this was shown to result from the movement into the nerve fiber of positively charged sodium ions. This model has led to a much clearer understanding of nerve function and to clarification of the mode of action of many drugs, such as the local anesthetics. But nervous tissue is not the only excitable tissue in the body; many other tissues develop electrical responses, including muscle fibers, the cells of the heart, the muscles of the intestines and blood vessels, and the retina. The Hodgkin–Huxley theory has led to a new understanding of all of these excitable tissues. Hodgkin himself and Silvio Weidmann showed that similar phenomena occur in the heart; carrying this type of experimental analysis further, Paul F. Cranefield, Brian F. Hoffman, and others have provided a deepened understanding of the electrical activity of the heart and its disorders and of the actions of many drugs that affect the rhythm of the heart.

Neurological research plays an important role in a wide spectrum of medical problems. All anesthesia, whether general or local, involves the use of drugs that act on the nervous system. The study of pain is a clearly neurological problem with universal medical applications and is currently being pursued intensively. While the study of obesity involves many types of research, one major aspect (especially during the past three decades) has been the study of those portions of the nervous system which control appetite. A large number of genetic disorders involve the nervous system; neurological scientists like Richard Sidman and his group have in recent years advanced our knowledge of the development of the nervous system and the mechanism of its disruption by abnormalities of genetic control. Much of the research on blindness and most basic research on deafness is neurological. Drugs of addiction are taken because of their effects on the nervous system, and in recent years there has been much new knowledge of the exact sites of action of some of these drugs, especially the morphine derivatives, in the brain.

One area of neurological research of almost universal interest is sleep. Although human beings spend almost one third of their lives in this state, there was almost no fundamental biological understanding of it until the last 25 years. Furthermore, some aspects of sleep, such as dreaming, appeared until only recently to be beyond the realm of biological investigation. The great breakthrough came when William Dement, following up earlier work by Nathaniel Kleitman, showed that it is possible to tell when someone is dreaming with a very high degree of accuracy. Sleeping subjects experience several prolonged periods each night in which their eyes move rapidly, although during most of the night the eyes remain at rest. If the subject is awakened in rapid eye movement (REM) sleep he will frequently report that he has been dreaming, while if awakened when the eyes are at rest he will usually not report dream experiences. Such objective criteria for identifying the stages of sleep have made possible animal experiments to clarify the structures of the nervous system involved in sleep and the biochemical properties of these structures. Many disorders, such as sleepwalking, narcolepsy (a disease in which patients suddenly fall asleep uncontrollably), and night terrors in children are now understood better. It has also been discovered that many physiological processes—for example, the release of growth hormones—occur during certain stages of sleep. Firm physiological grounds now exist for the development and evaluation of drugs to correct sleep disorders. The study of sleep is a dramatic example in which many years of basic and apparently esoteric research have had practical results in many areas.

Neurological researchers have also studied the systems in the brain involved in emotional behavior. John Flynn has mapped very completely those regions in the brain of the cat involved in attack behavior, and similar studies have been carried out on other types of emotional behavior. The importance of this type of work becomes clear when we realize that damage to such systems in man may lead to abnormalities of emotional response. It now seems likely that most of the drugs used for psychiatric treatment act at various locations in anatomical systems involved specifically in emotional responses. Research in this field is likely to deepen our knowledge of the biological aspects of many of these emotional disorders and improve their treatment.

One of the major functions of the nervous system is learning; most if not all learning is encoded in neural tissue. (It can be argued that certain types of acquired immunity should also be regarded as "learning.") Within the last quarter century there has been a marked increase in our knowledge of the special anatomical structures which are involved in memory. Very recent research in animals has been directed to identifying specific enzyme systems which are involved in certain types of learning. Although no practical application has yet resulted from these studies, we can look forward to the possibility of improving learning abilities in individuals of any level of intelligence.

The wide range of problems dealt with in neurological research is reflected in the variety of disciplinary backgrounds of investigators in the field. While some have a primary background in clinical specialties such as neurology, neurosurgery, and psychiatry, others are specialists in unexpected fields, for example, obstetricians who study the binding of female sex hormones to brain tissue. Another very large group includes scientists in nearly all basic sciences with a special interest in the nervous system: neuroanatomists, neurophysiologists, neuropharmacologists, neurochemists, neuroendocrinologists. Many important contributions have come from further afield, for example, from physiological psychologists who carry out research on animal nervous systems and their relationship to behavior.

Let us now turn to a consideration of two areas of neurological research, one already well established, one still in its early development. The first illustrates the benefits of research into the causes of neurological disease, the second the potential for correcting certain deficits resulting from damage to the nervous system.

Slow Virus Infection of the Nervous System

Infection of the nervous system by viruses has been recognized from almost the earliest days of the discovery of these remarkable organisms. All these illnesses were thought to be acute (of rapid onset and brief duration); and, although permanent after-effects might remain, it was presumed that survival from these diseases conferred lifelong immunity on the patient. In cases in which the disease proved fatal, changes detected through the microscope in the affected portions of the nervous system appeared to be quite uniform. The well-known viral illnesses were of two general varieties. Most common was acute viral encephalitis (inflammation of the brain produced by viruses). The patient with this disease suffered from a rapid onset of headache, stiff neck, mild fever, and drowsiness. Large numbers of these viral illnesses were described. Some of them, such as the viral encephalitis occasionally caused by the mumps virus, were mild and were followed by very good recovery. Others, such as equine encephalitis (in which the infective agent is transmitted from horses to man), were often fatal. Other forms of viral disease, in which the virus would attack highly specific portions of the nervous system, produced types of illness with very striking individual characteristics. The virus of poliomyelitis is an example, since it specifically attacks those cells in the nervous system which send out nerve fibers to control muscles. The rabies virus provides another dramatic example.

This virus probably has a special affinity for those regions in the brain of the dog which control biting activity. As the result of this highly specific effect, the dog begins to engage in aggressive biting attacks on other animals and thus ensures the transmission of the virus. But its remarkable predilection for these sites in the nervous system the virus facilitates its own propagation. (People usually do not transmit the virus, since in them it does not typically produce a real biting attack.)

The notion that neurological involvement by viruses might take other than acute forms was first considered over 40 years ago. Between 1918 and 1930 an epidemic of influenza spread across the entire world (see Chapter 6). The virus of this strain of influenza frequently attacked the nervous system to produce a dramatic illness called lethargic encephalitis, a form of sleeping sickness. The patient would sleep by day and often lie awake, confused, at night. This disease disappeared after 1930, although there is some question as to whether or not rare cases have been seen since. The changes seen under the microscope in the brains of those who died from the disease showed the expected appearance of an acute viral encephalitis in the affected portions of the brain. The subsequent clinical course of many survivors, however, presented features that had never been observed before. Some of these patients, after years of being stable, developed a slowly progressive neurological disorder which often got worse over many years. This illness is called postencephalitic parkinsonism, and has some resemblances to the more common disease, idiopathic parkinsonism (that is, parkinsonism of unknown causation). There are, however, certain striking differences between these two diseases. For example, patients with postencephalitic parkinsonism often suffer from curious attacks, called oculogyric crises, in which the eyes roll up; this type of attack occurs rarely, if at all, in parkinsonism of unknown cause. Even today, 35 years after the disappearance of acute epidemic encephalitis, many cases of progressive postencephalitic parkinsonism remain.

The discovery that an acute viral illness of the nervous system could be followed after a variable interval by the appearance of a newly progressive illness aroused enormous interest. This disease also taught the important lesson that new and previously unknown acute viral illnesses of the nervous system can appear unexpectedly; even if known serious illnesses are wiped out, other new ones may arise to affect large numbers of people. With the development of many laboratories with a special interest in the so-called neurotropic viruses, a monitoring system may eventually be perfected to detect new viruses of this type and control them before they have had a serious effect on the population.

Basic to the problem of controlling these diseases is the question of explaining the appearance of progressive illness after an interval of recovery. When cases of postencephalitic parkinsonism were first observed, several theories were advanced. The simplest argument was that cells that had been weakened in some way by the original illness later died prematurely. Another ingenious suggestion was that progressive postencephalitic parkinsonism represented persistence of viral infection in the brain; the virus that had produced an acute illness might remain dormant in the brain and produce a different type of slowly progressive disorder, quite unlike the usual acute viral infection, after several years. This suggestion, however, could not be adequately investigated with the virological techniques available at that period and therefore received little attention.

The entire concept of slow virus infections of the nervous system reappeared, however, after the Second World War. Certain diseases of animals, such as scrapie (a disease of sheep), appeared to result from viruses affecting the brain; but both the slow progression of these disorders and the lack of the usual microscopic appearances in several of them ran counter to the predominant concept of viral encephalitis. The most dramatic new data came from the discovery of a slowly progressive neurological disease, called Kuru, which occurs in only one human population, a small tribe in the Fore River Valley in New Guinea. Since this illness was found to be unique both clinically and in its appearance under the microscope, its presence in one confined population suggested at first that it was an inherited disease occurring in an isolated population with a special genetic constitution. The dramatic discovery was made, however, that chimpanzees inoculated with brain tissue from cases of Kuru also developed the illness. It was thus almost certain that Kuru was a viral infection of the nervous system and that a slow virus caused this slowly progressive illness. A great deal of evidence was brought forward to suggest that the disease was transmitted in the Fore River Valley by the custom of eating the brains of people who had died, many of whom had Kuru. With the decline of this type of cannibalism the disease has become less common.

It soon became apparent that such slow viral illnesses of the brain were not confined to this minute population. Investigations were made of the brains of patients who had died of Jakob–Creutzfeldt disease, an illness which affects patients in middle life or early old age and usually leads to death within two years. The cardinal features of this disorder are progressive intellectual deterioration and dramatic jerking of muscles (myoclonus). Brain tissue from such patients produced a similar illness when inoculated into the brain of the chimpanzee. Another remarkable illness, confined almost entirely to children but resembling Jakob–Creutzfeldt disease in other ways, goes under the name of subacute sclerosing panencephalitis (SSPE). Children afflicted with this disease also suffer intellectual decline and myoclonus and usually die within a year or two. It was discovered that the spinal fluid of these patients contains unusually high levels of antibodies against the measles virus. The current concept of this disorder is that measles virus remains in the brains of these children after an attack of measles in childhood. After a variable period the virus becomes active, leading to a progressive disease. It is quite possible that this course of events may occur more frequently in the brain than in other areas of the body; many of the immune processes which wipe out infection elsewhere in the body are probably considerably modified in the special environment of the nervous system.

While this chapter was being written reports appeared of yet another previously unknown condition of this type. It was discovered some years ago that infants born of mothers who had suffered infection with German measles (rubella) in the first three months of pregnancy were often born with abnormalities of certain portions of the nervous system. This discovery not only led to better understanding of some of the causes of birth defects but also established the important fact that viruses can pass from mother to fetus. Two groups of investigators have now reported that several of these children, after remaining stable for as many as twelve years, later developed a neurological disorder which worsened slowly over time. Rubella virus was found in the brain of one of these patients after death. Apparently this virus remains dormant in the brain from the time of the infection in fetal life and eventually produces a progressive illness.

Slow virus illness has also turned up in another unexpected area. Before the Second World War it was discovered that some patients with cancer develop neurological illnesses which progress over months or years and sometimes continue to worsen even after successful treatment of the carcinoma. These diseases are not the result of the spread of cancer to the brain (which is a common complication of many malignancies). In at least one of these curious syndromes, which is called multifocal leukoencephalopathy, there is strong evidence that a slow virus is the responsible agent.

The implications of these discoveries are of utmost importance for future neurological research. There are many nervous diseases of as yet unknown cause which progress over time; multiple sclerosis, idiopathic parkinsonism, amyotrophic lateral sclerosis, senile dementia, Alzheimer's disease, and Pick's disease (another form of gradual intellectual degeneration) cause an enormous amount of human suffering and exact a great economic toll. It now seems reasonable to assume that at least some of these are the result of viruses which have lain dormant for many years. The signs of the original infection of the brain may well have been mild or indeed inapparent. In some instances the virus may have passed from the mother to the fetus through the placenta. It even seems possible that some disorders thought to be hereditary are actually the result of viruses passed on in this manner; a disorder in cats known as cerebellar agenesis which was for many years regarded as hereditary is now thought to result from such maternal-fetal viral transmission. A similar mechanism may account for the occurrence of multiple cases of Jakob–Creutzfeldt disease in some families.

Obviously once it can be proven that a given disease is viral in origin the possibilities for prevention or treatment increase enormously, since research can be directed intelligently to the causes. Throughout the history of medicine, control of viral illnesses—notably smallpox, yellow fever, poliomyelitis, and measles—has led to major advances in human health. Furthermore, research into viral illness of the nervous system may have dividends other than the direct control of disease. Certain viruses which have affinities for very selected regions of the brain may become valuable tools in animal research for studying the functions and chemical peculiarities of these different regions. There may even be therapeutic uses of viruses. Since viruses change the metabolism of the infected cell, it is conceivable that some viruses could be used to correct genetic shortages of certain enzymes produced by lack of an essential gene. Clearly at this point we come to the highly speculative edge of future research. Yet the whole history of the slow viruses illustrates superbly what dramatic advances can be made from the ultimate combination of astute clinical observation, basic research carried on without consideration of its application to human disease, and applied research with specific aims. The omission of any of these would definitely have held up progress.

The importance of slow viral illnesses of the nervous system has been underlined by the award in October 1976 of the Nobel Prize to Dr. Carleton Gajdusek, who has made major contributions in this field.

Recovery from Aphasia

Let us now turn to another area of research, one in which there are fewer positive results to show but which nevertheless has major potential for the future and which illustrates some of the special methods of investigation that are almost unique to neurology. We have noted earlier that research can be designed to prevent or treat directly the original cause of neurological illness. The research on slow virus diseases is one example, since vaccination or antiviral agents might control such disorders; other types of preventive measures range from better design of automobiles and helmets for motorcycle riders (to minimize head injuries) to control of high blood pressure (a major cause of both occlusion of cerebral vessels and hemorrhage from them). A very different type of research is that designed to correct the disabilities produced by damage to the nervous system. Even if startling advances are made in the prevention or direct treatment of causes of neurological disease there will still be many thousands of patients who will suffer the destruction of portions of the nervous system. In some nonneurological illnesses restoration of function can be achieved despite loss of an organ. Lowered or absent thyroid function, for example, can be treated by means of thyroid hormones; and actual replacement of organs, as in kidney or heart transplantation, may be effective in a limited number of cases. The nervous system, however, presents special difficulties. In some instances replacement therapy can be helpful, for example, in the use of L-dopa to treat parkinsonism; this drug is converted in the nervous system to dopamine, which is the active agent in restoring normal function. But the difficulty that generally arises is that many portions of the nervous system control highly complex activities. If the cells of the brain controlling these activities are damaged, then there appears at first to be little hope for true restitution. Nerve cells, once destroyed, are not formed again. If a nerve fiber in the central nervous system is cut some distance from its cell body it will not grow again to span the break, although the peripheral nerves (those in the limbs) can regenerate across such discontinuities. Thus the prospects for recovery after gross damage to the brain have remained gloomy at best.

Consider, for example, the areas of the brain which are involved in language. It has been known for 100 years that these areas lie in most patients in the cortex of the left cerebral hemisphere, in which they probably occupy up to 20 percent of the total surface area. Destruction of all or part of this region leads to gross impairments in the use or understanding of language; sometimes these involve problems in speaking, writing, and comprehension of both spoken and written language, while in other cases with more selective damage only certain aspects of language may be defective. This type of language disorder is called aphasia. It has often been thought that major damage in the language areas of the brain leads to irreversible deficits; indeed there has always been a large number of permanently disabled aphasic patients, some of them widely known public figures. Lenin was totally disabled by severe aphasia for the last two years of his life, despite the extensive attentions both of his own doctors and of major figures called from abroad; needless to say, this disease probably had a major effect on the subsequent history of the Soviet Union. Joseph Kennedy, the father of John, Robert, and Edward, also suffered from severe aphasia for several years toward the end of his life. Cases such as these are understandably responsible for the common notion that destruction of the neural regions of the left hemisphere involved in language leaves the patient without hope of recovery.

A closer look, however, reveals that this pessimism may have been too hasty. From the earliest days of the study of aphasia, it has been known that some patients show excellent recovery despite massive damage to the speech region. Although the exact percentage of such recoveries is not known, studies made in the Soviet Union during the Second World War on patients who had suffered gunshot wounds in the speech areas found that 25 to 30 percent of such patients showed very good return of language functions after several months. A clue to the way such recovery occurs comes from studies in children who develop aphasia with damage of the left hemisphere. This is usually the result of occlusion of one of the major cerebral blood vessels, which is much rarer in childhood than in adult life. Such children develop aphasia but nearly always regain normal language function within three years. While such recovery occurs in nearly all cases up to the age of 10 or 12, the percentage who improve drops during later adolescence and early adult life.

The question arises, then, as to how the child recovers. Since recovery takes place even after massive damage on the left side it seems clear that the right hemisphere must be responsible for the recovery. Conceivably, the right side of the brain could be capable of relearning language after destruction of the left hemisphere. There is, however, an alternative hypothesis. It is possible that both hemispheres actually learn language in early childhood but that the right hemisphere is somehow prevented from using its store of knowledge, being literally dominated by the left. (The several possible physiological mechanisms by which this could occur are beyond the scope of this chapter.) If this hypothesis were correct, then recovery from asphasia would occur through the activation of the dormant store of language learning on the right side of the brain after damage to the left hemisphere. There is a considerable body of evidence to support this model. The child who becomes aphasic with left-brain damage may show a severe aphasia for two months, followed in the third month by a rapid return of all language capacities; this recovery occurs despite the fact that the child is often quite ill, is receiving no specific retraining, and often has little language interaction with others. Furthermore, his vocabulary generally includes many words that he could not have heard during his hospitalization. The speed of recovery and the preservation of old vocabulary argue strongly against the idea that a relearning of language takes place. These observations suggest in fact that a store of language learning was already present in the right hemisphere and became available within a few months of damage to the left.

This is a very encouraging result. If language learning is present but dormant in the right hemisphere at age 10, might it not still be there at age 50? The study of adults who recover spontaneously also supports the idea that at least some of them experience the revival of a previously existing store of learning. But then why do only 25 to 30 percent of older patients show spontaneous recovery? It is possible that in some instances the learning which is present on the right side in nearly all children has literally been lost in these adults; alternatively, the store of language learning may still be there but for some reason may remain suppressed. Since the reactivation of the old, submerged learning often takes many months in childhood, it is not surprising that in most instances in later life the liberation from very prolonged suppression may take place too slowly ever to be fully useful.

We have now, however, opened up entirely new possibilities for research into methods of facilitating recovery from aphasia. If there is indeed latent but unactivated learning in the right hemisphere, we should look for ways to bring about its expression. Before this can be accomplished, some highly specific biological questions must be answered. What are the exact regions on the right side that store this dormant learning? More important, how is it kept latent in the normal state of the individual? There are several possibilities. These regions may be chemically inhibited; nerve fibers ending on the nerve cells in the appropriate regions may release transmitter chemicals that keep the cells in the speech areas inactive. If this is the case, it should be possible to locate the regions of the brain containing the nerve cells which send out inhibitory fibers to the speech regions. It might then become possible surgically to destroy those areas that give rise to inhibitory fibers and thus to release the nerve cells in the speech region from their inactive state. An even better way to accomplish this objective would be to find a chemical antagonist to the inhibitory substance.

There are several other specific biological mechanisms that might be exclusively or jointly involved in maintaining suppression of the speech areas on the right. A detailed understanding of this suppression will probably lead eventually to effective means of treatment. Obviously research of this type presents great difficulties, since only human beings have well-developed language systems in the brain; many kinds of direct experiments thus cannot be carried out. When the problem is brought down to the level of suppression of cells, however, it becomes possible to carry out certain investigative studies in animals that should lead to findings applicable to people.

While many aspects of the function of the nervous system are still very poorly understood, modern laboratory techniques are beginning to clarify the causes of several types of neurological disorder in ways that would have been impossible only a few decades ago. Advances in the biochemical understanding of senile dementia may finally lead to the eradication of this nearly universal condition. It is hoped that continuing research into the viruses that cause progressive neurological diseases will facilitate the development of preventive screening and vaccination programs to control these viruses in the early stages of infection. A more precise understanding of the geography of the brain and the identification of areas responsible for specific functions will be of great value, not only in the treatment of diseases such as aphasia but also in the study of emotional and learning behavior. Research in neurological disease covers a wide spectrum; at one extreme it can concern itself with the neurotropic virus, and at the other it is involved in those highest levels of intellectual and behavioral activity that are unique or almost unique to human beings. In all cases, however, the problems faced can be phrased in biological terms that permit investigation at the laboratory bench, in the physiological laboratory, and in the clinic.

Diseases of
Organs and Systems

PART FOUR

The Heart
and Vascular System

THOMAS W. SMITH

12

Although providing two eyes, ears, lungs, and kidneys, nature in its parsimony bestowed on us only a single heart. Worse, damage to the heart is difficult to repair. Individual heart muscle cells that have been damaged fatally are not able to regenerate; like the brain and spinal cord (and unlike many other organs of the body) the heart must make do with the cells present at birth and must compensate as best it can for any decrease in the number of functioning cells. Since a loss of more than about 40 percent of one's functioning heart cells is inevitably fatal, it is crucial to prevent heart disease from developing or else to stop the progression of disease before too much irreversible damage has occurred.

Enormous strides have been made in the past several decades in our understanding of heart disease and our ability to diagnose, prevent, and treat it. When President Warren G. Harding died from a heart attack as recently as 1923, his physicians had no real idea of what had killed him; they ascribed his death to apoplexy brought on by "ptomaine poisoning from eating crabmeat tainted with copper in a month without an R in it." But in spite of the obvious progress that has been made since Harding's time, cardiovascular disease remains the predominant cause of death in the United States today. Heart and blood vessel diseases claim more lives in this country than all other causes of death combined; more than a million Americans die each year of heart attack, stroke, hypertensive heart disease, rheumatic heart disease, and congenital heart defects. Many more of the approximately 29 million Americans with some major form of cardiovascular disease are seriously disabled. Much of this death and disability strikes productive individuals in the prime of life. Partly for this reason, the economic cost to the nation of cardiovascular disease, including the cost of lost productivity, was an estimated 22.7 billion dollars in 1973.

In spite of the great national attention that has been given to heart and blood vessel disease, millions of people with the most common cardiovascular disorder—hypertension (high blood pressure)—do not even realize that they have it. Hypertension may go undetected for years; it is often referred to as a "silent killer" because there are no characteristic symptoms throughout most of the usually long course of the disease. Only 10 to 20 percent of the estimated 23 million hypertensive individuals in the United States are receiving effective treatment; and fully half are not aware that their blood pressure is higher than normal. But ignoring hypertension can be very dangerous. High blood pressure reflects an abnormally high resistance to blood flow in the blood vessels; the heart must pump harder than normal to propel the blood through these vessels, and the pressure created is higher as a result. This elevation of pressure puts a strain on both the heart and the blood vessels and may ultimately lead to stroke, heart failure, or kidney failure. In addition, hypertension is increasingly recognized as an important factor that increases the risk of developing coronary artery disease, an often fatal disorder of the blood vessels that nourish the heart.

Coronary artery disease is the most dramatic and widely publicized form of cardiovascular disease in our society; it has been termed the "twentieth century epidemic" by Paul Dudley White. Although virtually unknown in many primitive societies with profoundly different dietary and living habits from ours, symptomatic coronary artery disease afflicts about four million Americans; with an annual death toll of about 700,000, it leads all other causes of death by a wide margin. And recent research indicates that coronary artery disease may indirectly cause even more deaths than this. It is now believed that the vast majority of the more than 400,000 sudden deaths occurring each year in previously healthy individuals are caused by disturbances of the electrical activity that directs the pumping of the heart, and coronary artery disease is the predominant cause of such sudden disturbances of heart rhythm.

The prevention of coronary heart disease has been, and remains, a major focus of research in cardiovascular disease.

The Prevention of Coronary Artery Disease

The basic cause of coronary disease is now known to be atherosclerosis, commonly known as hardening of the arteries. This process consists of a deterioration in the lining of the arteries, with accumulation of deposits of fatty materials (such as cholesterol), cellular debris, and calcium. In addition to narrowing the channels through which the blood supplies nutrients, atherosclerosis also predisposes to formation of blood clot that further chokes off the blood supply to the heart. Since heart muscle requires a constant supply of oxygen and other nutrients carried by the blood via the coronary arteries, loss of adequate blood supply for a period of more than a few minutes results in the death of heart muscle cells and the symptom complex known as heart attack or, more precisely, myocardial infarction. Lesser degrees of coronary artery obstruction cause inadequacy of blood supply (ischemia) and consequent chest pain (angina pectoris) only when the demands on the heart are increased, as during physical exertion or emotional stress. Although symptoms of angina or myocardial infarction may have a sudden onset, the underlying process has usually been going on for years or, more likely, decades. Indeed, the early degenerative changes of coronary atherosclerosis are frequently observed at post-mortem examination in children dead of unrelated causes and were found in the majority of healthy young servicemen killed in the Korean War.

An important area of research during the past 20 years has been the identification of factors that predispose the individual to atherosclerosis or in other ways increase the risk of coronary artery disease. Although true causal relationships remain difficult to determine, coronary artery disease is definitely associated with hypertension, elevated serum cholesterol levels, a family history of coronary heart disease, being male, and smoking cigarettes. Additional associated factors found in some studies include obesity, circulating blood fats other than cholesterol, and certain personality traits. These risk factors are clearly additive. Cigarette smoking alone increases the risk of heart attack in a 45-year-old man by 59 percent, while cigarette smoking and a moderately elevated cholesterol level together increase the risk by more than 200 percent. If he also suffers moderately severe hypertension, a male cigarette smoker with high cholesterol runs five times the normal risk of heart attack and more than ten times the normal risk of stroke.

Control of elevated serum cholesterol levels is widely accepted as a worthwhile approach to preventing coronary disease, but the definition of an elevated level has proven elusive. Serum cholesterol levels are often considered normal up to values of 250 milligrams per 100 milliliters, yet it is clear that the risk of both heart attack and stroke starts to increase at cholesterol levels of 150 or less. It seems hazardous to base our concept of normality on the distribution of cholesterol levels found in our own population, which suffers one of the highest rates of coronary heart disease on earth. Perhaps we should rather consider as normal the cholesterol values near 100 that are typical in primitive societies where coronary disease is virtually nonexistent. In any event, the consensus among cardiologists and nutritionists today is that regulation of body weight and a diet low in cholesterol and saturated fats are of value in reducing coronary risk. For individuals who continue to have high blood levels of fats despite these measures, more stringent diets and drugs may be effective.

Although blood cholesterol can be controlled to some extent through proper diet, cholesterol intake in food is not the only factor controlling blood levels of this lipid. Cells of the human body also produce cholesterol for use in vital processes such as the construction of cell membranes. If the synthesis of cholesterol molecules is not properly balanced, elevated levels can exist even without excessive dietary intake. This is exactly what happens in families with a hereditary defect in the control of cholesterol production (see Chapter 4). Affected members of these families may have blood serum cholestrol levels of 1,000 milligrams or more per 100 milliliters and suffer angina and heart attack in their teens or even earlier.

It now appears that the hereditary defect that leads to these very excessive cholesterol levels is a disorder of cellular control mechanisms. Very recently, Michael Brown and Joseph Goldstein have delineated the mechanism by which mammalian cells use a specific receptor on the cell surface to control cholesterol production. Receptors are specific molecules or combinations of molecules that serve as sensing devices to detect the presence of substances like hormones and drugs and that mediate the response of the cell to such molecules. The interaction between the cellular receptor and the substance it reacts to is usually thought of as a sort of lock and key mechanism in which the shapes of the receptor and the molecule with which it interacts are complementary. Cholesterol receptors are needed to exert a feedback control on cholesterol synthesis, ensuring that the body will manufacture enough cholesterol to maintain vital processes but will shut off production before levels get too high and result in unwanted deposition in blood vessel walls. The situation is complicated by the fact that cholesterol, which is nearly insoluble in water, is transported in the blood by a specific carrier molecule known as low density lipoprotein (LDL). Thus, it is an LDL-cholesterol complex that must be monitored and held at appropriate levels by the cellular control mechanism.

Recent studies have shown that LDL receptors on the cell surface bind the LDL-cholesterol complex and transport cholesterol into the cell. Once inside the cell, cholesterol acts on the synthetic machinery to reduce the rate of further cholesterol production. The LDL receptor itself is regulated by a feedback mechanism so that it becomes less active as cholesterol accumulates within the cell. Cells normally acquire more cholesterol by increasing the number of receptor molecules and protect themselves against being overloaded with cholesterol by decreasing the production of LDL receptors.

This delicate balance is disrupted in individuals who have inherited a tendency to grossly elevated blood cholesterol levels and premature coronary heart disease. It is now evident that these patients suffer a hereditary absence of the normal LDL receptor on their cell surfaces. Lacking this vital link in the feedback regulation of cholesterol production, the cells never get the message that there is already too much cholesterol present; and they go on overproducing this fatty material until abnormal deposition occurs in blood vessel walls. Now that we have some understanding of the normal cholesterol control mechanism and of its disturbance in severe hereditary blood cholesterol elevation, investigators have important leads to follow in studying the more subtle abnormalities that must exist in patients with more moderate (but potentially harmful) elevation of cholesterol levels. Further advances in our understanding of these processes will be crucial to the development of new ways to prevent atherosclerotic heart and vascular disease.

Although hereditary risk factors can be identified and taken into account in the patient's treatment, they cannot be directly altered. But high blood pressure, high serum concentrations of fats (particularly cholesterol), cigarette smoking, obesity, and lack of exercise are all conditions that can be successfully changed by the patient and physician. The impact of preventive measures instituted before the onset of any symptoms is currently being evaluated in a large-scale multicenter Multiple Risk Factor Intervention Trial with the convenient acronym MR FIT. Supported by the National Heart and Lung Institute, this program has already screened more than 366,000 men between the ages of 35 and 57 and has enrolled 12,650 in a program designed to eliminate such risk factors as high blood pressure, smoking, and elevated blood cholesterol levels. Definitive information on the efficacy of these measures is expected in about five years. In the meantime, most physicians recommend treatment programs to minimize those risk factors that are subject to intervention.

A real problem in the implementation of these preventive programs has been the difficulty of getting patients to comply with their physicians' recommendations. Although the underlying cause of hypertension is still usually unknown, treatment with appropriate drugs can being the blood pressure under satisfactory control in nearly all cases; and recent large-scale studies have shown that lowering elevated blood pressure brings about substantial reduction of morbidity and mortality. Unfortunately, many of the drugs used to control blood pressure have side effects that patients find bothersome. One of the most difficult tasks faced by the physician is that of convincing patients who have not yet developed troubling symptoms to adhere to the recommended drug regimen. There is much current interest in the use of paramedical personnel, such as nurse practitioners or well-trained physicians' assistants, to discuss treatment programs with patients and explain their importance.

Even more difficult treatment problems are posed by the possibility that very basic aspects of the individual's life style may increase his risk of developing heart disease. The suggestion that certain behavioral patterns may predispose a person to coronary heart disease has stirred considerable controversy in recent years. Ray Rosenman and Meyer Friedman, who have published a book that has attracted much public attention (*Type A Behavior and Your Heart*), claim that the hard-driving, deadline-oriented "Type A" person may run an especially high risk of coronary heart disease. And some (but not all) studies indicate that people who exercise regularly have a lower incidence of symptomatic coronary disease than do people with a more sedentary existence. (In middle age or beyond, however, an exercise program may pose risks that should be evaluated by a physician before the program is begun.) Many physicians take issue with the claim that personality and behavioral factors increase the risk of heart disease. They feel that undue emphasis on these possible risk factors only serves to distract investigators, physicians, and the public from more important goals, like reducing cigarette smoking and achieving adequate detection and treatment of hypertension. More information is clearly needed to assess the part that behavioral patterns may play in the twentieth-century epidemic of coronary heart disease.

Researchers are examining a number of possible new approaches to coronary disease prevention. One recent suggestion—which is still highly speculative—is that regular use of aspirin may possibly reduce the risk of myocardial infarction. Aspirin is known to inhibit the activity of platelets, the small elements in the blood that promote clot formation; such inhibition lowers the likelihood of clotting in blood vessels, which can lead to heart attack. Other agents with anticoagulant activity have been used for many years to prevent clotting problems. Agents that alter the normal clotting mechanisms may be dangerous, however, because they also increase the risk of uncontrolled bleeding. The National Heart and Lung Institute is now studying the efficacy of aspirin in preventing coronary disease and is evaluating the safety of this approach.

Methods for the prevention of cardiovascular disease should continue to improve as the underlying causes of heart and blood vessel diseases are better understood. The potential impact of defining accurately the factors associated with a disease process is exemplified by the conquest of acute rheumatic fever during the first half of the twentieth century. When infection with the bacterial agent known as streptococcus was first recognized to precede acute rheumatic fever, a causal relationship was far from clear. In fact, the chain of steps leading from a streptococcal sore throat to rheumatic damage to the heart valves still remains unclear in many respects. Nevertheless, it is now certain that adequate treatment of the streptococcal infection with penicillin or another appropriate antibiotic will avert a subsequent attack of life-threatening acute rheumatic fever. This discovery has been one of the major advances in preventive medicine during the past several decades; and there is reason to think that a similarly painstaking analysis of the factors associated with coronary heart disease will provide clues to its prevention.

Treatment

While prevention is preferable to treatment, it is not always possible to achieve. Among the most pressing medical problems confronting patients and physicians every day is the necessity for relief of symptoms and prolongation of life after symptomatic cardiovascular disease has begun. Several important new treatment methods developed during the past decade deserve special attention.

Heart attack (acute myocardial infarction) is the most common cause of death in the United States, and much effort has been directed at lowering the death toll from this disease process. Since heart muscle cells that are irreversibly damaged by loss of their blood supply cannot regenerate, a massive loss of functioning heart cells leaves little hope for successful therapy. However, new reliable devices to monitor the electrical activity of the heart have shown increasingly that many deaths are caused not by an overwhelming loss of heart muscle cells but rather by disturbances of the electrical signals that direct the heart to beat. Many other-wise healthy hearts cease to pump effectively when damage to a very limited area of heart muscle results in a loss of coordinated electrical activity. The disturbance may take the form of heart block or cardiac standstill, in which the heartbeat slows or stops altogether. The resulting loss of effective circulation can cause irreversible brain damage if not counteracted immediately. Cardiac pacemakers have now been developed that can stimulate the heart to beat by sending a tiny pulse of electricity to the inner wall of the heart via a catheter electrode inserted through a peripheral vein. Such devices are often used temporarily until the heart recovers adequate electrical function. Battery-operated units can also be implanted permanently in patients who experience chronic heart block or recurrent episodes of marked slowing of the heart rate.

Cardiac arrest—the cessation of effective blood circulation—is usu-ally caused not by a total stoppage of electrical activity but by a condi-tion called ventricular fibrillation, in which electrical activity continues but becomes so disorganized and chaotic that no coordinated pumping action results. In this case, an electrical shock produced by a defibrillator, a relatively simple device placed on the patient's chest, often restores an effective heartbeat. Various drugs can then be given to prevent the recur-rence of ventricular fibrillation. Thousands of patients who have suffered cardiac arrest now enjoy active lives thanks to the development of these techniques.

These advances have been widely applied in coronary care units of hospitals throughout the country. Highly trained nurses often institute these measures, so that treatment can begin immediately even when a physician is not in attendance; closed-chest cardiac massage is also used to support circulation temporarily until other techniques can be applied. Hospitals with effective coronary care units have generally achieved a 50 percent reduction in mortality rates for acute myocardial infarction among the patients they treat. Confinement to bed following the acute episode is also less prolonged than was the case a generation ago; the total hospi-tal stay for a patient with an uncomplicated heart attack is now likely to be two to three weeks rather than four to six. As many as 80 to 85 percent of heart attack victims are able to return to work, and carefully super-vised exercise programs have been shown to improve cardiovascular function after myocardial infarction in 75 percent of properly selected patients.

Unfortunately, the effectiveness of hospital care is drastically limited by the fact that close to 70 percent of deaths due to coronary artery disease occur within seconds to minutes after the onset of symptoms; the patient may die before he can be rushed to the hospital. Several approaches to this problem can and must be taken if the death rate from coronary artery disease is to be reduced much further. The public must be educated to seek medical attention at the earliest appearance of symptoms suggesting heart attack. Mobile units with life-support equipment and skilled personnel must be available to respond swiftly to calls for assistance. And more effective drugs are needed to prevent severe cardiac rhythm disturbances in patients known to be predisposed to this problem.

Even if disturbances of heart rhythm could be prevented or effectively dealt with in all patients with coronary heart disease, an enormous toll of death and disability would remain as a result of mechanical "power failure" from loss of functioning muscle cells. Since the prognosis of a patient after myocardial infarction depends in large part on the amount of functioning heart muscle left, everything possible must be done to preserve those areas of marginally nourished muscle that are delicately balanced between survival and death. Figure 12-1 shows a heart with an obstructed coronary artery to a portion of the main pumping chamber (left ventricle) at greatest risk of damage from coronary artery disease. When a coronary artery becomes totally obstructed, some cells receive so little nutrient blood flow that they have no chance of survival. Other cells, however, receive enough flow through other pathways to be maintained, at least temporarily, in a borderline state; the ultimate fate of these cells is determined by the delicate balance between nutrient supply and cellular demand. Eugene Braunwald, Peter Maroko, and their colleagues have shown in experimental animal models that increasing the supply of oxygen and nutrients or reducing the energy demands of the heart will allow viable heart muscle to survive in these marginal areas. Preserving the function of such areas would be expected to improve both immediate survival and long-term prognosis of patients suffering myocardial infarction, and clinical trials are underway to test the validity of this concept. The drug propranolol, available only in recent years, blocks the stimulatory effects of hormones like adrenaline and thus decreases the heart's energy demands. For this reason, propranolol (now widely used for treatment of angina) may also find a place in the treatment of selected heart attack victims; but further studies are needed to define the proper role of this drug in the treatment of heart attack.

Progress in cardiovascular surgery, as outlined in Chapter 24, has been nothing short of spectacular during the past two decades. The earliest successes were in the treatment of congenital defects that could be cor-

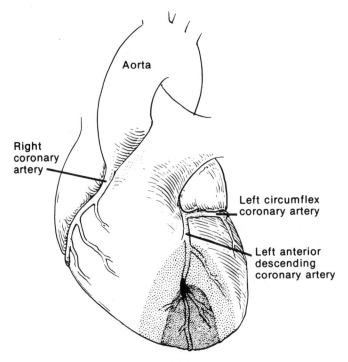

Figure 12–1. A heart with an obstruction in the left anterior descending coronary artery. The shaded area is heart muscle that has been endangered by
inadequate blood flow; dark shading indicates areas of the muscle that have
already died from lack of blood supply.

rected without interfering with the normal pumping function of the heart.
Soon, vigorous efforts were directed to the development of the heart-lung
machine, a device capable of taking over the function of the heart and
lungs while surgical correction of abnormalities inside the open heart
was carried out. With the technology that made open heart surgery possible, the surgeon became able to replace heart valves damaged in
rheumatic fever with artificial valves and to correct complex congenital
heart defects.

New cardiac surgeons have begun to attack directly the problem of
obstructive disease of the coronary arteries. Figure 12-2 shows a heart
with normal blood flow from the aorta through the coronary arteries to
the heart muscle; and Figure 12-3 shows a heart in which two of the three
major coronary arteries have been obstructed by atherosclerosis. One of
these obstructed areas has been bypassed surgically by implanting an

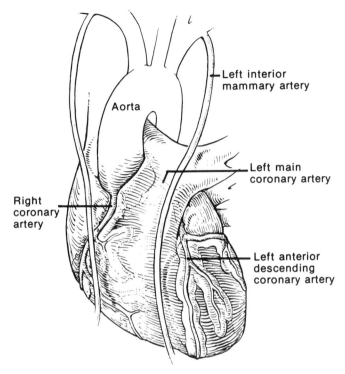

Figure 12–2. A normal heart with unobstructed coronary arteries.

artery (the left internal mammary artery) that normally runs along the inside of the breast bone; this vessel can easily be spared by the areas it normally serves, and its flow of blood put to the much more useful purpose of nourishing the heart muscle. The second obstruction, in the right coronary artery, has been bypassed by implantation of a segment of another nonessential blood vessel, a leg vein (the saphenous vein). This type of coronary artery surgery provides relief of the symptoms of angina in 80 to 90 percent of patients. The ultimate effect of such procedures on the patient's survival is less clear, but there is growing evidence that life is prolonged, at least in patients with marked obstruction of two or three of the main coronary arteries.

Research into heart transplantation, which has been well publicized, also continues to progress. As with kidney transplants, the surgical skills required to accomplish the heart transplant are well in hand; the principal problem remaining is to block the rejection of the transplanted organ. In order to overcome the patient's normal immune response, which recog-

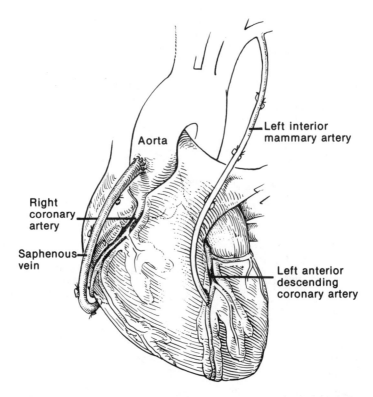

Figure 12–3. A heart with obstructions in two coronary arteries that have been by-passed surgically. The left internal mammary artery now supplies blood to the area normally supplied by the left anterior descending artery, which is obstructed. The saphenous vein has been taken from the leg and grafted between the aorta and a section of the right coronary artery, by-passing the obstruction in that artery.

nizes the transplanted organ as foreign and attacks it, drugs are given to suppress all immune responses. Unfortunately, these drugs also greatly weaken the body's defenses against infection. Clearly, what is needed is a way to produce specific tolerance to the transplanted organ without removing the immune defenses against the bacteria and viruses that the patient must be able to resist. Such specific immune tolerance has not yet been achieved; a basic scientific breakthrough will be required before this occurs.

A new, dramatic technique for aiding the circulation as the heart is recovering from surgery—or to support the function of hearts damaged by coronary artery disease—makes use of an innovative inflatable balloon device. Figure 12-4 shows how a long, flexible balloon can be introduced into the aorta (the main blood vessel leading from the heart) via an artery in the groin. Helium gas is pumped under pressure to expand the balloon rapidly just as the heart relaxes to take in blood carrying oxygen from the lungs. The expanding balloon gives the heart a boost by augmenting the flow of blood through the arteries that branch out to the body from the aorta; and the balloon is collapsed just as the heart con-

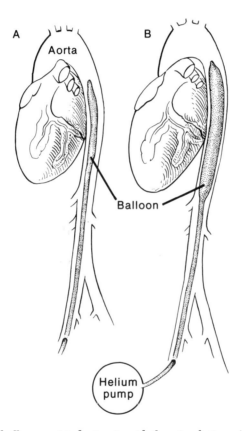

Figure 12–4. A balloon assist device to aid the circulation. As the heart contracts to pump blood, the balloon is rapidly deflated to reduce the work of the heart (A). As the heart relaxes to fill prior to the next pumping cycle, the balloon expands, augmenting the flow of blood through the arteries that branch out to the body from the aorta (B). The balloon is inserted through an artery in the groin. A helium pump external to the patient, shown schematically, supplies energy to inflate and deflate the balloon and thus to support a weakened heart.

tracts, to reduce the pressure against which the heart must pump and thus reduce the energy demands placed on the heart. This device can be used to support a patient through myocardial infarction while studies are performed to determine whether other measures might improve his chances for survival.

Basic biochemical research also promises to increase our understanding of heart disease and to lead to new methods of treatment. The normal cardiac muscle contraction that occurs in the pumping action of the normal heart is now becoming increasingly understood on the biochemical level. Unfortunately, we remain largely ignorant of the defects that may weaken the heart in the condition known as heart failure. Very sophisticated research at the cellular and molecular level, and involving basic scientists in several disciplines, is needed to elucidate the basic biological processes in heart failure. This condition, which is common to the late stages of virtually all forms of heart disease, results in the familiar symptoms of fatigue, shortness of breath, and the accumulation of salt and water. One approach to improved treatment of heart failure is through research in the use of digitalis, a drug that has been used to strengthen the failing heart for 200 years but that is still poorly understood.

My research with Edgar Haber and Vincent Butler has employed antibodies specific for digitalis to measure concentrations of the drug in the blood of patients treated with it. This antibody technique is exquisitely sensitive; typical doses of digitalis produce blood concentrations of only about one billionth of a gram per milliliter. Since the blood concentration of digitalis correlates well with its effects on the heart, measurement of blood levels of the drug has made it possible to use digitalis more effectively and to lower the incidence of toxic reactions, which are distressingly common because there is a narrow margin between the therapeutic and toxic doses of this drug. Antibodies to digitalis can be valuable beyond their use for monitoring drug levels; very recently, we successfully used these antibodies as a specific antidote in a near fatal episode of digitalis poisoning in a patient who took a massive overdose with suicidal intent. Perhaps antibodies specific for other potentially toxic drugs can be similarly used.

New Diagnostic Techniques

In the past three decades, methods for diagnosing heart disease have become increasingly accurate and safe. Of particular interest has been the recent trend away from invasive diagnostic methods (which require the introduction of instruments into the patient's body) to noninvasive procedures, which can be performed with less risk and discomfort to the patient.

Beginning in the 1940s, and throughout the 1950s and 1960s, rapid advances were made in the diagnosis and characterization of heart and vascular diseases through cardiac catheterization and new X-ray techniques. Smooth, flexible tubes (catheters) were developed that could be passed into the arteries or veins from an entry point in the arm or groin and thence into the great vessels leading to and from the heart and into the heart itself. Blood pressure and flow in these areas could now be directly measured, and the physician could make a precise diagnosis of circulatory abnormalities caused by malfunction of heart valves or congenital heart defects. Equally important were new techniques whereby fluids opaque to X rays could be injected and a series of X-ray pictures taken to delineate structures not well seen on conventional X rays. (This technique is known as angiography.) Rapid sequential films can even be taken to show the movement of such a special opaque dye with the blood through cardiovascular structures.

Without question, the major impetus for the development and refinement of these methods was the growing ability of the cardiovascular surgeon to correct congenital and acquired lesions of the heart and vessels (see Chapter 24). Hundreds of diagnostic laboratories across the country now perform coronary angiography daily, with specially designed catheters that are used to introduce opaque dyes directly into the coronary arteries. This procedure is usually done for the purpose of determining whether a patient with disabling angina pectoris might be helped by surgical bypass of obstructed coronary vessels.

These valuable diagnostic methods entail serious problems, however. One is the enormous cost of facilities and highly trained personnel to perform and interpret these sophisticated procedures; the cardiac catheterization process just described, together with the brief hospitalization it requires, may cost 1,500 dollars or more. Even greater drawbacks are the discomfort and small but real risk involved in procedures that require invasion of the cardiovascular system with catheters and dye injections. Recognition of these problems has led to intense interest in noninvasive methods for cardiovascular diagnosis. Familiar examples of noninvasive techniques in use for decades include the standard chest X ray and the electrocardiogram, procedures that entail no discomfort or measurable risk to the patient. The 1970s have been noteworthy for a number of exciting advances in the noninvasive approach to cardiovascular diagnosis, and certain examples are worth considering in some detail.

The most widely used of the new noninvasive techniques is echocardiography, a procedure made possible by wartime advances in technology. Demands for improved detection devices in submarine warfare during the Second World War led to advances in sound wave technology and the widespread application of sonar. The principle of localizing an object and defining its motion by bouncing sound waves off it is also the basis of echocardiography. As shown in Figure 12-5, a transducer held against the chest wall sends a beam of high frequency sound waves through the chest and receives the echoes returning from cardiac structures. A map of the returning echoes is recorded and delineates the location and motion (or lack of motion) of the muscular walls of the heart and of the heart valves. This conceptually simple approach takes

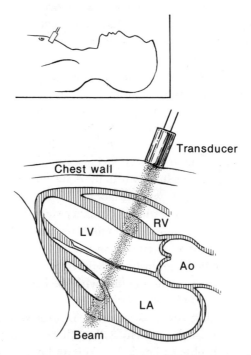

Figure 12–5. Echocardiography. A transducer held against the patient's chest sends high-frequency sound waves through the chest wall to the heart. These sound waves echo off the structures of the heart and bounce back to the transducer, where they are recorded and analyzed. LV-left ventricle; RV-right ventricle; LA-left atrium; Ao-aorta.

only about 15 to 30 minutes of the patient's time, involves no discomfort or risk, and is proving to be of great value in the assessment of rheumatic, congenital, and ischemic heart disease.

The echocardiographic method now in conventional use sends an essentially one-dimensional, pencil-like beam of sound waves through the chest wall and hence records the location and movement of structures only in a single dimension. Of still greater use would be a two-dimensional map approximating the anatomic appearance of cardiac structures. Two-dimensional echo scanners are under development in several laboratories. Current designs employ arrays of many transducers or a single transducer that moves rapidly through an arc to produce a large number of nearly simultaneous one-dimensional plots. When displayed together, these plots form a two-dimensional image of an acoustic "slice" through the patient's chest. These planar images can be recorded sequentially on videotape or movie film during the cardiac cycle to give a two-dimensional moving picture of the appearance and motion of cardiac structures. An even more advanced application of space-age technology—still well in the future—would be the use of ultrasound waves to produce three-dimensional images analogous to the holograms produced by lasers. Such highly sophisticated developments, if they prove feasible, will require extensive use of computer technology.

Another area of dramatic progress in the 1970s has been the use of radioactive tracers (isotopes) in cardiovascular diagnosis. Radioactive substances that are distributed in the bloodstream (and hence in the chambers of the heart) or that are taken up selectively by normal or abnormal heart muscle can be visualized by the use of scanning devices that pinpoint the location of radioactivity in the body. Following the distribution of these isotopes in the body provides useful diagnostic information with negligible risk or discomfort to the patient.

A current application of this approach involves the intravenous injection of a tracer that stays within the bloodstream. Early sequential images of the distribution of this material can reveal abnormalities of the direction of blood flow through the heart, as commonly occur in congenital cardiac defects. Crucial diagnostic information can thus be obtained with minimal risk or delay in critically ill "blue babies" (infants born with heart defects that result in inadequate oxygen content of the blood). A further refinement of this technique allows the "camera" or scanning device to collect information during specific phases of the cardiac cycle. When data are collected during a number of cardiac cycles, pictures emerge that allow the physician to compare the size and shape of cardiac chambers in contracted and relaxed states. Abnormalities in the pumping function of the heart can sometimes be evaluated adequately in this way, and the patient can be spared the discomfort, expense, and small but real risk of a conventional catheterization and angiographic procedure.

Some of the most promising new approaches employ selective localization of tracers in the heart muscle (myocardium). One such method can detect heart muscle damage due to loss of adequate blood supply; certain radioactive compounds are taken up selectively by damaged myocardium and appear in an image of the heart as a "hot spot." This technique can be of considerable value when information from conventional diagnostic methods is inconclusive, and it is likely that it will become still more accurate in the future.

One of the central diagnostic problems in the evaluation of patients suspected of having coronary heart disease is the assessment of blood flow in different regions of the heart muscle. Methods that measure total coronary flow are not very helpful, since total flow may remain near normal even when the distribution of blood flow is severely disturbed; and inadequate blood flow in even a small area can seriously damage heart muscle in that area. The conventional approach to this problem has been coronary angiography, with its associated drawbacks. Recently several laboratories, including my own, have been working to develop noninvasive ways to measure blood flow to different heart muscle areas. Radioactive potassium, or another ion containing a single positive charge and behaving like potassium, is injected intravenously and selectively taken up by normal heart muscle. Areas of reduced blood flow do not take up the radioactive substance and show up as "cold spots" in the images obtained. Patients with chest pains can undergo such diagnostic studies before and after exercise. If an area of relatively reduced myocardial blood flow appears after exertion, the patient is likely to have coronary artery disease, and further studies can be undertaken to clarify his condition. These procedures are quite safe; they subject the patient to trivial doses of radiation that often amount to less than the exposure from a conventional chest X ray.

The selective uptake of a radioactive substance has also been used to detect blood clots, particularly in the leg veins of patients at risk of developing phlebitis due to trauma, surgery, or prolonged inactivity. Detection of these clots is of particular importance, since aggressive treatment may be required to prevent potentially disabling or fatal consequences if the clot should break loose and travel in the bloodstream until it obstructs vessels to the lungs. The diagnostic approach used is to label fibrinogen, a protein in blood plasma that participates in clot formation, with a radioactive isotope of iodine. The labeled fibrinogen is injected intravenously; if it is incorporated into a forming or enlarging clot, its location and that of the clot can be determined.

Old diagnostic methods are also being updated by modern physicians. Although conceptually not new, exercise tolerance testing with monitoring of the electrocardiogram has undergone a resurgence of interest in the past few years. This increased application of an old technique undoubtedly stems from the growing importance of identifying patients with coronary artery disease, now that more effective therapeutic measures (including coronary artery surgery) are available. The procedure now used most frequently consists of increasingly vigorous exercise on a treadmill or stationary bicycle, with continuous recording of the patient's electrocardiogram as he reaches a maximum level of exertion. Typical changes seen in the electrocardiogram in association with chest discomfort can do much to confirm an otherwise equivocal diagnosis of coronary artery disease. Although exercise stress tests are by no means totally accurate, the information they yield is very useful when considered together with other available evidence.

Modern technology has been applied in imaginative ways to the diagnosis and treatment of cardiovascular disease. But in spite of these advances, the prevention of heart and blood vessel disease remains preferable to its treatment, for economic as well as human reasons. Methods of treatment may be extremely expensive, partly because they now involve such sophisticated techniques. For example, an uncomplicated coronary artery bypass operation now costs between $7,000 and $10,000 dollars, most of which goes to cover hospital expenses; and an estimated 150,000 Americans may be suitable candidates for these operations every year. One of the most pressing needs in cardiovascular research is the development of effective programs of prevention to minimize the toll of heart and blood vessel diseases. Effective prevention can only come through sophisticated understanding of the disease process; and that understanding, in turn, can only come from basic research. Through such research efforts, we are now beginning to approach an understanding of the fundamental processes that underlie cardiovascular disease on many levels.

The Respiratory System

EDWARD A. GAENSLER   13

The respiratory system differs in three important ways from other organ systems of the body. First, the lungs, like the skin, are constantly exposed to the atmosphere, to which they present a surface area about the size of a tennis court. This surface is exposed to approximately 70 million gallons of air during a lifetime. Second, mortality and disability from chronic lung disease, excepting tuberculosis, has increased constantly during the last 50 years, in contrast to chronic diseases of other organs which have remained the same or decreased over the same period. This increase has not been coincidental; it has been linked directly to the inhalation of noxious substances. Third, because most of these substances have been identified, the major causes of the most destructive lung diseases are known and preventable.

If all noxious substances were removed from the air that we breathe, most lung disorders would gradually disappear. Of course, there are many political and logistic obstacles to eliminating these air pollutants, whether they are of industrial origin or introduced into the lungs as a matter of personal choice (like cigarette smoke). But any approach to chronic lung disease must focus on prevention, which entails elimination of toxic agents, rather than on detection and cure. Prevention is vastly cheaper, less painful than diagnosis and treatment, and much more effective.

Chronic bronchitis and emphysema, the most widespread respiratory disorders, are still very difficult to treat after they develop, but both can be largely prevented by elimination of the major causative agent: tobacco smoke.

Chronic Obstructive Lung Disease (COLD)

Pulmonary emphysema was first described by R. T. H. Laennec in 1819. His description remains largely unchanged by modern definition. Emphysema is characterized by an abnormal enlargement of the peripheral air spaces of the lung, accompanied by destructive changes of their walls. This is an anatomic definition and is based on changes that can only be ascertained by direct investigation of the structures involved.

Chronic bronchitis, unlike emphysema, is now defined in clinical terms. It is characterized by excessive secretion of the mucus that lines the bronchi, the branched hollow tubes that conduct air through the lungs. The disorder is defined by a chronic or recurrent cough with sputum that lasts for three months a year for at least two successive years and which cannot be attributed to another cause.

Present information concerning prevalence, incidence, and mortality of both disorders is still unreliable. Since emphysema is defined in anatomic terms, it can only be evaluated by post-mortem examination. Standard autopsy procedure examines small blocks of tissue microscopically, a technique that is unsatisfactory for assessing the type and extent of emphysema. Special methods have been developed recently for examining the entire lung before it has been inflated and sliced into thin sections. These techniques require special interest, training, and instrumentation and hence are expensive and not generally available. Clinical and epidemiologic methods for assessing the prevalence of emphysema are unreliable because symptoms do not occur until the disease is relatively advanced. Moderate degrees of emphysema cannot be recognized by physical examination or chest X-ray, and even specialized lung function studies may not reveal the disease in the early stages.

The prevalence of chronic bronchitis is also difficult to establish. Most smokers accept moderate cough and sputum in the morning as normal. For this reason, the disease prevalence is difficult to determine through standard questionnaires.

Finally, the close relationship between these two diseases make differential diagnosis difficult. Since the major cause for both emphysema and chronic bronchitis is cigarette smoking, these disorders usually occur together, and the relative importance of each is difficult to assess by any means. Consequently, the term chronic obstructive lung disease (COLD) is used to make the distinction between the disorders unnecessary. COLD is defined simply as a disorder characterized by chronic, diffuse, irreversible airways obstruction.

In terms of both incidence and cost, COLD represents the most important public health respiratory problem in the United States; and most recent data suggest that it is increasing at an alarming rate as a major cause of death. The only increases in death rates from respiratory disease in the United States have been due to chronic bronchitis, emphysema, and malignancies; and even the large number of deaths from pneumonia often are related to underlying COLD. The increase in death rate for chronic bronchitis between 1958 and 1967 was 80 percent, and for emphysema was 172 percent. Estimates of the economic impact of COLD are subject to very large errors, but it is clear that this group of diseases represents a serious financial burden for the nation. For 1967, the estimated cost of morbidity and mortality due to COLD was 1.8 billion dollars. Of this amount the morbidity costs were 1.2 billion dollars, including an estimated 655 million dollars in lost earnings. The estimated cost for all chronic respiratory disease, excluding cancer, was 6.3 billion dollars for 1967.

Most deaths from respiratory disease occur as the result of COLD, which, in turn, is closely linked to cigarette smoking. The Surgeon General's comprehensive 1971 review of a large number of epidemiologic studies showed that the risk of dying from COLD is from 2.9 to 14.7 times greater for smokers than for nonsmokers.

Smoking has been very definitely linked to emphysema in older people who have smoked for a long time. The results of one of the most careful recent studies are summarized in Figure 13-1. Oscar Auerbach and his colleagues did post-mortem examinations of lungs from more than 1,500 persons, determined the degree of emphysema, and correlated the diagnoses with smoking histories. Significant emphysema was virtually unknown in nonsmokers but was found in 94.5 percent of all those who smoked more than 1 pack per day. Only a minute fraction of the heavy smokers—0.3 percent—was totally free of emphysema.

Smoking also increases the probability of respiratory infection through its effects on the lung at the cellular level. Animal experiments have shown that cigarette smoke inhibits the function of scavenger cells, which ingest and inactivate bateria. Tobacco smoke also interferes with the biological processes that normally keep the lungs clean and free of infectious organisms. Since particles in the air often carry bacteria, it is important that they be removed. The bronchi are protected by a coating of mucus; the cells that lie under this mucus have special hairlike projections, called cilia, that beat together rhythmically to propel the mucus in the direction of the throat and away from the lungs. Any particulate matter that has been inhaled, such as dust, sticks to the mucus until it

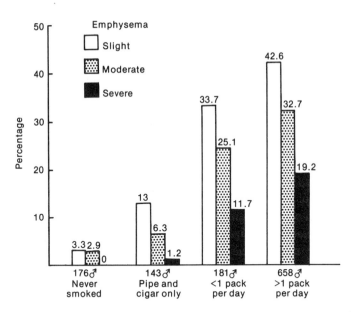

Figure 13–1. The correlation between cigarette smoking and emphysema. This graph shows the age-standardized percentage distribution of 1,158 males in each of four smoking categories according to degree of emphysema estimated semi-quantitatively from whole-lung (Gough) sections at autopsy. Findings in 388 women were similar. From O. Auerbach, E. C. Hammon, and L. Garfinkel, "Relation of Smoking and Age to Emphysema: Whole-Lung Section Study," *New England Journal of Medicine* 286 (1972): 853–857.

finally reaches the throat and is swallowed. In smokers, however, this cleansing system fails to operate effectively. Apparently tobacco smoke inhibits the activity of the cilia and hence slows the upward flow of the mucus blanket.

Young smokers were once thought to be unaffected by the adverse biological effects of cigarette smoke, but it now appears that this view was overly optimistic. Careful autopsy studies of accident victims killed in the third decade of life reveal that smokers, and only smokers, show inflammation of the bronchial walls. Tiny lesions in the smallest airways—the bronchioles—have been found in all of these youthful smokers. The bronchioles are narrowed by fluid, by inflammation, and by clusters of scavenger cells containing brown pigment from tobacco smoke. Autopsy studies have shown that in smokers inflammatory changes may reduce the cross-sectional area of the bronchioles by one half, and that the small airways may contain three times as much mucus as in normal controls.

The effects of "smoker's lung" may not become evident until the condition has progressed considerably, largely because the smallest airways are the first to be affected. Damage to these airways is hard to recognize because bronchioles, although small in diameter, are great in number. For this reason, the system of bronchioles offers less resistance to breathing than do the larger airways; together, the small airways account for only about 10 to 20 percent of the total airways resistance. An increase in the resistance of the bronchioles, such as occurs in smoker's lung, has little effect on the total resistance and may be difficult to detect clinically.

A number of new methods have been devised to measure small airways resistance. When a person breathes in maximally and then exhales as quickly as possible, the rate of air flow is determined by the condition of the airways. Studies of flow rates in college students have shown that smokers have significantly lower flow rates than nonsmokers, indicating that the airways are in poor condition. During full exhalation, some of the affected small airways close off completely; the volume in the lungs when this occurs, called the closing volume, can be measured by the inhalation of foreign gases. A number of groups have now reported unusually high closing volumes in young smokers, again suggesting obstruction of the bronchioles. Increasing stiffening of the lung during rapid breathing indicates that some parts of the lung are obstructed and inadequately ventilated. This, too, is more common in young smokers than in nonsmokers of the same age. Finally, because disease of small airways always affects some parts of the lung more than others, blood passing through one area receives less oxygen than blood passing through other areas. Discrepancies between blood flow and oxygen uptake can be measured by radioactive gases; such discrepancies are greater in smokers, almost all of whom show impaired oxygen uptake by the blood.

Tobacco smoking clearly causes measurable, progressive lung damage that may result in disease or even death. But while all smokers risk their health in a similar way, they do not all suffer the same consequences. A number of other factors besides cigarette smoking must affect the development of lung disease. Some variables that appear to be important are air pollution, occupational exposure, allergy, altered immunity, infection, genetic predisposition, sex, race, aging, and climate, as well as social and economic factors. All these are difficult to evaluate because of the overwhelming importance of tobacco smoking, but progress is being made.

Air pollution has been definitely identified as an aggravating factor. During every one of the famous air pollution disasters in London, the

Meuse Valley in Belgium, the small town of Donora, Pennsylvania, and in Osaka, Japan, it has been clearly documented that increased mortality occurs largely among elderly individuals with COLD. In Great Britain, a rise in death rate has been shown whenever both sulfur dioxide and particulate matter in the air are greatly increased. Clearly, air pollution aggravates illness from COLD; but its role in causation is less certain. Some studies, which have shown no difference in the prevalence of COLD between nonsmoking city and country dwellers, suggest that urban air pollution alone is not a prominent cause of COLD.

Occupational exposure also seems to play an aggravating rather than a causative role. The prevalence of chronic bronchitis and emphysema is no greater in nonsmoking coal workers than in other nonsmokers. Coal workers who do smoke, however, are even more likely to suffer COLD than are nonminers who smoke.

The most exciting recent discovery has been that genetic factors in some people are related to the development of emphysema. Carl-Bertil Laurell and Sten Eriksson, in 1963, while studying blood donors, discovered that a small number of people lacked a protein in the blood containing alpha$_1$-antitrypsin. This deficiency is inherited through a recessive gene and was soon found to be strongly associated with a type of emphysema that occurs at an early age even in nonsmokers.

Several theories have been proposed to explain the connection between this inherited disorder and emphysema. The most plausible hypothesis explains the link on the basis of the fact that alpha$_1$-antitrypsin inhibits the activity of trypsin, a powerful protease (substance that breaks down protein). One theory holds that certain cells in normal lungs regularly produce proteases which, under normal conditions, are inhibited by antitrypsin. Where the individual's blood lacks this inhibitor, or if concentrations of the inhibitor are too low, then the proteases could damage lung structure and ultimately cause emphysema.

Although hereditary alpha$_1$-antitrypsin deficiency seems to be a definite cause of emphysema, it accounts only for a small fraction of all cases. No more than one half of 1 percent of the population is totally deficient in alpha$_1$-antitrypsin, but chronic obstructive lung disease is very common. Nevertheless, the study of inherited alpha$_1$-antitrypsin deficiency has provided valuable insight into the processes that may cause emphysema when it is not hereditary. One suggestion has been that emphysema may result when proteases from outside the body are introduced into the body in amounts that cannot be inhibited by normal amounts of alpha$_1$-antitrypsin. Bacteria or tobacco, for example, may contain such proteases. This theory has been strongly supported by the discovery of Paul Gross in 1965 that various known proteases introduced into the trachea of animals can produce emphysema. While his model cannot be considered precisely equivalent to human emphysema, it and other experimental models have increased our understanding of the physiology and biochemistry of emphysema. Meanwhile the search for other predisposing genetic factors continues.

Although a great deal is known about the causes of COLD, no cure has been found. Emphysema, by definition, is not reversible; destruction of the lungs is permanent. Chronic bronchitis may be partially reversible; most patients experience a marked decrease in cough and sputum after they stop smoking. There is some suggestion that the early changes in the small airways of young smokers may be reversible but there is less evidence as to whether or not the late functional abnormalities resulting from chronic bronchitis are equally correctable.

Our ignorance in this respect is explained, in part, by the frustrating fact that few long-term smokers can be persuaded to give up smoking. Also, definitive evidence could only come from large-scale, long-term studies comparing continuing smokers with similar people who have stopped smoking. And few investigators have been able to attract long-term funding because most agencies are geared to short-term grants for quick results.

The benefits of smoking cessation may best be demonstrated by mortality rates among British physicians. During the past 25 years, one half of these doctors have stopped smoking. Between 1961 and 1965, there were 24 percent fewer deaths from COLD among British doctors than there had been between 1953 and 1957, while in the rest of the British population—whose smoking habits did not change appreciably over the same period—deaths from COLD decreased by only 4 percent.

There is no question but that the most effective way of preventing COLD is to avoid smoking or to stop before serious disease develops. While genetic and environmental factors may make some individuals especially susceptible to respiratory disease, cigarette smoke is by far the most important direct cause of COLD.

Lung Cancer

The study of British physicians also demonstrates the causative role cigarette smoke plays in another serious lung disease: lung cancer. While death rates from bronchogenic carcinoma (cancer arising in the bronchi) decreased among British physicians by 38 percent between 1953–57 and 1961–65, mortality from lung cancer increased by 7 percent among the British population in general. In America, too, this deadly disease is increasing at an alarming rate.

Changes in incidence and mortality rates for lung cancer—although not for emphysema and bronchitis—can be studied through reliable statistics collected over an extended period of time. The frightening data compiled in the United States, presented in Figure 13-2, show the growth of this health problem. In 1930 lung cancer was a relatively rare tumor with an age-adjusted death rate of only 2 to 3 per 100,000 and rates for both sexes were about the same. During the next 40 years, while rates for most cancers remained about the same or declined, mortality from lung cancer in males rose to 50 per 100,000, an increase of approximately 1,700 percent. It is now estimated that 73,000 American men and 20,000 women will develop lung cancer each year. The problem is not limited to the United States; similar observations have been made in all industrialized nations, with even higher rates found in Great Britain, Finland, Czechoslovakia, and the Netherlands. Lower rates are reported for many less developed countries, but detection and reporting are less reliable in those areas.

It is interesting to study Figure 13-2 in the light of changes in cigarette smoking habits. Smoking became widespread among American males around 1900, and 30 years later the death rate from lung cancer began to increase sharply. By contrast, cigarette smoking among women was uncommon until 1930, when George Washington Hill, the late president of the American Tobacco Company, began his famous advertising campaign to make smoking fashionable for ladies. The lung cancer incidence for women remained level until 1960, again about 30 years later, and then began to increase markedly. Today, lung cancer incidence rates for males and females are increasing at approximately the same speed.

The link between smoking and cancer was first documented in "Tobacco Smoking as a Possible Etiologic Factor in Bronchogenic Carcinoma," a study of 684 proven cases published by Ernest Wynder and Evarts Graham in 1950. Tragically, Graham, the first surgeon to remove a lung because of cancer, succumbed to the disease himself some 25 years later. Quick confirmation of the study came from Richard Doll and A. Bradford Hill in Great Britain, and these reports—plus an enormous amount of subsequent statistical and experimental work—led to the first

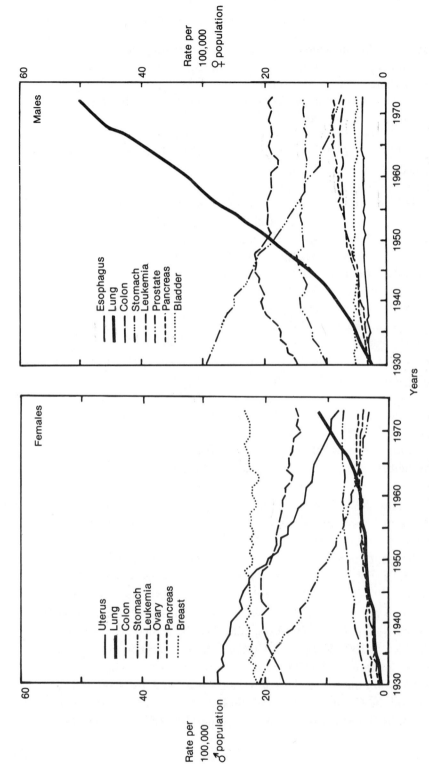

Figure 13–2. Age-adjusted cancer death rates for selected sites, United States, 1930–1973. Death rates for females are shown on the left, for males on the right. Data come from the U.S. National Center for Health Statistics and the U.S. Bureau of the Census and have been standardized on the basis of the age distribution of the 1940 U.S. Census Population. From "Cancer Statistics, 1976," *CA: A Cancer Journal for Clinicians* 26 (1976), 2–29. Redrawn by permission of the American Cancer Society.

report of the Surgeon General on smoking and health in 1964. The conclusions were as follows:

> Cigarette smoking is causally related to lung cancer in men; the magnitude of the effect of cigarette smoking far outweighs all other factors. The data for women, though less extensive, point in the same direction.
>
> The risk of developing lung cancer increases with duration of smoking and the number of cigarettes smoked per day, and is diminished by discontinuing smoking. In comparison with nonsmokers, average male smokers of cigarettes have approximately a 9- to 10-fold risk of developing lung cancer and heavy smokers at least a 20-fold risk.
>
> Cigarette smoking is much more important than occupational exposures in the causation of lung cancer in the general population.

Innumerable epidemiologic studies since 1964 have reinforced these conclusions, and similar findings have been reported from around the world. Recent results of a prospective study of more than 200,000 Japanese males are shown in Figure 13-3. It appears that the irritation of cigarette smoke first manifests itself by irritation and inflammation of the bronchial walls, which ultimately may lead to cancer. This concept of the effects of cigarette smoke was first proposed by Oscar Auerbach and others on the basis of a study of the cells lining the trachea and bronchi of more than 750 persons. The relationship of the amount smoked to disease was confirmed in dogs trained to smoke. Almost all dogs that smoked the equivalent of two packs, 13 percent of those that smoked 1 pack, and 6 percent of those that smoked filter tips showed evidence of emphysema, while none of the nonsmoking dogs developed this disease. The cells lining the bronchi showed a wide spectrum of pathological changes, and several dogs developed invasive cancers.

Smoking is not the only determinant of lung cancer, although it is the most important factor. As with COLD, occupational and environmental variables may also come into play. A number of occupations are clearly associated with an increased incidence of lung cancer. This was first demonstrated in pitchblende miners in Joachimsthal, Czechoslovakia, at the beginning of this century. The greatly increased incidence of lung cancer was first attributed to arsenic; only later was it traced to the radioactive uranium dust in pitchblende. With the greatly increased demand for uranium during the last 30 years, rates of lung cancer have also risen among "yellow-cake" or carnotite miners in Utah and Colorado. It is now well established that radioactive dust stored in the lungs is carcinogenic. Other agents that may cause lung cancer include nickel and nickel carbonyl, chromium, coal tar, pitch and soot, bis (chloromethyl) ether, and arsenic. The last has been a special problem for vineyard workers

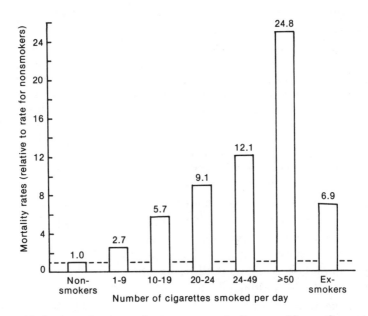

Figure 13–3. A study currently in progress in Japan adds to the weight of evidence supporting a causal relationship between cigarette smoking and lung cancer. It is the first large-scale prospective study to be conducted in a population characterized by genetic, dietary, behavioral, and cultural influences distinctively different from those in previously examined Western populations. The three-year preliminary data for lung cancer from this population of 265,118 adults in Japan demonstrate overall effects and dose-response relationships similar to those observed in previous studies. From T. Hirayama, "A Prospective Study on the Influence of Cigarette Smoking and Alcohol Drinking on the Death Rates for Total and Selected Causes of Death in Japan," *Smoke Signals*, July 1970, pp. 1–8. Copyright © 1970 by Narcotics Education, Inc. Redrawn by permission.

and sheep dippers (who may dip sheep in arsenic-containing liquids to destroy their parasites).

Currently of most serious concern is the increased incidence of lung cancer among asbestos workers. Approximately 15 percent of all cigarette-smoking insulation workers die of lung cancer—roughly 5 to 10 times the rate among smokers who are not exposed to asbestos. Interestingly, the incidence of lung cancer in nonsmoking asbestos workers is very low, no larger than that of other nonsmokers. It is thought that the effect of cigarette smoke is potentiated by the mechanical irritation of the asbestos fibers on the lining of the bronchi.

Entirely unrelated to smoking, there is a further carcinogenic risk related to asbestos exposure which is a subject of present concern. J. C. Wagner in South Africa first demonstrated the development of a normally rare but highly malignant tumor, mesothelioma, in individuals who had been exposed to asbestos some 20 to 40 years earlier; 80 percent of all people with this tumor had been exposed to asbestos at some time in their past. Perhaps the worst aspect of this new finding was the discovery that mesothelioma may develop in individuals whose exposure to asbestos was very slight: people who have lived near asbestos factories which they have never even entered, and wives of asbestos workers whose only contact with the substance was through their husbands' clothes, also run an increased risk of developing this tumor. The facts that mesothelioma can be stimulated by a very slight amount of asbestos and that the use of asbestos has increased greatly since the Second World War suggest that this previously rare tumor—which is almost invariably fatal—may reach epidemic proportions in the near future.

It may be difficult to identify the many different causes of lung cancer so as to prevent the disease completely; but at the state of present knowledge, prevention, not treatment, is the only rational approach. Progress in therapy, to the extent that any has occurred, has been slight. It was thought that early detection might improve the chances of survival but, unfortunately, large-scale annual X-ray screening studies such as have been carried out in Philadelphia have not had the hoped-for results. This failure is related in part to the rich blood and lymphatic supply of the lung, which promotes early spread of the cancer, and in part to the reluctance of people to submit to early surgery after screening. At present, routine Papanicolau (Pap) smears of sputum in high-risk groups are again in vogue, but the effectiveness of these tests in reducing mortality awaits confirmation.

Surgery is still considered the only curative method for lung cancer, but the results have not significantly improved during the last 25 years: the proportion of patients with successful lung resection who remain free of disease for at least five years has remained at 20 to 35 percent. Unfortunately, in more than half the patients who develop lung cancer the disease when first detected has already progressed too far for surgical intervention. Thus the overall five-year survival rate is only 7 to 9 percent. New aids to surgery, such as preoperative radiation or "radical resection," have failed to alter the outcome. For inoperable situations and with certain especially malignant tumors, the introduction of a variety of cytotoxic (cell-killing) agents, million-volt therapy, and betatrons and linear accelerators for radiation have increasingly resulted in better palliation of disease. Research in these areas appears to be more promising than more radical surgical approaches.

Environmental Lung Disease

Great strides have been made in recent years in the reduction or prevention of lung diseases that stem from occupational exposures. The most common and most widely publicized diseases relating to occupations have been recognized since antiquity and have decreased in importance, thanks to long-standing and increasingly effective legislation, well-established limits to exposure, and effective monitoring and industrial hygiene. Also, the number of individuals at risk for these diseases has been decreasing both in relative and absolute terms because of mechanization and the substitution of new materials in industry. Anthracosilicosis or coal worker's pneumoconiosis (black lung)—notwithstanding all the recent publicity and political pressures—has been a good example of a decreasing occupational disease.

Unlike black lung, asbestosis—a severe and sometimes fatal inflammation of the lung caused by inhalation of asbestos fibers—has been of increasing concern both because of its seriousness and the number of individuals it affects. The dangerous effects of asbestos fibers actually have been known for some time. Asbestosis has been recognized since the 1920s, when the premature deaths of spinners and weavers of asbestos cloth were first described in Great Britain. Excellent epidemiologic studies in Italy and the United States in the 1930s confirmed these findings, and standards were established to limit the exposure of workers in the asbestos industry.

But these measures proved ineffective in controlling the effects resulting from the enormously increased use of asbestos during the last 30 years. The crash program of ship construction during the Second World War led to virtually uncontrolled exposure of hundreds of thousands of men and women who worked in the vicinity of asbestos pipe coverers or walked all day in the debris of old pipe covering that had been removed during refitting. After the war, asbestos was introduced into thousands of products that virtually surround us every day. Kitchens were fitted with asbestos-insulated ovens and asbestos mats, floors were covered with vinyl asbestos and asphalt tiles, houses were covered with asbestos siding and roofing, and asbestos brake lining, undercoating, and clutch facings were used in automobiles. Cars' air and oil were filtered through asbestos paper, and similar filters were used to clarify wine and beer. High-rise buildings had their steel beams lagged with asbestos, and hospital and school buildings had asbestos ceilings installed for safety. The workers who handled these vast quantities of asbestos were often uninformed of the potential dangers of their jobs.

It now seems that asbestos exposure is even more dangerous than was originally thought. Asbestosis progresses relentlessly after the individual has been exposed to the mineral, and the disease usually does not manifest itself until decades have elapsed. Many people who worked in shipyards for a few months 20 to 30 years ago are developing asbestosis today. Recent recognition of the problem has led to a downward revision of the limits for asbestos exposure on two occasions during the last five years, and a further revision is being contemplated; but unfortunately, we will have to wait another 20 to 30 years to determine the effectiveness of these new measures. Present research deals largely with methods for early diagnosis and prevention because there appears to be little hope in neutralizing or removing the asbestos fibers once they have been inhaled.

There is now much interest in the need to evaluate the effect on workers' health of new synthetic materials and new processes. Industrial research leads to the development of a large variety of substances that are propelled from the test tube to the production of thousands of tons with incredible speed. Many such materials are manufactured and distributed before their health effects on workers and consumers are fully known, and some eventually prove to be harmful. Many examples have been well publicized. The introduction of beryllium 30 years ago into the manufacture of X-ray tubes, into the research and development of the atomic bomb, into the coating of fluorescent light bulbs, and into the electronics industry led to widespread berylliosis, a chronic lung inflammation stemming from exposure to beryllium. The tragic results of the use of beryllium were compounded by ignorance of the foreign medical literature, by misleading statements of the Public Health Service, and by a conspiracy of certain industries and insurance companies.

The beryllium story illustrates well that workers can be adequately protected without decreasing industrial productivity; industrial hygiene measures introduced after the effects of beryllium were acknowledged have virtually eradicated berylliosis, while the production of beryllium has continued to increase (Figure 13-4). Clearly, occupational pathogens like beryllium and other chemicals must be identified and demonstrated to cause disease before basic hygiene measures to prevent disease will be introduced. For example, chemicals used in the synthetic ureafoams that

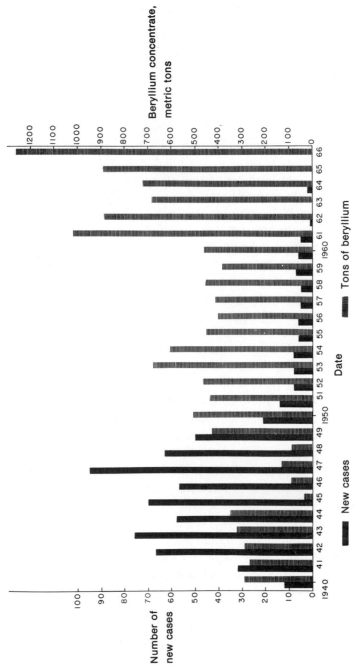

Figure 13–4. A diagram that illustrates the effectiveness of industrial hygiene measures concerning a highly toxic material. The number of cases of berylliosis from new exposure that were reported to the Case Registry are shown for the years 1940–66. There has been a rapid decrease and now virtual disappearance of the disease in spite of the fact that production of beryllium concentrate, estimated from shipment figures of the two major manufacturers in the United States and from beryllium ore imports, has constantly increased since 1946. From R. A. Redding, H. L. Hardy, and E. A. Gaensler, "Beryllium disease: A 16-Year Follow-Up Case Study," *Respiration* 25 (1968), 263–276. Reprinted by permission of S. Karger AG, Basel.

have replaced more expensive natural foam rubbers have been shown to induce asthma. Dangerous substances continue to accompany industrial progress, and these substances must be identified and workers protected from their effects.

While certain types of factory worker clearly run special risks related to their occupation, the problem of environmental substances that can cause lung disease is not confined to these workers. A number of respiratory disorders that were once linked to specific occupations are now being recognized among larger groups of the population who are preferentially exposed to certain environmental agents. The development of berylliosis in people who lived several blocks away from the factories is one of the earliest examples of such "neighborhood" cases.

One important disease of environmental origin, and one that has only recently received widespread attention, is hypersensitivity pneumonitis. This disorder was first recognized in 1932 by J. M. Campbell, a general practitioner who noted that chills, fever, and shortness of breath often followed exposure to the white dust of moldy hay. Because of the source of this disorder, he called the syndrome "farmer's lung." Sporadic reports continued until, by 1953, a clear-cut relationship between inhalation of various kinds of molds and lung disease was established. Researchers in Wisconsin isolated certain fungi whose growth was stimulated by the heat generated within moldy hay and other similar material, and which seemed to be related to hypersensitivity pneumonitis. Finally, in the 1960s, it began to appear that the disease was a kind of allergic phenomenon that resulted in inflammation and injury of the lungs.

Some ten years ago, it became evident that hypersensitivity pneumonitis was not restricted to farmers and others whose work might bring them into contact with moldy organic material. Cases of "bird breeder's lung" were reported; this allergic reaction was similar to that of farmer's lung, but the offending allergen proved to be dried protein contained in bird droppings rather than fungal or bacterial contaminants. This disease is not restricted to people with massive occupational exposure to avian droppings and feathers; it also threatens thousands of hobbyists who keep pigeons and parakeets in their homes.

Jordan Fink and his coworkers have identified another type of hypersensitivity that places an even larger population at risk. Hypersensitivity pneumonitis has now been related to the contamination of humidifiers and certain air conditioners by bacterial and fungal organisms similar to those that cause farmer's lung. The microorganisms which cause an allergic reaction are released into the home environment on invisible droplets propelled by the fan of a forced-air heating or cooling system.

It will be difficult to eliminate biologic dust disease by modifying humidifiers that spread it, and other methods of fighting the disorder are being sought. In addition to seeking new possible causes of the disease and investigating the allergic mechanisms involved, researchers are also developing more specific methods of testing people who are at risk for hypersensitivity pneumonitis. The ideal test would be one which identified specific antibodies in the blood of all patients with hypersensitivity pneumonitis, yet which was negative for people without the disease. Unfortunately, no such test yet exists. Also, our understanding of the allergic mechanism involved is still incomplete. The recent development of a model of hypersensitivity pneumonitis in laboratory animals may help investigators to unravel these complex issues.

The case of hypersensitivity pneumonitis illustrates an important point: the distinction between occupational and environmental causes of disease is becoming increasingly blurred. Hobbyists are made ill by the pigeons that they fancy or by the glues and foams that they use for their sailboats. The entire family may become sick from attempts to increase the comfort of their homes by humidification or air conditioning. Workers in unrelated occupations are exposed to asbestos by pipe coverers working near them, and even the wives of asbestos workers may develop mesothelioma.

The magnitude of these public health problems is difficult to estimate; epidemiologic information concerning the prevalence of environmental disease and its impact on community health is largely lacking. But these problems clearly present an increasing challenge to physicians, to public health officers, to industrial hygienists, and, in the end, to lawmakers who must often sift through uncertain, insufficient, or contradictory evidence. The urgent need for careful cross-sectional and longitudinal studies has been stressed in the preambles to two pieces of recent legislation, the Federal Coal Mine and Safety Act of 1969 and the Occupational Safety and Health Act of 1970. Unfortunately, neither OSHA, the agency created by the latter act, nor its research arm, the National Institute of Occupational Safety and Health, has ever been funded adequately to do its job.

Respiratory Distress Syndrome

Respiratory distress syndrome, which may occur in newborn infants or in adults, is the most acute, most rapidly progressive, and most highly fatal of the lung diseases. Yet this disorder has been characterized only in the past two decades. Part of the delay in its recognition has been due to the fact that the syndrome is associated with a malfunction in a component of the lung that has only recently been identified. This is the surface-active material, or surfactant, that lines the lung's tiny air cells, or alveoli.

The existence of lung surfactant, which is now known to be essential to normal function, was first postulated in 1929 by a Swiss tuberculosis physician, K. von Neergaard. His study of the mechanics of breathing and his observation of the differences between air-filled and fluid-filled lungs when inflated and deflated led him to conclude that the inner surface of the lung must be coated with a chemical that alters surface tension. His discovery received little attention until the 1950s, when this substance was identified.

It is now clear why a pulmonary surfactant is necessary. The lungs consist of 300 million minute gas bubbles, essentially a stable emulsion of air in blood. Ordinarily, when bubbles of air are surrounded by a thin film of fluid, the surface tension at the interface tends to reduce the surface area by collapsing bubbles. The surfactant lowers surface tension, prevents the bubbles from collapsing, and gives the lung stability. A complex mixture of lipids, protein, and carbohydrates comprises the surfactant system. Serious problems result when this system malfunctions due to deficient production, mechanical disruption, or contamination of the surfactant layer. The lung becomes unstable and collapses irregularly, fluid leaks into the airspaces, and breathing becomes difficult. The clinical manifestation of a deficiency of surfactant is the respiratory distress syndrome.

Respiratory distress syndome of the newborn (RDS) is the most serious lung disease in infants; it affects more than 100,000 babies per year and causes 27 percent of all neonatal deaths. It is a disorder due to immaturity of the lung and is characterized primarily by formation of hyaline membrane—a clear, structureless material lining the air sacs and smallest air passages—and by diffuse uneven collapse of the lung. Cyanosis, or a blue appearance of the skin, results from inadequate oxygen uptake in the blood of infants with this disease. The microscopic picture of RDS was first described by K. Hochheim in 1903 and the often-used term "hyaline membrane disease" derives from his description of the peculiar membranes found lining the interior of the lungs of infants who died shortly after birth. The cause is most likely an impaired ability to synthesize or secrete adequate amounts of the pulmonary surfactant. The onset of respiratory distress occurs within 8 hours of birth, and death usually occurs within 72 hours.

Present therapeutic measures require highly skilled teamwork in specialized facilities. Important measures include temperature control, correction of blood acidity, and supplying oxygen in the environment at the lowest effective level with transfusion of fresh frozen blood plasma and albumin. The application of constant positive air pressure (CPAP), a recent development, may save the infant's life by helping to stabilize the structure of the lung and by minimizing leakage of fluid.

Until a better understanding of lung development makes it possible to begin preventive measures before delivery, the best prevention of respiratory distress syndrome will depend upon prenatal diagnosis, possibly with selective abortion of high-risk infants, and on the availability of sophisticated neonatal intensive care during labor, delivery, and in the immediate postpartum period. The development of the lung and of its surfactant can now be gauged by measuring levels of the phospholipids, particularly lecithin and sphingomyelin, in amniotic fluid. Lung maturation can be assessed by the measurement of the lecithin/sphingomyelin (L/S) ratio or by testing the stability of surfactant bubbles. Although the L/S ratio is normally dependent on gestational age, certain abnormal conditions such as high blood pressure, toxemia, diabetes, certain drugs, stress, and temperature may all affect the rate of fetal lung maturation.

Different clinical problems are posed by the adult respiratory distress syndrome (ARDS). Since the discovery of the X ray, it has been known that the terminal state of a variety of apparently unrelated conditions is associated with opaqueness of the lungs to X rays, apparently because they become filled with fluid. This situation, characteristic of ARDS, is now also referred to as the stiff lung syndrome because of the associated breathing difficulty and the demonstration of actual stiffening of the lung. Until recently this condition was attributed to terminal heart failure leading to accumulation of fluid in the lung. But improved methods for monitoring cardiac function have shown the condition to be unrelated to heart function; instead, like RDS, it seems to result from conditions that disrupt the surfactant system.

ARDS was first seen extensively during the war in Vietnam, when helicopter evacuation made it possible for the first time in military medical history to transport grievously injured soldiers rapidly to superbly equipped and staffed base hospitals. Often, extensive injuries not involving the chest could be repaired, and the patients appeared to be well on the way to recovery when, on the third or fourth day, they began to experience serious respiratory distress that could end in death. In 1968 the National Research Council convened a conference about the effects on the lungs of trauma to other parts of the body; and since then, investigation into the problem has been energetic. ARDS is now observed most commonly by surgeons dealing with sepsis, burns, extensive trauma, and hemorrhagic shock. It often occurs in patients with no history of previous lung damage. And it is associated with a large variety of other conditions ranging from malaria to heroin intoxication.

ARDS is a severe problem that now preoccupies virtually every intensive care unit. Why, then, was it not seen until 15 years ago? It is possible that the syndrome was simply not recognized before then. But it is also possible that the prevalence of ARDS has actually been increased —paradoxically enough—by newer forms of medical treatment.

Serious trauma, sepsis, burns, and hemorrhagic shock all share at least one thing in common: they all lead to the need for replenishing losses of the formed elements of blood, plasma, and minerals. The exuberant use of therapeutic replenishing solutions, while preserving kidney function, may lead to fluid accumulation in the lungs. Circulation in the very small blood vessels of the lungs may also suffer from infusion of banked blood that is too old or is inadequately matched with the patient's blood.

The therapeutic administration of oxygen may be another contributor to ARDS. Until 15 years ago oxygen generally was administered in tents or through nasal catheters; the concentration of oxygen that reached the lungs was never higher than 40 to 50 percent. More recently oxygen has been administered by pressure breathing machines that can deliver pure oxygen. Such high oxygen concentrations are quickly fatal to some healthy animals and may well injure an already compromised human lung. Also, until 15 years ago assisted ventilation was uncommon and, when absolutely necessary, was given in an iron lung, which worked by creating a partial vacuum around the patient's body. Since then, it has been customary to apply positive pressure, often high pressure, at the mouth rather than negative pressure around the body. This high positive pressure may also contribute to lung injury.

There is ample evidence that agents formed within the body and circulating in abnormal amounts can seriously alter lung structure and function. These substances may injure the cells that produce long surfactant, either through inflammation or by direct chemical interaction. When lung surfactant is lost in this way, the results are not unlike the respiratory distress of the newborn. The lung becomes stiff and blood does not take up adequate oxygen. The patient may require breathing assistance, first with air and later with increasing amounts of oxygen, until a state is reached at which pressure breathing even of pure oxygen can no longer sustain life.

One new method that quickly found widespread acceptance in this situation has been the application of PEEP (positive end-expiratory pressure). A degree of positive pressure is maintained during expiration; this tends to keep the lungs inflated despite loss of surfactant and it pneumatically restores lung stability. Unfortunately, this method sometimes results in a fall in heart blood output and it frequently leads to escape of air from the lung into the chest cavity, which requires emergency treatment.

Today, when all methods of improving the patient's breathing have failed, the possibility of extracorporeal membrane oxygenation (ECMO) is considered. Artificial membrane lungs have now reached a stage of development that makes it possible to use them to supply oxygen to the patient's blood for up to two or three weeks. The aim, of course, is to allow the lung to heal naturally. There are now eighteen reported survivors from 150 patients so treated. Although the technical problems appear to be largely solved, there remains a dilemma. At present the only patients subjected to ECMO are those who clearly would die without such assistance. Experience has shown that in such severely ill patients ECMO can provide some additional days of survival. But almost always, instead of the lung healing, there is progressive deposition of scar tissue and the situation becomes irreversible. ECMO may have been started too late for these very ill patients. However, if less ill patients were to be selected for ECMO, then the group to be considered for this exceedingly expensive form of therapy (which requires an enormous amount of highly trained manpower) would be too large to be economically supportable. Future researchers will have to clarify the criteria for deciding that a patient should be placed on ECMO.

Diagnosis of Lung Disease

The political, sociological, and personal factors involved in effective prevention of lung disease have led many researchers to focus on developing new methods of diagnosis and treatment. Some truly impressive strides have been made in these areas in the past several years.

Many unique features of the respiratory system offer special opportunities both for the study of structure and function and for the diagnosis of disease. The constant tide of air moving in and out of the lungs causes sounds that can be heard with a stethoscope; the products of external respiration can be measured easily and instantly by connecting simple instruments to the mouth; and since breathing can be altered at will, lung sounds and the capacity for breathing can be measured during voluntary overbreathing or breathholding. The conducting airways, the trachea and bronchi, are normally open and can thus be readily examined by various procedures. Also, the lungs do not block X rays, since they contain mostly air and their fine detail therefore can be readily visualized. The accessibility of the respiratory system has great advantages for diagnostic purposes and has led to the development of many fascinating new methods of investigation. But ease of access also presents certain problems. A number of diagnostic methods have been used excessively in relation to the public health benefits that may accrue.

Modern respiratory diagnosis really began in 1816, when Laennec first explored breath sounds. In that year, at the Hospital Necker in Paris, he was consulted by a young woman in whom "percussion and the application of the hand were of little avail on account of a great degree of fatness." Furthermore, application of the ear was "rendered inadmissible by the age and sex of the patient." Faced with these clinical obstacles, Laennec constructed a hollow tube with an earpiece to hear the sounds of respiration better. The stethoscope, as he called his device, has remained virtually unchanged to this day. While it has been relied on less and less since the advent of the chest X ray, interest in breath sounds has recently been revived by the suggestion that certain abnormal sounds may signal the development of some types of slowly developing pneumonias, particularly those associated with asbestosis. Breath sounds are now being recorded and analyzed electronically. This approach holds the promise of providing a method for simple, rapid, noninvasive health surveillance in industry.

In 1902 Edison's invention of the electric light bulb made it possible to look at the lungs as well as to listen to them. The bronchoscope, invented in that year, is a rigid tube that can be inserted through the mouth and larynx and used to inspect the vocal chord, trachea, and bronchi. Initially, the instrument was used mainly to remove foreign bodies that had been inhaled; with the development of chest surgery, it was used more commonly for the localization of tumors and structural abnormalities as well as for the removal of tissue samples for microscopic examination. The principal limitations were its rigidity and its large diameter. Recently, these drawbacks have been overcome with the development of fiberoptic instruments similar to those used for examination of the gastrointestinal tract (see Chapter 16). Ten years ago, Shigeto Ikeda of the National Cancer Center Hospital in Tokyo first demonstrated a flexible bronchofiberscope made with a bundle of glass fibers. Thanks to the relatively small diameter and great flexibility, it can be introduced through the nose of a comfortably seated patient and used to inspect much more distant areas of the lung. The image obtained is also much clearer and brighter. Tiny brushes can be introduced to collect secretions and small tissue samples for analysis; a fluoroscope is used to guide these brushes to the area of the lung being sampled.

The stethoscope and bronchoscope are important diagnostic tools, but more reliance has been placed on the chest X ray. Chest radiography remained basically unchanged for some 50 years after Conrad Roentgen's description in 1895 of the powerful, invisible rays. Such photographs, taken first on glass plates, were the principal tool in the fight against tuberculosis. They also led directly to the development of the specialty of chest surgery.

Although the ready visualization of the lungs by radiography clearly has been of enormous benefit to mankind, it has also led to certain problems. Small lesions are easily visualized—a feature that is important for the early detection of cancer or potentially dangerous infection—but so are small healed scars and unimportant anomalies of no clinical significance. When these are seen they become a cause for concern, and the patient may undergo unnecessary, expensive, painful, and sometimes dangerous diagnostic exploration. Conversely, a normal chest X ray may give rise to a false sense of security and the unwarranted conviction that the lungs are free of disease; conventional chest X rays are not always precise enough to show the presence of very fine diffusely dispersed lesions, which may go undetected. Finally, the chest X ray is a static picture that obviously cannot reflect the impairment of dynamic events, such as the slowing of the airstream due to airways obstruction—the main feature of chronic bronchitis and emphysema.

Radiology is now a rapidly changing field (see Chapter 25), and many technological advances have improved methods of respiratory diagnosis in the last 20 years. Image amplification, now used together with television techniques for direct visual examination by fluoroscopy, provides a sharper image and reduced radiation dosage. Cinefluorography permits the radiologist to film rapidly occurring events within the chest for later study without posing the hazard of high radiation dosage. Tomography is an increasingly useful and constantly developing technique that allows selective visualization of a "slice" of lung tissue without interference from the structures lying in front or behind.

The bronchial tubes, which are generally not visible because there is no contrasting density difference between these air-filled tubes and the air-containing surrounding lung, can now be made visible through bronchography. A material opaque to X rays is instilled by nose or mouth and outlines the bronchi. Sometimes the opaque material interferes with breathing or causes an adverse reaction. Therefore the recent introduction to bronchography of powdered tantalum metal, which does not have these side effects, is a further exciting advance.

The blood vessels, like the bronchial tubes, are not easily seen on a conventional chest X ray. Injection into the bloodstream of radio-opaque material permits visualization of the arteries of the lung; this technique of angiography, a relatively recent development, is now used extensively for detection of blood clots and in many preoperative situations. Finally, small quantities of radioactive material can be injected or given by inhalation to outline abnormalities in the circulation or ventilation of the lung. One radioactive substance, ^{67}Gallium, has been found useful in the detection of cancer cells (which grow at an abnormal rate) because this material is taken up preferentially by growing cells.

In all these radiographic techniques there is ample room for technical development with respect to image size and quality, miniaturization of equipment, computer-produced image enhancement, selective contrast improvement, and perhaps even image recognition. Unfortunately, several major electric and electronic manufacturers have abandoned this field entirely because the potential market is small compared to the market for industrial and consumer products; and the National Institutes of Health and universities have shied away from this area because of the enormous expense of radiologic instrumentation research. The recent development of CAT (Computerized Axial Tomography) scanners is an example of both the rewards and the great cost of such advances.

Future Research

Speculations on the future of medical research usually conjure up visions of great new theoretical breakthroughs in the understanding or treatment of a disease or group of diseases. There is some feeling in the scientific community and elsewhere that an illness can be eradicated only when the underlying pathological processes are fully understood, whether the disease stems from a microorganism, a virus, a chemical, or even a faulty gene. But medical history has shown many times that this basic level of theoretical comprehension is not always necessary. Ignatz

Semmelweiss eliminated the dread childbed fever from his wards in Vienna many years before bacteria were discovered, simply by ordering general cleanliness and scrubbing of the hands between pelvic examinations. And chimneysweeps were saved from their usual early death from cancer of the scrotum by adopting the simple expedient of wearing leather pants during their work, this some 200 years before the first cancer cell was recognized. A similar situation exists with respect to the major lung diseases today. While often the physical and biological processes underlying their causation are incompletely understood, the agents that cause them have been largely identified.

With the conquest of tuberculosis and the virtual elimination of the complications of untreated pneumonia, 90 to 95 percent of all chronic lung disease has become attributable to emphysema, chronic bronchitis, or lung cancer. The relationship of these diseases to cigarette smoking has been established beyond doubt, even though no one has clearly identified the specific physical and chemical agents in smoke that cause disease, and the cellular processes leading to these disorders are still unknown. Virtually all research efforts in recent years have been devoted to the study of the type and nature of the lung malfunctions that result from smoking, to studies that attempt to reproduce the diseases and study their causation in animals, to improving methods of therapy, and to repetitive epidemiologic studies that merely confirm the known facts. While some of these approaches are important, a much more valuable step, and much more effective, would be the elimination of the causative agent, tobacco. But neither the agencies that fund research nor the scientific community are able to deal with this approach. The task of discouraging people from smoking is a matter for public policy, which has been slow to change in response to scientific knowledge. Nowhere is the gap between scientific knowledge and legislation more dismaying than in the case of the cigarette.

Of course, dissuading people from smoking is no easy matter. History has shown that attempts to change the habits of confirmed, and perhaps addicted, middle-aged smokers are doomed to failure. To appreciate the degree to which tobacco can be addicting, one need only think of pictures of prisoners fighting for a thrown-away cigarette butt, or of early postwar Germany, where a carton of cigarettes was the monetary standard for which people gladly traded their food, jewels, and household goods. A significant reduction in smoking could be achieved only by highly funded and effective educational programs at the grammar school and junior high school levels, when cigarettes have not yet been tried, and by massive federally funded advertising campaigns aimed at the young. However, many other means could also be employed to discourage smoking: decreased availability of cigarettes, sales by state stores only, increased taxation to the extent of making cigarettes unaffordable by the young, preferential life insurance rates for nonsmokers in recognition of their increased longevity, and other similar measures. Motivational and psychological research are also important to gauge the most effective ways of convincing people not to smoke.

The problem of widespread smoking is by no means simple, nor is it on the verge of solution. All of the possible ways to discourage tobacco use that have just been mentioned are beyond the scope of the agencies that provide conventional research funding. And, of course, there are huge political and economic considerations involved. The tobacco industry is a big industry, involving large amounts of money. Effectively curtailing that industry would have to presuppose a national consensus to supply significant financial concessions to tobacco farmers, importers, and manufacturers that would make it profitable for them to switch to other ventures.

The obstacles involved are as great as those that face conventional research scientists who grapple with obscure biochemical processes in the laboratory in the attempt to understand disease. But the best knowledge we have indicates that the current epidemic of lung disease must ultimately be fought in the legislature, not in the laboratory.

The Kidneys

JOHN P. MERRILL

14

Until recently, the kidney and its diseases have not been popular subjects for medical discussion. This may be because the kidney has been thought of in the past purely as an excretory organ, and the formation of urine is not generally considered a subject for polite conversation. It is true, of course, that urine was only minutes before an integral part of the blood; but still, the kidney has not had the appeal for the investigator, the philosopher, or the layman that the heart has. For example, no one has ever seen a kidney on a valentine. Isak Dinesen has been one of the few writers to appreciate the beauty of the kidney; in her *Seven Gothic Tales*, she describes an Arab sailing off the African Coast in the moonlight and musing, "After all, what is man but an intricate and ingeniously devised apparatus for turning the red wine of Shiraz into urine."

The excretory function of the kidney is its most obvious role and was the first aspect of renal activity to be studied thoroughly. In 1917 A. R. Cushny, an English physiologist, published his monograph supporting an earlier suggestion that urine was probably formed by the filtration of blood plasma through the glomerulus, an intricate maze of intertwined capillaries at the head of the nephron, or functioning unit of the kidney (Figure 14-1). Each human kidney contains a million nephrons, each with its own glomerulus; together, these glomeruli filter some 180 liters (190 quarts) of fluid per day. If all this filtrate were excreted as urine, the individual would be totally desiccated within half an hour. Since this does not occur, some reabsorption of the filtrate must take place. The pioneering work of A. N. Richards and Arthur Walker, who devised an

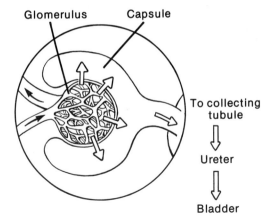

Glomerulus   Capsule

To collecting
tubule

Ureter

Bladder

Figure 14–1. A glomerulus. The blood (black arrows) enters this web of capillaries. Fluid containing wastes from the blood (white arrows) filters through
the glomerular capillaries into the surrounding tubular capsule. The filtrate
then travels to a collecting tubule, to the ureter, and finally to the bladder.
Much fluid and various blood components are reabsorbed from the collecting
tubule into the blood before the filtrate reaches the ureter and bladder.

intricate apparatus for puncturing single nephrons in the frog, demonstrated that this was the case. In the early thirties Homer Smith began to
outline patterns of filtration and reabsorption for the various components
of the blood and began to investigate the factors controlling these oppos-
ing processes.

But the functions of the kidney go far beyond the mere excretion of
poisons and wastes. This organ controls the production of substances that
maintain blood pressure and facilitate the production of red blood cells.
It also helps regulate blood levels of insulin and therapeutic drugs, the
volume and composition of the body fluids, the metabolism of blood
sugar, and even the production of an integral component of muscle. Since
the kidney performs so many essential functions, renal failure can clearly
have multiple consequences. For this reason the extent of disease and
death resulting from kidney dysfunction is difficult to evaluate. It is
usually estimated that there are some 10 to 20 thousand deaths a year
resulting directly from excretory failure; but when one realizes that kidney disease may be a major factor in the genesis of hypertension (which
in turn is the primary cause of stroke), such mortality figures become
meaningless. The available statistics on kidney disease are impossible to
clarify, and appear to be totally unreliable. It is obvious, however, that

kidney disorders are a greater cause of sickness and death than has generally been realized.

The Artificial Kidney

One of the first and most dramatic breakthroughs in the treatment of kidney failure was the development of a dialysis machine to take over the excretory function of the kidney. J. J. Abel, a professor of pharmacology at Johns Hopkins University, developed a crude apparatus for dialyzing the blood plasma of experimental animals as early as 1913. More than three decades later, Wilhelm Kolff constructed the prototype of the first successful artificial kidney for human use. In contrast to contemporary American kidney researchers, Kolff, working in Nazi-occupied Holland, had to build his machine with his own resources. His apparatus was crude and fraught with problems but the basic principle behind it was sound, and it did work. Kolff's machine dialyzed the patient's blood through a cellophane membrane; his original device used an ordinary sausage casing. The pores of this dialyzing membrane were large enough to permit small waste molecules, such as urea, uric acid, and creatinine, to pass through and thus be removed from the blood; but the pores were small enough to block the passage of essential elements such as blood proteins and red and white blood cells, which were retained in the plasma (Figure 14-2). In 1947, after the end of hostilities in Europe, Kolff visited the Peter Bent Brigham Hospital in Boston and very kindly lent the blueprints of his apparatus to Carl Walter, a surgeon-engineer. Walter and his colleagues, George Thorn and I, improved the apparatus by constructing it of newly available plastics, steel, and modern electronic devices. It became widely available to patients and was used extensively throughout the Korean War. Once the outlook for patients with acute kidney failure had been improved by this device, accelerated interest and research resulted in a vast improvement in methods for treating all types of acute renal failure. Especially important was the development of peritoneal dialysis, a simple and effective procedure for removing wastes by introducing a rinsing fluid directly into the abdominal cavity.

Through the early fifties the use of the artificial kidney was largely restricted to the treatment of acute kidney failure, since separate surgical procedures were required to reach the blood vessels used to conduct blood to and from the dialyzing membrane. In 1960, however, Wayne Quinton, Belding Scribner, and their colleagues solved this problem by devising a plastic tube for semipermanent implantation into the blood vessels of the forearm which "shunted" blood from artery to vein. When

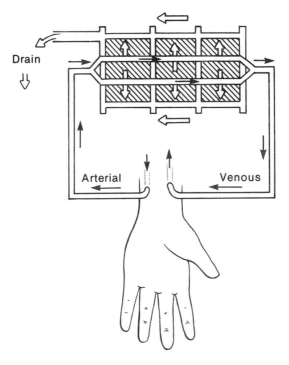

Figure 14–2. Basic design of a dialysis machine. Blood from an artery (black arrows) is pumped through tubes of a dialyzing membrane immersed in liquid. Molecules of waste substances flow out through pores in the dialyzing membrane (white arrows); but the pores of the membrane are small enough to keep the essential blood components within the tubing, which eventually leads back to the patient's vein. The liquid containing waste products is drained from the machine.

the patient was connected to the artificial kidney, this shunt was temporarily disconnected and blood flowed from the arterial tube through the machine and, after being cleansed, flowed back into the patient through the tube in the vein. After each dialysis treatment, the shunt was reconnected and kept open by the continuing flow of blood between artery and vein. More recently, direct surgical connections between the artery and vein, known as fistulae, have largely replaced plastic shunts. These simple devices for connecting the blood vessels have opened a new era in the treatment of kidney failure. Patients whose kidneys have totally failed or have been removed can now be maintained in satisfactory health for years with frequent dialysis treatments. A series of so-called satellite centers for dialysis has been established where the patients are treated largely by paramedical personnel at less cost than in the hospital. And it is possible for the patient to treat himself or be treated by a companion at home. Marked improvements have been made in the design of various types of dialyzers, thanks to research supported by the National Institutes of Arthritis and Metabolic Diseases of the National Institutes of Health, the National Kidney Foundation, and the American Heart Association. Recently, too, the economic obstacles to dialysis treatment have been made less formidable by congressional legislation authorizing the use of Medicare funds to pay for chronic dialysis and kidney transplantation regardless of the age of the patient.

Kidney Transplantation

Valuable though the artificial kidney is, it is not a perfect solution to the problem of kidney failure. Dialysis machines can only replicate the excretory function of the kidney; they can do nothing to fulfill its metabolic functions. Clearly, the transplantation of a normal kidney capable of supplying these extra functions would be preferable to maintenance on dialysis.

In the early 1950s a team from Peter Bent Brigham Hospital (where the artificial kidney was first used in the United States) undertook a series of kidney transplantations in people who were in terminal renal failure and being maintained on the artificial kidney. Cadavers were the source of kidneys; not infrequently, the organs for transplantation came from patients who had died in the operating room during the early pioneering days of open heart surgery. Previous animal experiments had shown that organ and tissue transplantation was feasible (see Chapter 24), but to our great surprise the human kidney actually functioned better than any of the animal models. In 1954 the first successful transplant of a kidney from one identical twin to another was accomplished. Although this was an exciting surgical feat, it left unsolved the basic biologic problem of tissue rejection, which is the main obstacle to successful transplantation. (Since identical twins are born of the same fertilized egg, they have genetically identical tissues, and therefore one twin will not reject the tissues or organs of another.) It was not until 1959 that the first successful tissue graft between genetically different individuals was accomplished at the Peter Bent Brigham Hospital. Following this operation, in which the patient received a kidney donated by a nonidentical twin, the rejection problem was eventually overcome through the use of X irradiation and cortisone.

X irradiation soon proved to be much too crude and dangerous a tool, and was superseded by the immunosuppressive drugs, which are con-

siderably easier to manage. But these drugs pose very real hazards themselves. While suppressing the immune response to transplanted kidneys,
they also suppress the response to bacteria, to viruses, and to fungi, thus
making the individual vulnerable to severe and life-threatening infections. The incidence of spontaneously occurring cancer is also considerably higher in patients using these agents; proponents of the immune
surveillance hypothesis of cancer have suggested that immunosuppressive
drugs disrupt a built-in mechanism by which the body normally recog-
nizes and destroys malignant cells.

In spite of these problems, kidney transplantation has progressed to
the point today where it is an effective and life-saving form of treatment
in properly selected cases. More than 27,000 kidney transplants have now
been performed, often with dramatically beneficial results. Yet as Table
14-1 shows, the success of these operations does not seem to be improving. (In fact, the postoperative prognosis for survival of a transplanted
kidney actually appears to have worsened slightly between 1970 and
1972.) Further advances in kidney transplantation depend on the discovery of a method for preventing the immune response against the
transplanted organ without leaving the individual unprotected against
infections and spontaneous cancers. This has already been accomplished
in experiments with specially bred animals, and there is much hope that
current research efforts will lead to the clinical application of these experimental findings in the near future.

Apart from its direct importance to such problems as the kidney

Table 14–1. Percentage of first transplants functionally surviving

Donor source	Year of transplant	1 year	2 years
Sibling	1970	81.1	78.2
	1971	73.7	69.6
	1972	79.9	73.7
Parent	1970	73.8	68.3
	1971	73.7	66.8
	1972	71.7	61.1
Cadaver	1970	55.3	47.2
	1971	53.1	45.7
	1972	50.6	42.6

Source: "11th Report of the Human Renal Transplant Registry," *Journal of the American Medical
Association* 226 (1973), 1197–1204.

transplant, the vast amount of research that has been done on transplantation in general has had tremendous impact on the study of other human diseases. Research into the analysis of human tissue types has led to a whole new system for describing the antigenic properties of human cells. One of the interesting by-products of this work has been the correlation of many diseases, such as psoriasis and ankylosing spondylitis, with specific antigens found on the surface of white blood cells (see Chapter 7); these observations may increase our understanding of the etiology and treatment of these diseases. Recently, the study of cell-surface antigens has yielded new clues to the aging phenomenon. And, as mentioned before, the investigation of cellular immunology has considerably deepened our understanding of cancer.

Glomerulonephritis

Neither dialysis nor cadaver kidney transplantation in their present forms are satisfactory methods of therapy for all patients with end-stage renal disease. While much kidney disease is not treated until it reaches this stage, it would clearly be preferable to prevent the disease which destroys the kidney in the first place and thus make such treatment unnecessary. Remarkable strides have been made in the diagnosis and antibiotic therapy of the infectious diseases, which account for 13 percent of all cases of kidney failure. However, less success has been achieved in the treatment of glomerulonephritis, the inflammatory disorder that causes more than two thirds of the end-stage renal failure seen in the United States. Successful control of this disease would obviate the need for the majority of artificial kidneys and kidney transplants. It would not even be necessary to prevent the disease; normal, healthy life would be possible if the disease were arrested even after 50 or 60 percent of the kidney tissue had been destroyed. The study of glomerulonephritis is thus a major focus of contemporary kidney research.

We have considerable knowledge about spontaneously occurring glomerulonephritis in the animal model, and it seems likely that this knowledge applies to the human disease as well. The vast majority of spontaneous cases observed in experimental animals result from the deposition of antigen-antibody complexes in the kidney. These complexes induce inflammatory changes in the glomeruli (the filtering beds of the nephrons); the eventual result is scarring and destruction of the functioning renal tissue. The disease process is essentially the same as that which occurs in rheumatoid arthritis and the other inflammatory diseases (see Chapter 7).

Much work has focused on characterizing the antigen that causes the inflammation of glomerulonephritis. When the antigen has been identified in animal studies, it has always been found to be a virus or part of a virus. This is consistent with the results of some attempts to determine the antigens responsible for human glomerulonephritis. The hepatitis virus, for example, has been found to act as such an antigen. And in the nephritis of lupus erythematosus, the antigen is deoxyribonucleic acid (DNA), an essential ingredient of many types of viruses. (DNA is also a vital component of human cells, however, and the DNA acting as an antigen in this disease may actually be of human rather than viral origin.) Especially interesting is the fact that a specific antigen found in cancer of the colon has also been found to cause glomerulonephritis in some patients with this cancer. Further advances in the study of antigenic determinants of glomerulonephritis may come from observation of kidney transplant patients, in whom the disease may recur after transplantation; these individuals provide a unique opportunity to study the disease prospectively rather than retrospectively. As more of the antigens causing this disorder are identified and the formation of antigen-antibody complexes is better understood, the prevention and treatment of glomerulonephritis should improve greatly.

The Kidney and Hypertension

Apart from its excretory function, the most important action of the kidney is probably its role in the control of blood pressure. R. Tigerstedt and Norman Bergman discovered in the late nineteenth century that the kidney secreted a substance responsible for raising blood pressure, but it was only decades later that the factors controlling the release of this substance began to be understood.

A key to the study of the kidney's role in hypertension came in 1934, when Harry Goldblatt and his colleagues published the results of their pioneering animal experiments. These investigators found that impairing the blood supply to the kidney with an arterial clamp resulted in an increase in blood pressure. They determined that this rise in pressure was due to a substance, renin, released by the kidney when its supply of oxygen decreases (as occurs when blood supply to the kidney is restricted). Years of subsequent work showed that renin interacts with a protein manufactured by the liver to form angiotensin, which is the substance directly responsible for raising the blood pressure.

We now know that human hypertension can be caused by conditions very much like those simulated in the experiment of Goldblatt and his coworkers. Injury to the renal vessels, or the process of arteriosclerosis, may diminish the function of one or both of the arteries that supply the kidney with blood; renin is released in response to the low blood supply, and hypertension results. This condition can be diagnosed by actually measuring the amount of renin coming from both renal veins at the same time. If one kidney is delivering three or more times as much renin into the blood as is the other kidney, and if X rays show that the main renal artery (or occasionally one of its branches) is constricted, then hypertension is likely to be caused by dysfunction of the arteries, which may be corrected by surgery. It now seems quite possible that many cases of sustained high blood pressure may be due to abnormalities of the blood vessels in the kidney; such cases include those which seem to occur naturally with the aging process. But hypertension, even when it is known to result from disease of the renal blood vessel, does not necessarily have to be treated surgically. Some cases respond very well to newer medications which act to suppress the secretion of renin and thus of angiotensin, the substance that actually raises the blood pressure.

The kidney malfunctions that can lead to hypertension are not always as obvious as constriction of the renal arteries. High blood pressure may have its origins in a specific functional defect in the blood vessels of the kidney particularly related to the excretion of salt. Since the research of Arthur Merrill, Homer Smith, and other investigators working in the late forties and early fifties, many types of heart failure have been known to be associated with the abnormal retention of salt and water by the kidney. The investigation of this phenomenon continues, along with research into the nature of the renal hormones controlling blood pressure.

While great strides have been made in the prevention and treatment of kidney disorders in the last few decades, the problem of renal disease are far from solved. Glomerulonephritis remains poorly understood and difficult to prevent. The methods for treating kidney failure when it does occur are fraught with problems; dialysis is inconvenient and expensive, while kidney transplants are difficult and not guaranteed of success. And although the excretory function of the kidney is thoroughly understood, the production and release of the several renal hormones remain mysterious in many ways. But although the advances made in kidney research during the last half century may not have been final victories, they are certainly a series of very promising beginnings.

The Blood

DAVID G. NATHAN **15**

Clinical hematology and hematology research are relatively new disciplines which had their beginnings in the late nineteenth century in Europe and England. Paul Ehrlich, by applying the so-called Romanowsky stains created by the German dye industry to smears of human blood, became the first to describe the various cells of the blood and relate their appearance and prevalence to human disease. The major categories of blood disease—anemia, leukemia, and the bleeding disorders—began to be recognized and characterized as separate entities. In later years, the introduction of physiological and biochemical techniques deepened the understanding of the various types of blood cells and of their normal and abnormal function. While much remains to be discovered, a great deal is known today about the formation of blood cells in the body, their role in the life of the healthy individual, and their disruption in disease.

Hematopoiesis

Production of the components of the blood, hematopoiesis, takes place only in the marrow of the vertebrae and pelvis of adults, although it also occurs in the arm and leg bones of children. The process begins with a single type of cell, the stem cell, that can reproduce itself or change its structure to become a differentiated cell that will give rise, after more divisions, to red cells, white cells, or platelets. Red cells contain hemoglobin, which carries oxygen through the body. White cells are capable of destroying bacteria and serve as the body's primary defense against infection. Platelets are the essential elements in the stoppage of bleeding; when a blood vessel is damaged, platelets block the flow of blood by collecting in the wound, then release a substance initiating a biochemical chain reaction that leads to blood coagulation.

Perhaps the most remarkable aspect of stem cell differentiation is its precise responsiveness to the body's needs. When the pool of white cells becomes depleted in combating an infection, the marrow increases its production of white cells. When the number of platelets decreases after serious bleeding, more platelets are released. And when red cells are lost through bleeding or destroyed by disease, the marrow may even expand through the arm and leg bones to assure an adequate yield of these vital cells.

The chemicals that control the marrow remain largely unknown and are the subject of much current hematologic research. The first such chemical to be identified and studied was erythropoietin, which can be isolated and purified from plasma and urine. This substance has been shown to increase stem cell differentiation into red cell precursors, but the exact way in which erythropoietin does this remains unclear. Control of the production of erythropoietin itself seems to reside with the kidney; apparently the kidney measures the amount of oxygen circulating in the blood and releases increasing amounts of erythropoietin when the oxygen level falls below normal. (Since red cells are responsible for oxygen transport in the body, augmenting the number of red cells increases oxygen circulation.)

The controlling factors in the production of white cells and platelets have only recently been studied and remain less well characterized than erythropoietin. A substance called colony-stimulating factor appears to play an important role in regulating production of granulocytes, a kind of white cell. Another material even less well characterized is thrombopoietin, which appears to regulate platelet production. As the chemicals that control the production of all the blood components are better understood, it should become easier to cure illnesses that result from dysfunction of these control mechanisms.

Many types of serious disease result from abnormalities in the production of the different kinds of blood cells and platelets. Failure to form red cells may be caused by kidney failure leading to decreased erythropoietin levels; it may happen when antibodies—for no apparent reason—are formed against the differentiated cells that are precursors of red cells; or it may occur for no known reason. One discovery that holds promise for the treatment of these disorders has been that large doses of androgens, male sex hormones, can be converted by the body into compounds which stimulate erythropoietin production and hemoglobin synthesis.

Some patients suffer from decreased production of neutrophils (a type of white cell) and may develop serious infection as a result; no specific treatment for this condition has yet been found. There is some evidence that a factor in plasma can be used to treat certain failures of platelet production which occur in rare instances in children, but the specific nature of the factor has yet to be determined.

Aplastic anemia is a condition in which bone marrow production of all of the blood components decreases drastically. The etiology of this disease is unclear. It may follow ingestion of certain drugs or viral infection, especially with infectious hepatitis. In rare instances, children may be affected by a congenital form of aplastic anemia. Some patients with aplastic anemia respond to androgen therapy, and others even recover spontaneously, but most have required intensive support with red cell, white cell, and platelet transfusions. Recent research by E. Donnell Thomas and Reiner Storb in Seattle, and by several physicians at Children's and Peter Bent Brigham Hospitals in Boston, has led to the development of techniques for the treatment of aplastic anemia through bone marrow transplantation. Such therapy requires massive suppression of the patient's immune system. Marrow is then aspirated from the bones of a donor who is immunologically similar to the patient (usually a sibling) and is given intravenously to the patient. When the procedure is successful, the transplanted stem cells settle in the marrow and grow into perfectly normal marrow cells. This technique has already been used effectively to treat several cases of aplastic anemia that would otherwise have proved fatal.

At the opposite end of the spectrum, disorders that result in an excess of blood cells can be just as dangerous as those entailing insufficient production. The leukemias are a group of diseases characterized by the uncontrolled, cancerous growth of white cells. In these disorders the blood stream becomes flooded with immature white cells while marrow production of red cells and platelets decreases correspondingly; red cell deficiency and an increased tendency to bleed usually lead to the patient's death. When leukemia was first identified in the mid-nineteenth century, it was thought that the white cells that filled the bloodstream were pus cells responding to some type of infectious agent. While this simple hypothesis was quickly refuted, the possibility remains that leukemia may originate in viral infection. It is also possible that the disease is caused not by the presence of a pathogenic agent but by the absence of some substance that is essential to normal blood cell development. One theory holds that leukemia is actually due to a failure of white cells to mature properly, and that the result is the abnormal accumulation of immature white cells in the body. If this is the case, then the disorder may be due to the absence of some chemical factor essential to the process of maturation. At present, treatments for leukemia are still in early stages of development. Marrow transplantation is being investigated in the treatment of this disease as well as in the treatment of aplastic anemia.

Other disorders of excess production have a clearer etiology. Certain types of congenital heart disease are known to result in a disproportionately low flow of oxygen to the kidney, which in turn releases massive amounts of erythropoietin. This substance increases red cell production to a dangerous level (a condition known as polycythemia); the blood becomes extremely thick, and the patient may suffer strokes as a result.

Disorders of Red Cell Metabolism and Function

Red cells lack a nucleus and thus are simpler than other cells (in fact, the absence of a nucleus means that they are technically not cells at all); but they are still complex enough and certainly important enough to merit extensive study. Basically, the red cell is made up of a membrane enclosing a viscous solution saturated with hemoglobin. The application of modern biochemistry and physical chemistry to hematology has increasingly clarified the interrelationship of the metabolism, membrane, and life span of the red cell, often with important practical results. One example is the recent discovery of the role of organic phosphate, particularly 2, 3-diphosphoglyceric acid, in red cells; the recognition of the vital importance of maintaining this compound in stored blood has made it possible to develop methods for prolonging red cell preservation and improving the quality of blood given to the patient. Research has also led to an understanding of metabolic disorders of the red cell, such as pyruvate kinase deficiency and of abnormalities like excessive permeability of the membrane to sodium and potassium. But perhaps the greatest contribution of red cell research has been in the understanding and prevention of the various anemias, diseases characterized by abnormally low concentrations of functioning red cells in the bloodstream.

Infectious disease was the primary cause of anemia worldwide until the early twentieth century. Tuberculosis, malaria, and schistosomiasis, each in a different way, may produce profound anemia. Although these diseases are generally under control in the developed countries, they remain major health problems in many areas of the world today.

In the United States, with the gradual disappearance of the infectious diseases that could cause anemia, attention turned in the 1920s and 1930s to the study of anemia resulting from nutritional deficiency. Iron deficiency, which had been established as a cause of anemia for over a century, was intensively investigated; many different causes of iron deficiency were identified and characterized. But real conceptual breakthroughs came from the investigation of pernicious anemia.

Pernicious anemia, a disorder seen mostly in northern Europeans, damages the nervous system and is fatal if untreated. George R. Minot and William P. Murphy, working in the Thorndike Memorial Laboratory of the Boston City Hospital and the Peter Bent Brigham Hospital, discovered that this disease could be effectively treated with a diet of liver. Further investigation showed that liver contained a specific therapeutic ingredient, vitamin B_{12}. William B. Castle followed the work of Minot and Murphy by examining the mechanism by which vitamin B_{12} is absorbed in the small bowel; he found that a substance called intrinsic factor, produced in the stomach, was necessary to this process. The resulting study of the mechanisms by which intrinsic factor and vitamin B_{12} affect bone marrow function signaled the introduction of physiological and biochemical techniques into hematologic research. These approaches have been essential to the understanding and treatment of many types of blood disorders.

One of the most important applications of biochemical techniques was the study of sickle-cell anemia (see Chapter 4). This serious disease results from an inherited abnormality in the red blood cells; under certain conditions, these abnormal cells become sickle-shaped and cannot function properly. As a result, the individual suffers acute attacks of pain, and many of the body's organs may be damaged (Figure 15-1). Once sickle-cell anemia was known to result from abnormalities in the hemoglobin molecule itself (rather than in the red cell membrane), Linus Pauling and his coworkers undertook the biochemical study of sickle hemoglobin. Through years of research by Pauling and others, and particularly by Vernon Ingram at the Massachusetts Institute of Technology, the disorder in sickle hemoglobin was finally traced to the presence of one incorrect amino acid at a crucial spot in the hemoglobin molecule; this molecular error makes sickle hemoglobin relatively insoluble, especially when it is not carrying oxygen. Basic research into sickle-cell anemia continues and is especially directed at methods of treatment and cure;

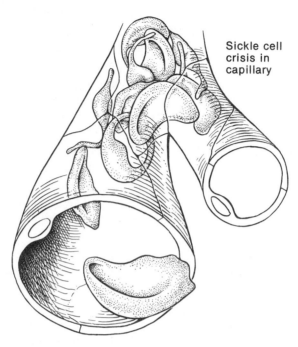

Sickle cell
crisis in
capillary

Figure 15–1. Sickle-cell crisis in a capillary. The sickle-shaped blood cells are unable to travel through the small blood vessels like normal cells. Instead they bunch together, as shown here, and blood flow through the body is disrupted.

since the 1960s, a national program for the study of this disease has been carried out by the National Institutes of Health. Some very encouraging progress has been made. Recently, new techniques have been developed that may make it possible to detect sickle-cell anemia prenatally in the fetus. (Similar methods have been utilized for the prenatal diagnosis of Cooley's anemia, another inherited disorder of hemoglobin that can have severe consequences.)

Both vitamin B_{12} and sickle hemoglobin were finally understood through the use of basic research techniques to investigate a specific disease that was already being studied clinically. Other breakthroughs have come through the application to clinical problems of previously available knowledge from basic research. Probably the greatest triumph of this type of approach has been the development of treatments for erythroblastosis fetalis, or Rh disease of the newborn.

Rh is a factor in the human red cell membrane. Most individuals have Rh in their red cells and are called Rh positive; some, however, lack it and are Rh negative. When an Rh negative mother carries an Rh-positive fetus, a few of the fetal cells may find their way into the maternal circulation and stimulate Rh antibodies; these antibodies may then cross the placenta into the fetus and destroy its Rh-positive red cells. This severe destruction releases an immense amount of hemoglobin, much of which is broken down into a compound called bilirubin that causes brain damage in the fetus. Since about 10 percent of the population is Rh-negative, erythroblastosis fetalis was a serious problem until an effective therapy was developed.

The problem in treating and preventing Rh disease was to find a means of preventing the immune response of the mother to fetal cells. Through basic animal studies, researchers had already developed the concept of antibody suppression, a technique for interrupting the natural immune response to a substance by giving the animal antibodies to that substance. This basic concept was applied to the treatment of Rh disease; through clinical trials, it became possible to prevent the immune reaction that causes Rh disease by giving the mother specific human antibodies (immune globulins). Where this procedure is inapplicable or ineffective, the fetus or newborn infant can be transfused with Rh-negative blood (which is unaffected by Rh-positive antibodies). Thanks to these two methods of preventive treatment, erythroblastosis fetalis, once a major public health problem, has been virtually eradicated.

Granulocyte Function

As biochemical and biophysical studies of the red cells became increasingly productive, attention began to turn to the class of white cells known as granulocytes. Of special interest have been the mechanisms by which these mysterious cells locate and kill bacteria. Apparently granulocytes move toward their prey by using a system of contractile proteins very similar to those found in the muscle; they kill the bacteria with hydrogen peroxide after they have found them and ingested them. Chronic granulomatous disease, a rare hereditary disorder of childhood, is associated with deficient hydrogen peroxide production by granulocytes; the granulocytes of individuals with this disease can ingest bacteria but not kill them. Further study of this illness should clarify the mechanisms by which this type of white cell normally produces the toxic chemicals essential to its function.

One aspect of granulocyte activity remains very mysterious, however: how does the cell locate the bacteria it is to destroy in the first place?

It is thought that each bacterium sends out some sort of chemical signal which stimulates the granulocyte to move in its direction. This type of process, known as chemotaxis, is still very poorly understood. Poor transmission of chemotactic signals in certain individuals may result in increased susceptibility to infection; however, this is still a theoretical speculation.

Bleeding Disorders

The biochemical mechanism of human blood coagulation, initiated by the platelets, is too complex a chain of reactions to be described here in detail. This very complexity made bleeding disorders extremely difficult to treat for many years. Recently, however, research has opened new avenues for the treatment of several of them.

Hemophilia is a hereditary disease (see Chapter 4) that is best known for its affliction of Queen Victoria's descendents, including the last tsarevich of Russia; it remains the commonest of the hereditary bleeding disorders today. It has been known for some time that hemophilia results from an inherited inability to produce Factor VIII, a substance essential to blood clotting. The past few years have brought enormous advances in our understanding of biochemical aspects of the production, structure, and function of this molecule. Especially important has been the development of methods for concentrating Factor VIII from plasma; these concentrates have for the first time made it possible to perform major surgery in hemophiliacs. Also under study are methods for storing Factor VIII in a dried form that can be made available to hemophiliacs. In certain patients Factor VIII can be injected regularly to prevent the painful joint bleeding that is so common in this disease. A remaining problem is that the supply of Factor VIII is limited, so that all patients cannot yet be treated regularly with it.

Hemorrhagic disease of the newborn, characterized by spontaneous internal or external bleeding between the third and sixth days of life, was a major cause of infant mortality until its etiology was clarified. It is now known that this disease is caused by a deficiency of vitamin K, a fat-soluble vitamin essential to the synthesis of prothrombin and other vital proteins which induce the plasma clotting mechanism. Routien treatment of newborns with Vitamin K has virtually eradicated this disease in the United States.

Platelet deficiency characterizes certain immunologic disorders in which platelets are rapidly removed from circulation and diseases of the marrow in which platelet production ceases (for example, leukemia and aplastic anemia). Modern techniques of bloodbanking have made it possible to treat, but not cure, these conditions through platelet transfusion. Several types of congenital abnormalities in platelet function are being studied; in some individuals, certain common drugs, such as aspirin, can dangerously interfere with the accumulation and agglutination of platelets in damaged blood vessels. Further identification and investigation of such hereditary disorders should increase our knowledge of normal platelet function as well as facilitate treatment for the individuals affected.

Future Hematologic Research

Assigning priorities to different research approaches to the blood diseases is a difficult and controversial task. Not least among the many factors which must be taken into account are the ethical and legal issues involved in human experimentation. Because of the relative ease of drawing blood from subjects, hematologists have been able to do research on human subjects more easily than investigators in most areas of medicine. And many effective therapeutic procedures—including bone marrow transplantation, leukemia chemotherapy, granulocyte and platelet transfusion, and the use of coagulating agents—have been developed through experimental treatment programs using subjects likely to benefit from these innovative techniques. Much more controversial, however, is the use of human subjects who will not themselves be benefited by the research being done but who are essential to the success of a given research program. For example, techniques for the prenatal diagnosis of hemoglobin disorders cannot be perfected without comparative studies of normal fetuses at similar stages of development. The ethical and legal problems involved in the nontherapeutic use of human subjects are sensitive issues, and human research is now carefully restricted. Much essential research can be carried on in accordance with the regulations that exist, but effective development of certain methods for prenatal diagnosis has been hampered and delayed.

At least as important as these ethical issues is the evaluation of the possible benefit to be gained from a given area of research. To begin with, one naturally asks whether clinical or basic research is more likely to yield a solution to a given medical problem. But in hematologic research (as in many areas of medical research) there is often no clear-cut answer to this question. The most crippling of the red cell disorders—pernicious anemia, sickle-cell anemia, and Rh disease—were all understood through the careful integration of clinical and basic research approaches. Neither approach alone would have been able to solve the problems posed by these diseases.

Just as different levels of research are necessary, so may complementary research in different areas be essential to the understanding of the various blood disorders. Future developments in hematology will certainly come from a research approach that integrates clinical medicine with genetics, molecular biology, biochemistry, and physiology. The prenatal diagnosis of genetic blood disorders like sickle-cell anemia and Cooley's anemia is a major research priority. Biochemists and molecular biologists will continue to study the specific proteins involved in coagulation and the role those proteins play in thrombosis (abnormal clotting within the heart or blood vessels) and hardening of the arteries. And physiologists will be required to perfect the technique of marrow transplantation, which could be of enormous benefit in the treatment of congenital blood disorders, leukemia, and aplastic anemia. Very recently, hematology has begun to benefit from the participation of specialists in yet another discipline: engineering. Diagnosis of blood disorders has been facilitated by instruments that can rapidly count the number of different types of cells in blood samples; and machines that separate white cells from blood and return red cells and plasma protein to the donor have decreased the risk of infection for patients receiving white cell transfusions.

A truly interdisciplinary approach is necessary, both to increase our theoretical understanding of the blood disorders and to enhance the hematologist's clinical effectiveness.

The Gastrointestinal System

KURT J. ISSELBACHER

16

Gastrointestinal disorders are among the most common, the most distressing, and the most costly of all illnesses. One out of every nine Americans has suffered from a chronic or recurrent digestive ailment, while one third of all patients undergoing surgery other than tonsil removal and normal obstetrical delivery is operated on for a digestive disorder. Although gastrointestinal diseases are more often chronic than fatal, they account for nearly one out of every ten deaths in the United States; more than half of these deaths are caused by cancer of the digestive organs. The economic cost of digestive disease is also enormous and is continually increasing. The annual cost of treating these disorders increased from 12.5 billion dollars in 1968 to 16.5 billion in 1973, with about a quarter of these funds going to treat cancer of the digestive system.

Digestion is a complex process that occurs in several stages. It begins with the breakdown of food by hydrochloric acid secreted in the stomach, sodium bicarbonate and enzymes produced by the pancreas, and bile from the liver. Digestion is completed in the small intestine, and nutrients are absorbed into the bloodstream through the intestinal walls. This process of absorption is concluded in the large intestine, or colon, which also regulates fecal elimination. Just as it performs many different functions, the gastrointestinal system is subject to several kinds of disease. The secretion of acid and digestive enzymes is normally controlled by a complicated hormonal feedback system to ensure that these substances are produced in proportion to the amount and type of food in the digestive tract; if this feedback system malfunctions, these chemicals may be excessively or insufficiently produced, with dangerous results. Toxic agents ingested orally, such as certain types of chemicals and alcohol, may have especially devastating effects on the digestive organs. And, like all other organ systems, the gastrointestinal system may be damaged by infection or cancer. All these factors contribute to the high incidence of digestive disease seen in the United States every year.

Disorders in the Secretion of Digestive Acids and Enzymes

Peptic ulcers are very common; they occur in 8 to 12 percent of our adult population. Such ulcers affect both the stomach and a portion of the intestine just beyond the stomach called the duodenum. They begin when hydrochloric acid production increases or when the stomach's or duodenum's resistance to acid decreases; either of these changes can lead to destruction of surface tissue and finally to ulceration of these organs. Considerable progress has been made in understanding what controls the secretion of hydrochloric acid. One of the notable achievements in this century has been the identification of the hormone gastrin, the chemical agent whose release leads to increased acid production. Histamine, a chemical that plays a central role in inflammation, has also been found to stimulate the production of acid by the stomach. Many researchers are now trying to discover the biochemical mechanism by which these substances induce acid secretion and are working to develop drugs that can inhibit such secretions; for example, antihistamines similar in many ways to those used in treating the common cold have recently been studied for their possible use in the treatment of ulcers. The complex regulatory role of the nervous system in gastrin release is another very important area for future research. Many investigators are studying the nature of the stomach's remarkable native resistance to ulceration and the ways in which this may be affected by alcohol, pain-relieving drugs, excessive smoking, and—perhaps most important—by psychological stress. Finally, the possible role of genetic factors in the causation of peptic ulcers is being examined.

A process of self-digestion similar to that which causes ulceration in the stomach and duodenum may also occur in the pancreas. When this organ is damaged, it may release increased amounts of its powerful digestive enzymes; these enzymes, in turn, can cause more destruction to the pancreas itself, leading to serious, chronic pancreatitis. We still need to discover how pancreatitis is produced initially and how it can be prevented from becoming chronic. At present, two common causes of the initial damage leading to this disease seem to be excessive alcohol intake and gallstones.

Gallstones themselves are formed as the result of another type of error in the production of the digestive juices. Here, however, the disorder is not one of overproduction, but of the liver's underproduction of certain bile components. The scientific understanding of gallstone formation began only ten years ago, when new chemical methods for studying the constituents of the bile were developed. Thanks to a concentrated research effort, we now know that most gallstones are formed when cholesterol crystallizes out of the bile in the liver's ducts or the gallbladder. There are two components of bile, namely the bile salts and certain kinds of fats known as phospholipids, which normally keep cholesterol in solution. When the proportion of cholesterol to the other two substances increases, cholesterol will tend to come out of solution and crystallize into gallstones. Our understanding of this process has led to the development of techniques for dissolving gallstones with certain forms of bile acids. An extensive national cooperative study is under way to study the problems of dosage and duration of treatment in this type of therapy and to bring these new advances to the American public in a safe and effective manner. Gallstones, which presently affect between 10 and 12 million Americans annually, constitute a major public health problem.

Adverse Reactions to Digested Material

Since it is the first of the body's organ systems to come into contact with food, drink, and drugs taken by mouth, the gastrointestinal system may be the first to be damaged by these substances. Perhaps the most vulnerable organ is the liver, which serves the function of eliminating toxic materials from the body. Some of the substances with which we come into contact, such as food additives, drugs, chemicals, and anesthetics, may damage the liver during its attempts to render them harmless; certain people may suffer serious liver disease resulting from allergic reactions to these materials. Our understanding of the biochemical nature of such reactions is still very incomplete. Much more is known about liver damage resulting from chronic alcohol use.

Alcohol can damage other organs of the digestive tract besides the liver; excessive drinking may be a causative factor in chronic pancreatitis, and alcohol can interfere with the absorption of nutrients by the intestine, leading to impaired nutrition. But its effects on the liver are probably the most dangerous consequences of chronic alcohol intake. Cirrhosis (scarring) of the liver is the seventh leading cause of death in the United States; and alcoholism is one of the major causes of cirrhosis of the liver. While it was once thought that a proper diet would protect the heavy drinker from liver damage, this is now known to be false; in fact, it appears that anyone who drinks excessively over a sufficient period of time runs a high risk of liver cirrhosis.

This scarring is dangerous because it leads to changes in the blood circulation; the resulting detours in the blood supply can have many devastating, life-threatening consequences. Since the essential component of these scars is the protein known as collagen, much research has focused on finding ways to interfere with the deposition of collagen on the liver or to dissolve it once it has deposited. However, much more work is necessary before these investigations can begin to yield clinically applicable results.

Infectious Diseases of the Gastrointestinal System

Liver disease may also result from different kinds of viral infections. Hepatitis, or inflammation of the liver, is a serious disorder that often leads to chronic liver disease and cirrhosis. Recent research has shown that there are actually at least two different types of viral hepatitis, and that each of these is caused by a different virus; hepatitis A virus is responsible for infectious hepatitis, while serum hepatitis is caused by a virus known as hepatitis B. (There may also be a third type of viral hepatitis, nonA nonB; see Chapter 6.) The identification of the A and B viruses has been an essential first step in the control of hepatitis. Tests have already been developed to detect the presence of hepatitis B in the blood; these tests can be used to screen blood donors and thus minimize the risk of transmission of serum hepatitis in blood transfusions. And there is every indication that vaccines will be developed in the next five years for the prevention of type A and type B viral hepatitis. If such vaccines could be administered routinely in youth (as polio vaccines are given now), the incidence of hepatitis could be drastically reduced.

Interestingly enough, the enormous progress that has recently been made in our understanding of hepatitis began with the work of a geneticist who was not initially investigating the disease at all but who was energetically studying certain blood constituents in a tribe of Australian aborigines. His discovery of the hepatitis viruses was a totally unexpected result of this work. Such fortuitous discoveries often happen in science and medicine, frequently with major benefits to society, and are a testimony to the value of basic research in fundamental biology, chemistry, and related fields.

Such basic research has also been important recently in improving our understanding of diarrhea and related disorders. While most of us only know of diarrhea as an annoyance, it can become a serious medical problem; diarrheal diseases are the world's leading cause of infant mortality and a major cause of disability for the military of all countries. The fact that these illnesses can have many different causes has made them especially difficult to study. But recently, our knowledge of diarrhea has been greatly augmented by American research into the biochemistry of cholera.

Although cholera is virtually unknown in the United States, research into this disease has had immediate benefit for Americans. Studies of the toxin produced by the cholera organism have greatly expanded our understanding of the way in which fluids are absorbed and secreted by the intestine. Moreover, the mechanism by which the cholera toxin disrupts these functions seems to be very similar to the process causing many forms of diarrhea that are seen in the United States. It is now certain, for example, that "traveler's diarrhea" is due largely to toxins produced by a variant of one type of bacterium commonly found in the intestinal tract; these toxins cause the intestine to secrete water, salt, and other substances. Further study may lead to the development of oral vaccines against some of these bacterial infections.

Meanwhile, other approaches to the treatment of diarrhea are being investigated. Another offshoot of cholera research has been the development of a simple and effective method for treating diarrhea by replacing the body's fluids orally (rather than intravenously); this has now become a standard clinical procedure. And in the past three years, several hormones causing intestinal secretion have been identified. These hormones, which are produced by the stomach, the pancreas, and the intestine itself, can be triggered by states of abnormal stress, especially in association with certain malignancies. As we learn more about these substances, it may become possible to control diarrhea by altering the action of these hormones directly.

Gastrointestinal Cancer

While everyone is aware of the medical problem and personal threat posed by cancer in general, few realize that fully 30 percent of all cancer deaths are caused by cancer of the digestive tract. It is obvious that gastrointestinal cancer must therefore be a subject of major and immediate medical concern. Fortunately, recent work has begun to break some important new ground in the understanding and treatment of this prevalent type of cancer.

One theory of cancer holds that the disease is caused primarily by a malfunction of the immunological system. Many researchers believe that cancer cells are always arising spontaneously within the body but that a normally functioning immune system is able to recognize those cells as "foreign" and destroy them before a malignancy develops. There is now increasing evidence that gastrointestinal cancer may be related to an immunological abnormality that allows cancer cells to grow. Inflammation, which is itself an immunological problem, is a common precursor to cancer of the digestive tract. Ulcerative colitis, a chronic and debilitating type of inflammation that primarily affects young people, may be followed by cancer of the colon; gastritis is found to precede stomach cancer; and celiac disease (intestinal intolerance to the protein gluten) may be complicated by the later development of intestinal malignancy. As the relationship of these inflammatory disorders to the later development of cancer is clarified, our ability to prevent these kinds of cancer is certain to improve.

Cancer prevention may also be facilitated by the development of blood tests for the early detection of gastrointestinal cancer. Abnormal blood proteins are known to accompany cancer of the intestine and to disappear when the malignancy is removed. Tests to detect these abnormal proteins have already been developed, and it is hoped that a similar blood test for cancer of the pancreas will be devised in the near future. Early detection is essential in pancreatic cancer, since this disease usually does not produce noticeable symptoms until it has progressed well beyond the point where it can be cured. Moreover, because cancer of the pancreas has been increasing in incidence (for reasons that remain unclear), its immediate control is now all the more desirable.

The Future of Gastrointestinal Research

Recent advances have opened whole new areas in the prevention, diagnosis, and treatment of gastrointestinal disorders.

Several investigators have begun to examine the possible role of dietary fiber (roughage in the diet) in the causation of certain types of digestive diseases. The low fiber content of a typical Westerner's diet appears to slow down the movement of food through the intestinal tract.

Some have hypothesized that this low rate of intestinal transport may allow potential carcinogenic agents to remain in contact with the surface cells of the colon for a prolonged period of time, thus making the individual more susceptible to cancer of the colon (see Chapter 3). Low dietary fiber content has also been suspected as a causative factor in such common ailments as hiatus hernia, appendicitis, and outpocketing of the colon (diverticula). The importance of dietary fiber is a provocative subject that may have great implications for preventive medicine.

The diagnosis of gastrointestinal disease has been revolutionized by the development of fiberoptic instruments. These flexible bundles of light-carrying glass or quartz fibers can actually be used to examine almost the entire intestinal tract directly. The fiberoptic probe that carries a visual image of the intestine outside the body can also be equipped with instruments that allow the physician to take fluid and tissue samples or remove small lesions while examining the intestine visually. Fiberoptic instruments have brought about tremendous advances in the early diagnosis of diseases of the esophagus, stomach, duodenum, bile ducts, and colon; they have also made it possible to detect gastrointestinal cancer much earlier than could be done before (Figure 16-1).

In the future, it may become possible to insert fiberoptic instruments directly into the abdominal cavity through a small incision to visualize the contents of the abdomen and probe organs that still cannot be readily viewed by this technique, such as the liver and gallbladder. The pancreas, which lies deep in the abdomen, has been virtually inaccessible to study in the past; but fiberoptics and new X-ray technology have made it possible to examine even this hidden organ. The physician can now determine the size of the pancreas, locate damaged areas and tumors on the organ, and outline the pancreatic ducts, which secrete its important enzymes. As they are further refined in the future, the new methods for visual diagnosis will doubtless become even more widely used.

Technological innovations will probably make major surgery for gastrointestinal disorders increasingly unnecessary. Already, surgery can often be avoided through the use of fiberoptic techniques; one main advantage of this approach is that it does not require hospitalization and can be done on an outpatient basis. The use of lasers to stop gastrointestinal bleeding by coagulating the blood vessels is also being investigated; it seems likely that lasers will be used in the near future to treat bleeding ulcers or bleeding areas in the stomach. When surgery is inevitable, intravenous alimentation (intravenous nutrition) can assure that the patient is well nourished before undergoing surgery and can facilitate

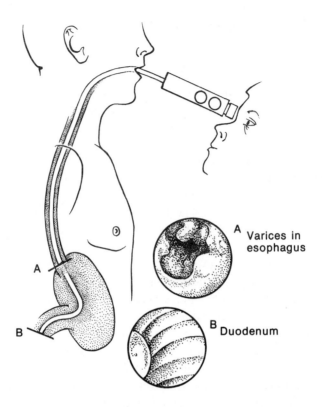

Figure 16–1. The use of a fiberoptic probe. The physician inserts the fiberoptic tube down the patient's throat and into the gastrointestinal tract. Light travels directly up the fiberoptic tube to the eyepiece to give a direct view of the inside of the patient's gastrointestinal tract. With the probe stopped at point A, as it is in this drawing, the physician could examine the patient's esophagus. The upper insert is taken from a photograph of a fiberoptic image of the esophagus; it shows an esophagus with varices (dilated and tortuous veins). Lowering the probe to point B enables the doctor to examine the duodenum; if the patient's duodenum were normal, he would see an image like that shown in the lower insert.

the recovery from digestive disease. Thanks to special techniques for introducing solutions of sugars and amino acids into large blood vessels, it has become possible in the past decade to maintain patients for prolonged periods of time on intravenous diets averaging 4,000 calories per day.

Intravenous nutrition, in fact, has advanced to the point where it is a major treatment method in its own right, as well as being an important aid in surgery. In people with severe intestinal inflammation, intravenous alimentation can be used to bypass the intestine entirely until it has functionally recovered. This technique is even applicable to patients with chronic disease; they can now be fed intravenously for a period of years, much as individuals suffering from kidney failure can be maintained on dialysis. Just recently, techniques for the safe intravenous administration of fats have been developed, and patients can now be maintained on intravenous alimentation for even longer periods of time. The so-called "artificial gut" has already saved many lives and has proven a revolutionary development of gastrointestinal and nutritional research.

While these major technological advances have improved the treatment of all kinds of gastrointestinal disorders, equally impressive results have come from the careful study of specific diseases. Great strides are being made in the treatment of liver disease. It is very likely that preventive vaccines against the major hepatitis viruses will be developed within the next year or two. The pancreatic hormones insulin and glucagon may be used to speed the regeneration of liver tissue that has been damaged by disease (like severe hepatitis); and researchers are investigating ways to prevent or dissolve the scar tissue which is responsible for cirrhosis of the liver. Agents are being developed to dissolve gallstones without surgical intervention. Recent clinical trials suggest that peptic ulcers may be treated by drugs that block the tissue response to histamine, a substance that plays a key role in inflammation (see Chapter 7); apparently these drugs stop the production of acid in the stomach. Even the inflammatory bowel diseases, which are still a major clinical problem, may soon be treated by drug therapy.

Basic and applied research, aimed both at improving medical technology and increasing the understanding of specific disorders, has already greatly improved the control of gastrointestinal disease. If present trends are any indication, there is every reason to hope that our ability to diagnose and treat these serious illnesses will continue to improve in the future.

Diabetes

GEORGE F. CAHILL, JR.

17

Our knowledge of diabetes dates back thousands of years; ancient Egyptians and scholars in India described it as a disease associated with copious urination. The discovery that this urine contained large quantities of a sugar (glucose) led the Roman physician Aretaeus to label the disorder diabetes mellitus; "diabetes" is the Greek word for "siphon," and "mellitus" is a Latin adjective meaning "like honey." The Indians were aware of the hereditary nature of the disease, as they were of the two general forms that diabetes takes. The first, now known as maturity-onset type diabetes, was characterized as being associated with "torpor, indolence and corpulence"; the juvenile type, in contrast, was accurately identified by its effect of metabolic starvation, or, in Aretaeus' words, the "melting down of the flesh into sweet urine."

In the late 1800s, German scientists found that surgical removal of the pancreas, the principal digestive gland of the intestine, produced a state resembling diabetes in the dog. This finding suggested that some malfunction of the pancreas might be responsible for the spontaneous occurrence of diabetes in people. At the turn of the century an American pathologist, E. L. Opie, discovered that the disease was in fact associated with a disturbance in the beta cells, which are found clustered together in tiny islets of tissue scattered throughout the pancreas (Figure 17-1). The real breakthrough came in 1921, when the young Toronto surgeon, Frederick Banting, and his medical-student assistant, Charles Best, used these new discoveries to develop a method of treatment for diabetes. Working through the summer on a nonexistent budget, in a laboratory

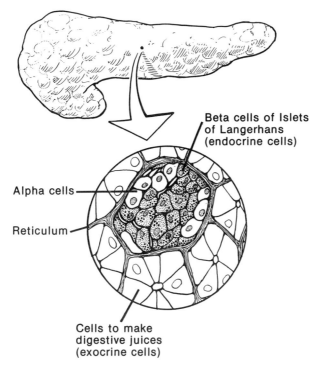

Figure 17–1. The pancreas and an islet with beta cells. The beta cells contain small crystals of insulin, shown here as dots.

loaned to them temporarily by a vacationing professor, these two researchers were able to prepare extracts of pancreas that actually lowered the glucose level of diabetic dogs. Within months, this extract was made available for human use under the names it still bears today: iletin and insulin. It proved a lifesaver. Diabetic children who were wasting away through metabolic starvation regained strength days after they began to take the pancreatic extract. For a while it seemed that the problem posed by diabetes mellitus had been solved.

But in the 1940s and 1950s, it became all too clear that this was far from the case. By this time, many of the children whose lives had been saved by insulin had grown up and were in their thirties and forties; they had already been kept alive by insulin injections for many years. The vast majority of these patients were now plagued by complications of diabetes mellitus. These complications had rarely been seen in juvenile diabetics before the advent of insulin, as most of the children affected had died before the complications had had a chance to develop. But now the complications began to be a much greater problem than the threat of immediate death, which could easily be prevented by insulin therapy.

The complications of diabetes remain the major threat to diabetics today. Half of all juvenile diabetics now alive are expected to die of kidney failure, while 10 to 20 percent will probably become blind. Maturity-onset diabetics can also expect to suffer from complications affecting the retina or the kidney, although to a lesser degree than juvenile diabetics; they may also develop disorders of the peripheral nerves. Diabetes, especially the maturity-onset type, is associated with accelerated atherosclerosis; it doubles the risk for stroke and increases the probability of death due to heart attack two to three times. Diabetics are also especially subject to problems affecting peripheral blood vessels, particularly in the feet, where gangrene and infection readily develop; they experience these disorders fifty times more often than do nondiabetics. All these factors combine to make the life expectancy of the diabetic only two thirds that of the normal individual.

These statistics would be bad enough if diabetes were restricted to a tiny fraction of the population; but in fact it may affect as many as 10 million people within the United States alone. Diabetes still kills several hundred thousand annually, as well as being the leading cause of new blindness in this country.

Since the time of Banting and Best, a great deal of research has been focused on the metabolic role of insulin both in healthy people and in diabetics. To understand the complex factors leading to the development of diabetes, one must first be familiar with the normal action of insulin in the body.

The Function of Insulin

Insulin, in simplest terms, is the hormone that controls the body's storage and mobilization of fuels taken in as food to ensure that these fuels are maintained at relatively constant levels in the bloodstream. The synthesis, storage, and release of insulin are mediated by the beta cells of the pancreas.

When a normal person eats, chemical substances capable of stimulating the beta cells are sent out from the intestinal wall. These chemicals (which have not yet been identified) are apparently released in proportion to the amount of food eaten; the larger the meal, the more the beta cells will be sensitized to release insulin into the bloodstream, particularly as levels of glucose and amino acids increase. Once released into the blood, insulin remains there for only a few minutes, due to its rapid removal by certain tissues. During that time, it performs the essential function of signaling the body's tissues to store the fuels from the meal that has just been eaten. Insulin stimulates liver tissue to store circulating glucose as glycogen or as fat; the fat synthesized by the liver is then released and circulates in the bloodstream in small droplets, along with fat ingested as food. Insulin signals fat tissue throughout the body to remove these droplets from the blood and store them, thus preventing their dangerous accumulation in the walls of the blood vessels. Muscle tissue also stores circulating glucose, although it may use some of this sugar for immediate energy; for example, glucose is the sole fuel used by heart muscle after a carbohydrate-containing meal. Finally, circulating insulin levels help control the replenishment of muscle protein, which is synthesized from amino acids circulating in the bloodstream.

When a person is not eating, blood levels of glucose and amino acids fall, the intestine sends out no chemical signals to the beta cells, and insulin levels in the bloodstream decrease. The relative absence of insulin serves to signal the liver, muscle, and fat tissues to mobilize the fuels that they stored after the body's last meal. The liberation of these fuels is essential to life; the brain gets all its energy from glucose and requires 100 to 150 grams of this sugar daily whether one is eating or not. Low insulin levels signal the liver to produce glucose from its stored fuels to meet this basic energy requirement; they also signal the release of fat from the fat tissue, so that various tissues, such as the heart muscle, can use fat as a fuel instead of glucose. Some of the fat is also broken down by the liver into organic acids known as ketones, ketone bodies, or keto-acids; these also serve as fuel for muscle, and, with prolonged starvation, for the brain as well.

The normal individual alternates between two metabolic states: the fed state, characterized by high levels of circulating insulin, and the fasted state, characterized by low insulin levels. But what about the abnormal individual? What are the consequences of disorders in the complex systems that regulate the synthesis and release of insulin? The most frequent consequences are the diverse illnesses grouped together as diabetes mellitus.

The Etiology of Diabetes Mellitus

While diabetes may take many forms, they all have one thing in common: all are characterized by an absolute or relative deficiency in insulin. The abnormally low levels of insulin seen in this disease make it impossible for the beta cells to signal the body's tissues to store fuels, particularly glucose; thus diabetic glucose levels rise higher than normal and remain elevated for extended periods of time. In mild insulin deficiency, fasting levels of glucose may be normal, with elevated glucose appearing only after a meal or a test dosage of sugar. But with more severe degrees of deficiency, even the basal insulin needs of the fasting state may not be met. In such serious cases the fasting glucose level may rise above the concentration at which the kidneys can retain glucose, particularly after meals; the sugar then spills over into the urine and is excreted, while the liver, signaled by the body's low insulin levels, makes more and more glucose at the expense of the body's protein. This is the basis for the process of metabolic starvation that can cause the "melting of the flesh into sweet urine"; it is a dangerous process, made worse by the dehydration and loss of minerals that accompany such voluminous urination. In these markedly insulin-deficient states, too, the liver's production of ketoacids from fats reaches a dangerously high level, resulting in acidosis. This entire clinical picture of insulin deficiency, which generally leads to a state of shock, is termed ketoacidosis, or diabetic coma. Before the advent of insulin therapy, it almost always ended in death.

The severity of the insulin deficiency found in diabetes correlates very well (although not absolutely) with the age of onset of the disease. Insulin-dependent or ketosis-prone diabetics, who suffer from severe insulin deficiency, first show the disease at an average age around the time of the adolescent growth spurt; for this reason, they are also called juvenile diabetics. Maturity-onset diabetics, in contrast, usually do not develop the disease until the fifth or sixth decade of life and suffer from insulin deficiencies that are generally less severe than those experienced by the juvenile diabetic. Although the maturity-onset diabetic may need injections of supplemental insulin, ketoacidosis and death will usually not occur if this exogenous insulin is withheld. Maturity-onset diabetics are also referred to as "stable" or insulin-independent.

Both juvenile and maturity-onset diabetes result from the inability of the beta cells to produce enough insulin for the body's needs. There is much evidence, however, to indicate that this failure of the beta cells has very different origins in the two different cases.

Clues to the nature of the beta cell dysfunction in juvenile diabetes have come from the study of the puzzling time course this disorder follows. The disease usually develops very rapidly, within days to weeks, and may result in ketoacidosis if not treated quickly. But once a diagnosis has been made and insulin therapy is given for a short period of time, the patient may continue for weeks or months with little or no need of additional injections. After this period of remission, the child may develop a type of diabetes similar to that seen in maturity-onset patients, with a single daily injection of insulin being sufficient to maintain normal glucose levels. This "honeymoon" phase of juvenile diabetes, as it has been termed by Priscilla White, can last for several years. Arthur Rubenstein and Donald Steiner in Chicago have shown that juvenile diabetics continue to produce reduced quantities of their own insulin during these periods. When the child reaches the age of sixteen or eighteen, his condition may worsen again. Glucose levels become much harder to control, even with two daily injections of insulin, and the patient runs a greater risk of developing the symptoms associated with glucose levels that are either too high or too low.

The rapid onset of juvenile diabetes has long suggested to researchers that a virus might be the direct cause of this disease. While anecdotal reports of cases of diabetes following mumps, measles, or even colds have been recorded for years, these observations found their first statistical support in the work of David Gamble and Keith Taylor. Studying juvenile diabetes in England in the mid-1960s, these investigators found that clusters of new cases often appeared in conjunction with Coxsackie B virus. Similar findings were reported in the United States in Buffalo and St. Petersburg. John Craighead, a virologist and pathologist in Burlington, Vermont, has further shown that a strain of encephalomyocarditis virus can cause acute diabetes in mice and even in some subhuman primates. All this evidence strongly suggests that a virus may be responsible for the initial attack on the beta cells in juvenile diabetes.

But if juvenile diabetes begins with a viral infection, then what is the explanation for the period of remission and the honeymoon phase? Apparently the initial infection only destroys some of the beta cells, yet sets in motion some sort of destructive process that eventually kills virtually all these cells. Much evidence suggests that juvenile diabetes may result from an immunological disorder like those described in Chapter 7; the beta cells may finally be killed by the patient's own immune system. Like hypersensitivity and other immunological disorders, juvenile diabetes is characterized by inflammation. The Belgian pathologist Willy Gepts analyzed two dozen autopsies of juvenile diabetics who died soon after developing the disease; in two thirds of these, inflammatory cells were found surrounding the beta cells. Individuals who are prone to autoimmune diseases (in which the body's defenses attack its own cells) also seem to run a higher than normal risk of contracting juvenile diabetes.

Research of the past few years has shown that this type of diabetes appears with unusually high frequency in families whose members have suffered from thyroid or adrenal failure traceable to antibodies directed against the tissues of those glands. More striking is the recent finding that many juvenile diabetics have antibodies against human pancreas tissue circulating in their blood. It is possible that the cells of juvenile diabetics are especially prone to destruction by such antibodies; juvenile diabetics may have abnormalities of the cell-surface antigens, which mediate such immune responses as the rejection of transplanted tissue. Workers in Canada, Liverpool, and Copenhagen have shown that certain types of these antigens are more prevalent in juvenile diabetics than in the general population. (The cell-surface antigens of maturity-onset type diabetics, in contrast, are indistinguishable from those of nondiabetics.) It is possible that these special surface antigens on the beta cells make them more susceptible to virus invasion or permit an autoimmune destructive process to begin after a viral attack.

Further understanding of the chain of events that follows viral infection in juvenile diabetes should make it possible to interrupt the process before the beta cells are destroyed. If certain viruses are found to be consistently associated with this disease, then prior immunization may be attempted. But since juvenile diabetes affects only about one in 6,000 children annually, prior immunization may prove less efficient than methods of intervening after the disease has been diagnosed but before large numbers of beta cells have died.

Any treatment aimed at replenishing the body's supply of beta cells will have serious difficulties, however, since beta cells have only a limited ability to replicate themselves. Unlike mature brain and muscle cells, beta cells can divide and reproduce, as shown by the electron microscope studies of the Boston pathologist Arthur A. Like; but unlike the cells of the blood and the skin, beta cells cannot replace themselves indefinitely. Beta cells must be strongly stimulated before they will divide. And John Logothetopoulos in Toronto, William Chick in Boston, and workers in Geneva and Sweden have all suggested that the beta cell is probably capable of only one or two divisions during its lifetime.

The poor replicating potential of the beta cell is not only a complicating factor in the treatment of juvenile diabetes; it may be the explanation for the development of maturity-onset diabetes as well. Unlike the beta cells of the juvenile diabetic, those of the maturity-onset diabetic often appear relatively normal, although they may be decreased in number. It appears that maturity-onset diabetes may be due not to an actual disease process attacking the beta cells but rather to an acceleration of the aging process in these cells leading to early cell death. Aging results in deficient beta cell function even in nondiabetics; most nonagenarians resemble diabetics in their deficient ability to metabolize glucose. Since beta cells are in limited supply, the aging and death of these cells result in their permanent loss.

What factors could cause the beta cells to be inadequate in maturity-onset diabetics? One factor could be obesity. Obesity increases the body's need for insulin, for reasons that are not yet entirely understood, and can stimulate beta cells to divide to meet that increased need. Among nondiabetics, fat people have more beta cells than thin people. Since beta cells are poor dividers, obesity, by causing a need for more insulin, may force the cells to use up the replicating potential that otherwise would be used to replace beta cells dying of old age. But many fat people do not become diabetic; therefore, other factors must be involved. At present, the most likely explanation seems to be that maturity-onset type diabetics suffer from a generalized deficiency in cellular replication. This concept has gained much support from the work of Samuel Goldstein, and of John Littlefield and Stuart Soeldner, who has shown that skin cells from diabetics age more rapidly in tissue culture than do cells from nondiabetics grown under identical conditions.

One would expect that such a generalized defect in the ability of cells to divide would be hereditary; and indeed, maturity-onset type diabetes does seem to be genetically determined. Marise Gottlieb and the late Howard Root found that the identical twins of maturity-onset diabetics almost always developed the disease; since this was not true for fraternal twins of diabetics, this correlation must be due to genetic rather than to environmental factors. Interestingly, juvenile diabetes was *not* found to be genetically determined to the same extent as the maturity-onset type; only half of the identical twins of juvenile diabetics also suffered from the disease. The English researchers Robert Tattersall and David Pyke further discovered that all the twins of juvenile diabetics who did become diabetic did so within two to three years of the onset of the first twin's disease. These findings suggest that both genetic and environmental factors are basic to the etiology of juvenile diabetes. This is consistent with the concept that juvenile diabetes is initiated by viral infection but only develops in individuals genetically predisposed to certain types of autoimmune disease.

While the problem of the etiology of diabetes is extremely complex, theoretical explanations of the initiation and progress of this disease are beginning to emerge. Current research efforts in Boston, St. Louis, Minneapolis, London, and elsewhere are directed to improving our understanding of the causes of diabetes so that better programs of prevention and early intervention may be designed.

The Complications of Diabetes

While the various complications of diabetes mellitus have been well characterized, their relationship to low insulin levels and high quantities of circulating glucose remains a subject of much debate. Are these complications a direct result of the diabetic's abnormal metabolism, or are they an independent expression of an underlying disease process that also affects the beta cells? This question is clearly of primary importance in devising treatment programs, and much research has attempted to answer it.

The changes seen in the small blood vessels in diabetes have been extensively studied, as they seem to underlie the eye and kidney disorders suffered by diabetics. It has been known for decades that a part of the blood vessel wall, the basement membrane, is thicker in diabetics than in nondiabetics; this was demonstrated conclusively by the late pathologist Paul Kimmelstiel. Recently, Joseph Williamson of St. Louis has found that this abnormal thickness is correlated with the duration and probably with the severity of the illness. The increased thickness of the blood vessel wall seems to be symptomatic of a disease process that results in the basement membrane becoming leakier and weaker; these pathological changes, in turn, eventually affect the functioning of the kidney and the eye. Workers in Knud Lundbaek's group in Aarhus, Denmark, have found that abnormalities in the filtering bed of the kidney, the glomerulus, appear within four or five years of the development of diabetes. In time, the capillaries of the glomerulus become increasingly leaky, and large portions of it are destroyed. Finally, the filtering bed becomes like a sieve that has lost most of its area and has had big holes punched in the remainder; it is totally unable to function as a filter, and the kidney fails as a result. In the eye, diabetes is accompanied by the formation of bubbles in the small blood vessels. When these rupture, they release blood into the retina, often leading to blindness unless this process is reversed. David Cogan and Toichi Kuwabara have noted that certain cells surrounding the blood vessels of the eye appear to die prematurely; this early cell senescence may also play a role in causing the eye disorders that accompany diabetes.

Although the small blood vessel changes seen in diabetes are still poorly understood, the evidence increasingly indicates that these pathological alterations are the direct result of insulin deficiency. Clinical observations have indicated that reductions in their abnormally high glucose levels diminish the rate and severity with which diabetics develop diseases of the retina and the kidney; these observations have been supported by very recent animal studies, in which accurate correction of elevated glucose levels in dogs and rats was shown to stop the development of complications in the kidney and eye. Researchers have begun to investigate the possible biochemical basis for the pathological effects of excess glucose on the small blood vessels. Robert and Mary Jane Spiro have shown that the blood vessel walls of the rat kidney undergo biochemical changes in diabetes; the enzymes that attach sugars to these walls become increasingly active when the rats are made diabetic, and return to their normal levels of functioning following insulin therapy. These studies offer some insight into the mechanism by which abnormal insulin and glucose levels may directly affect the small blood vessels.

The factors leading to the accelerated atherosclerosis that accompanies diabetes are less clear. The University Group Diabetes Project (UGPD) has established that alterations in glucose levels achieved through the application of insulin or of oral antidiabetic agents have little or no effect on the progression of atherosclerosis in the diabetic. What, then, could be the cause of this disorder? Three explanations have been proposed. The first is that the abnormally high circulating levels of fuels, particularly fats, may lead to accelerated incorporation of these substances into the blood vessel walls in diabetics. A second hypothesis is that alterations in the small blood vessels lead to increased leakage of proteins and fats in the blood vessel walls and hence to atherosclerosis. The final possibility, and perhaps the most interesting, is that the cells of the blood vessel walls may be subject to the same premature aging that affects the beta cells and may consequently suffer from early and progressive damage. Further research will be necessary to determine which of these three explanations comes closest to the truth.

Methods of Treatment

Much evidence suggests that the complications of diabetes, at least those affecting the kidney and the eye, could be theoretically prevented by normalizing insulin levels in the body. But the question of how those levels can best be controlled has been a subject of extensive debate since commercial preparations of insulin first became available. The problem, of course, is that injections of insulin cannot possibly match the exquisitely accurate feedback system that so precisely regulates glucose concentration in nondiabetic individuals. The situation of the diabetic receiving injections of insulin is analogous to that of a refrigerator in which the thermostat is broken and the cooler must be timed to run fifteen or twenty minutes out of each hour regardless of whether the machine is too hot or too cold; precise control simply becomes impossible.

In an attempt to overcome these inherent difficulties, certain physicians, particularly the late Elliott P. Joslin, urged juvenile diabetics to match their intake of food and insulin as precisely as possible; this meant weighing food, testing the urine for sugar several times daily, and maintaining a strict schedule of meals, exercise, and sleep. Joslin and his colleagues, who become known as advocates of "tight-control" treatment, claimed that their patients developed small blood vessel complications less severely and at a later time than did patients on less strict schedules. But many physicians have pointed out that great numbers of tight-control patients developed complications in spite of their rigid treatment schedules; thus the possible benefits of tight control may not actually outweigh the inconveniences of the treatment.

The basic problem seems to be that even tight-control patients may have to live with glucose levels that are almost twice the normal, since any attempt to lower sugar levels beyond this point runs the risk of overshooting the mark. Abnormally low glucose concentrations can pose just as immediate a threat as high concentrations, since the brain relies on glucose as its only source of fuel. When glucose levels start to fall below normal, adrenaline is released in defense, resulting in feelings of hunger, anxiety, and restlessness; as the levels continue to fall further, the patient may suffer confusion, unconsciousness, and even death. The dangers of the insulin reaction are perhaps the greatest hindrance to effectively lowering the glucose levels of the body to normal through insulin injection.

In spite of the problems associated with it, tight-control treatment still has its advocates; and there is some new evidence for its effectiveness. G. Tchoubroutsky in Paris has recently demonstrated through controlled experiments that precise regulation of blood glucose levels through multiple daily insulin injections and frequent testing of glucose levels does in fact slow down the progress of the retinal complications of diabetes.

Another approach to normalizing diabetic insulin levels has been the attempt to improve the beta cells' production of insulin. This is the purpose of the oral antidiabetic agents that have been used extensively in the treatment of maturity-onset diabetes. (These agents are not useful in the treatment of juvenile diabetes.) But the UGDP has found that these drugs may not only be ineffective but may actually be dangerous to patients using them over a long period of time. Nearly a decade of careful study in twelve hospitals and universities showed that patients using the oral antidiabetics phenethylbiguanide and tolbutamide were far more likely to die suddenly than were control patients receiving insulin therapy or placebos.

The UGDP study immediately became the subject of an intense controversy. First, the validity of the study was questioned. Previous studies, which had been smaller and less elegantly designed, had failed to find any increased mortality rates in patients taking oral antidiabetic drugs; and it was suggested that a statistical quirk might simply have put sicker patients into the group receiving these drugs than into the control group in the UGDP study. But for those who believed that the UGDP results had at least a good probability of being accurate, the study raised many more difficult questions. If these drugs were in fact dangerous, should they be banned completely? Or did their possible benefits justify their continued use in certain cases?

The questions raised were not limited to the use of tolbutamide and biguanide, since many other drugs currently in use and planned for future use could easily be found to be just as dangerous if accurate studies were done. Although such studies might yield vital information about many pharmacologic agents, the UGDP study alone cost about nine million dollars; who would pay the cost of studying every potentially harmful drug this thoroughly? In addition to money, time was also a problem. Long-term studies of drug effects take at least five to ten years; would this much delay in making proposed new drugs available cause more harm than good? Finally, the UGDP study highlighted the serious ethical issues involved in studying the effects of potentially dangerous drugs on human subjects. The patients studied, while technically maturity-onset diabetics, were symptom free; and many questioned whether these asymptomatic patients should have been receiving any therapy other than diet in the first place. The work of the UGDP thus became the focus of many issues in a raging debate between governmental regulatory agencies, researchers, practicing physicians, the pharmaceutical industry, and consumers.

Most knowledgeable researchers, including an expert panel of statisticians who reviewed the UGDP study, agree that its results were probably (although not certainly) valid. It also appears that the number of diabetic patients on oral drugs in the United States was definitely excessive. The best medical practice now seems to be to limit the use of these agents to patients with diabetic symptoms for whom dietary control is inadequate or ineffective and who could not easily be maintained on insulin therapy.

The UGDP study has clearly had a valuable impact. But many of the questions it raised remain, and professional opinion on these issues is still as divided as ever. One can only hope that new and better therapeutic approaches will soon make the problem of oral antidiabetic drugs a matter of past history.

Some success has already been achieved in circumventing the problem of controlling insulin levels by instead treating the complications of diabetes directly. Especially notable progress has been made in therapy for the complications of diabetes in the eye. As described earlier, retinal disorders begin in diabetics when the small blood vessels develop out-pocketings which burst and bleed. Intense light or laser beams can now be used to coagulate these lesions and prevent their bursting or spreading. Moreover, therapeutic coagulation of multiple scattered small areas throughout the eye in normal as well as diseased areas of the retina appears to inhibit the overall disease process. The long-term efficacy of this procedure has just been evaluated in a large-scale, multi-university study supported by the National Eye Institute; a significant improvement in treated eyes was observed when compared to untreated eyes.

Directions of Future Research

While the technique of photocoagulation is invaluable in many cases, it is not an ideal solution to the problem posed by the retinal complications of diabetes. The best solution to this and other complications would be some method of preventing them from developing in the first place. This has been the focus of much recent work that has just begun to yield positive results.

Since so many of the complications of diabetes appear to be directly related to increases in glucose levels, the direct effects of glucose on the body's tissues have been studied in the hope of developing methods of interfering with those glucose effects that lead to diabetic complications. Albert I. Winegrad in Philadelphia and Kenneth Gabbay in Boston have been investigating drugs and other agents that may be capable of inhibiting the effects of diabetes on various tissues, particularly nerve tissue. This research has led to experimental treatment methods that have proven effective in reversing damage of nerves to the extremities in diabetic rats, and it is possible that clinical trials of these techniques may be initiated in the near future.

The abnormally high levels of glucose found in diabetes originate because low insulin levels signal the liver to produce glucose and signal the tissues of the body to utilize the sugar inappropriately. If the action of insulin on body tissues could be understood, it might be possible to signal them artificially to store or burn glucose rather than liberate it. To this end, workers under Jesse Roth at the National Institutes of Health in Bethesda are intensively investigating the mechanism of the effect of insulin on the peripheral tissues, particularly focusing on its action on the cell membrane. This work may eventually yield very valuable results; but at present, it remains highly theoretical. Many researchers have chosen to tackle the more immediate problem of how to maintain insulin in the diabetic at approximately normal levels.

The most straightforward way to correct the pancreatic dysfunction seen in diabetes would be to replace the pancreas, and several research teams have investigated the possibility of transplanting this organ. Since 1966, about forty diabetics have received total or partial pancreas transplants. One of these has lived for over three years with normal levels of blood glucose following surgery by Marvin Gliedman and his team at Montefiore Hospital in New York. But there are multiple problems associated with these operations. In the first place, the digestive juices produced by the pancreas must be drained somewhere. (Gliedman solved this problem by draining them into the urinary system.) Second, as in any organ transplant, there is the strong likelihood that the pancreas tissue will be incompatible with the patient's immune system and will be rejected. So far, pancreas transplants have been performed only in diabetics who had previously received kidney transplants and were already receiving immunosuppressive treatments. Finally, surgeons must deal with the problem of finding donors while they are still alive. Most of the organs used in these operations were donated by patients dying of brain tumors or extensive injuries. Clearly, any attempt to perform a pancreas transplant poses tremendous logistic problems.

Other researchers have investigated the therapeutic possibilities of injection of beta cells, in an attempt to avoid some of the problems associated with whole organ transplantation. The late Arnold Lazarow, Paul Lacy, William Chick, Holbrook Seltzer, and others have corrected diabetes in rats and mice with injections of islets or beta cells grown in tissue culture. All the animals used in these experiments were from pure inbred strains; thus rejection by the immune system was not a problem, as the animals receiving the injections had the same hereditary tissue transplant antigens as did the beta cells from the tissue culture. But immunorejection remains an obstacle to the clinical application of this technique. Even if this problem is overcome, transplantation will continue to be a limited approach until large masses of beta cells can be grown in tissue culture. Several researchers, notably the surgeon John Najarian in Minneapolis, are currently trying to develop methods of using beta cell injection to treat human diabetics.

A final approach to the problem of insulin regulation is the mechanical route. Cardiac pacemakers are now a standard part of life; so why not an artificial pancreas? Michael Albisser and his colleagues in Toronto have devised a machine that can control glucose levels even more precisely than a functioning human pancreas can. The heart of their device is a glucose analyzer, which receives blood samples from a catheter placed in a vein; this analyzer is connected to a computer that regulates insulin injection back into the patient. Unfortunately, this machine requires constant blood sampling and weighs hundreds of pounds. The main challenge of miniaturization is the problem of developing a tiny device to measure glucose levels. Stuart Soeldner in Boston and Samuel Bessman in Los Angeles are working with electrodes that can generate electric current proportional to glucose concentration. Some of their devices have worked for several months when implanted into experimental animals, although their overall success has been limited and variable. The mechanical pancreas may yet provide the best solution to the problem of insulin control in the diabetic; it is no longer a fanciful hope but is now a straight bioengineering problem being approached in a truly scientific manner that should yield applicable results within the next five to ten years.

Other approaches are also likely to lead to improvements in the treatment of diabetes in the near future. Further study of the role of viral infection and the initiation of an autoimmune reaction in juvenile diabetes should make it theoretically possible to reverse this process; and with better identification of tissue transplant antigens, those at risk for developing juvenile diabetes will be able to be identified and possibly immunized. These advances could well take place within the next decade. As the biochemistry of insulin function and the development of diabetic complications become more clear, direct preventive measures can be perfected. (However, much more basic research will have to be done before this is accomplished.) Finally, general research into atherosclerosis should facilitate the treatment and prevention of this complication of diabetes, since diabetic atherosclerosis is unique only in the speed with which it develops.

These new ideas are still in early stages of development. But as interest in diabetes research increases, the outlook for the control of this disease is becoming better now than it has been at any time in the past.

The Reproductive System

KENNETH J. RYAN **18**

The issues involved in reproductive medicine are quite different from those of any other health care field. Most branches of medicine focus on the treatment of well-defined diseases presented to the physician through patient complaints. In contrast, reproductive medicine is primarily preventive in character. Contraception, prenatal care, and fetal monitoring are all used to prevent the birth of unwanted or abnormal children; and the treatment of postmenopausal women has been centered on the attempt to prevent the disorders that may follow the end of female reproductive life.

Our ability to control the human reproductive system has increased enormously since 1950, largely through the application of knowledge and techniques derived from basic research. At the same time, new medical problems have arisen as unforeseen consequences of interfering with the reproductive system. Today we face the double challenge not only to control the reproductive process but to control it accurately and safely at all stages of reproductive life.

Family Planning

Mechanical and surgical means of preventing conception, available in one form or another since antiquity, have gone through revolutionary changes in the last few decades. The modern intrauterine device has been made possible by advanced technology in material processing and manufacture, as well as by research in the local factors that control the implantation of a fertilized egg and the beginning of pregnancy. (There are still certain medical problems with the use of IUDs, such as infection and misplacement; these will have to be solved through basic research and clinical study.) Permanent sterilization has also been made much easier through the minor surgical operations of vasectomy and the tying of the oviducts. But the greatest conceptual breakthrough in family planning—and the one that has had the greatest social implications to date—was the development of the birth control pill.

The pill came about as the result of the confluence of two different streams of basic research, one biological and the other pharmacological. Biological research had demonstrated that the release of the gonadotropins, the pituitary hormones that control ovulation, was controlled by blood levels of the steroid hormones estrogen and progesterone. High levels of these steroids inhibit gonadotropin release and thus prevent ovulation and pregnancy. It was suggested that estrogen and progesterone taken by women might therefore prevent pregnancy; but without synthetic steroids, it was impossible to test this idea in a practical way. At the same time, however, researchers for the Syntex drug company in Mexico were perfecting methods of synthesizing potent organic steroids. Once these synthetic steroids became available for testing, the birth control pill could be developed. Today, the major problem that remains with the use of the pill is that of preventing the rare but important side effects its use can cause: thromboembolism, coronary disease, and stroke. In general, the risk that a woman will develop these medical problems is decreased by lowering the dosage given and screening out patients at potentially greater risk.

The pill was developed at a time when techniques for measuring hormone levels were still in very early stages of development. Since that time reproductive medicine has been revolutionized by the technique of radioimmunoassay, which makes it possible to measure hormone levels in very small blood samples through the use of antibodies to the hormones being measured. This technique can now be used to detect the hormonal changes that indicate pregnancy before a single period has been missed. More important, radioimmunoassay has been instrumental in the development of new techniques for the diagnosis and treatment of infertility.

Until the past decade, it was very difficult to diagnose the cause of female infertility because the release of the gonadotropins, essential to ovulation, is controlled by so many factors. Gonadotropin release is modulated by blood levels of steroid hormones, and interference with this control mechanism is the basis for the action of the birth control pill.

But before gonadotropin release can occur at all, the pituitary must be stimulated by substances called releasing factors produced in that part of the brain known as the hypothalamus (Figure 18-1). The existence of these factors was known for some time, but their identity eluded researchers until the advent of radioimmunoassay and other sophisticated experimental techniques. While substances thought to be the releasing factors could be given to patients, it was impossible to determine whether or not those substances were actually stimulating gonadotropin release until radioimmunoassay made it possible to measure changes in blood levels of gonadotropins quickly.

Once the releasing factors were found, it became much easier to

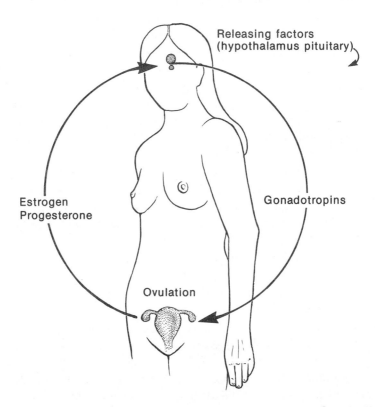

Figure 18–1. The reproductive hormone system in women. Releasing factors produced in the brain's hypothalamus stimulate the pituitary gland to produce gonadotropins. Gonadotropins, in turn, trigger the release of estrogen and progesterone, the steroid hormones that are essential to ovulation. Finally, these steroid hormones modulate the secretion of gonadotropins and releasing factors and thus complete the feedback loop shown here.

understand the causes of infertility. Infertility is often due to a failure of gonadotropin release, since gonadotropins play an essential role in stimulating ovulation in the female and maintaining an adequately high sperm count in the male. But since the pituitary release of gonadotropins is in turn controlled by the hypothalamus, it is not enough to determine that gonadotropin release is deficient; one must determine whether that deficiency is caused by a dysfunction of the pituitary or of the hypothalamus. The site of the dysfunction can now be diagnosed by giving the patient releasing factors and measuring the effects on gonadotropin release. If gonadotropin levels rise when the releasing factors are given, then the pituitary is clearly able to produce gonadotropin, and it is the hypothalamus which is at fault; in contrast, a failure of gonadotropin levels to respond to the releasing factors indicates probable (although not certain) pituitary dysfunction. After a diagnosis has been made, the gonadotropins or releasing factors may be given to the infertile individual therapeutically to improve fertility.

With these advances in contraception and the treatment of infertility, pregnancy has become a matter of choice rather than chance. But conception is only the first step in the reproductive process. As important as the control of conception are methods of improving the care of both the mother and the fetus once pregnancy does begin.

Prenatal and Perinatal Care

At one time, death in childbirth was a major cause of female mortality. But over the years, and especially since the Second World War, the risk to the mother during childbearing has decreased dramatically in the developed nations. Many major causes of death in childbirth are no longer significant. Infection can now be treated with antibiotics. Hemorrhage is treated by administering blood and blood substances. The complications attending toxemia of pregnancy (such as convulsions) were once a major cause of maternal death and are now largely preventable. And the legalization of abortion, along with improved methods for terminating pregnancy, has made that procedure much safer for women who choose it.

Certain specific diseases of pregnancy have also been effectively combated through medical advances. Hypofibrinogenemia, a disease common to pregnancy that is caused by depletion of a blood clotting factor, can be readily cured or prevented. And choriocarcinoma, a cancer of pregnancy, can now be detected early; the cancer is characterized by certain patterns of gonadotropin release which can be measured by radio-immunoassay. Once detected, choriocarcinoma can be cured with specific medicines that have replaced the ineffective surgical procedures that were once employed.

As maternal mortality has decreased, attention has turned increasingly to the care of the fetus while in the womb and at the time of birth. The United States is still ranked behind many European countries, including the Netherlands and Scandinavia, in perinatal mortality; the risk is especially great for Americans in lower socioeconomic groups. Nevertheless, new techniques for fetal monitoring during pregnancy and delivery promise to reduce infant morbidity and mortality rates substantially.

The growth of the fetus can now be monitored safely and effectively through ultrasonography, which works on the same general principle as sonar; a sound wave is transmitted over the mother's abdomen and the echoes recorded, giving an accurate picture of the infant's size and hence of its maturity (Figures 18-2 and 18-3). Before this technique was developed, fetal growth could only be ineffectively measured through the use of X rays, with all the hazards such radiation entails.

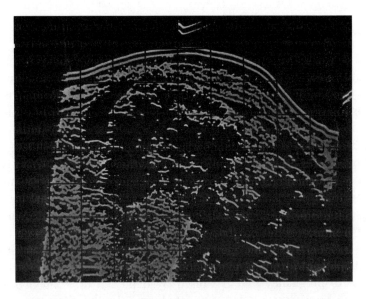

Figure 18–2. An ultrasonic representation of the fetus within the uterus. Photograph courtesy of Kenneth Scheer, Boston Hospital for Women.

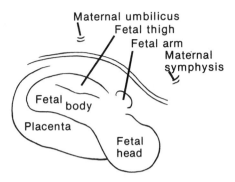

Figure 18–3. Diagram identifying the various structures of fetal and maternal anatomy as they are represented in Figure 18–2.

Amniocentesis is another very useful technique for monitoring the health of the developing fetus. In this procedure, a needle is inserted through the abdominal wall and uterus into the fluid-filled amniotic sac that surrounds the infant, and a small amount of amniotic fluid is withdrawn. This fluid can be analyzed directly or fetal cells in the fluid can be cultured and studied. Amniocentesis can be used to detect Rh disease in the fetus; once detected, this disorder can be effectively treated by intrauterine transfusion (see Chapter 15). Over fifty genetic causes of disease and mental retardation can now be identified by amniocentesis. Examination of the cells can reveal genetic defects such as Down's syndrome and various metabolic diseases as early as the eighteenth week of pregnancy and can provide a basis for deciding whether or not to abort in these cases (see Chapter 10). New tests for determining the health of the fetus through amniocentesis are being developed. Recently, for example, it has become possible to measure the maturity of the fetal lung by examining the levels of certain lipids in the amniotic fluid; when the lecithin/sphingomyelin (or L/S) ratio reaches an acceptable level, the infant can be delivered with less fear of respiratory distress (see Chapter 13).

As monitoring techniques make it possible to determine the optimum time for delivery of the infant, methods for controlling the timing of labor and delivery are also developing rapidly. While the causes of premature delivery remain largely unknown, different substances can be used to delay labor and prevent premature birth, which can seriously endanger the life of the newborn infant. The use of alcohol to delay labor was pioneered in Denmark; apparently alcohol inhibits the release of the hormone oxytocin and thus delays the time of birth, although the efficacy of this treatment is now questioned. Labor can also be delayed with drugs which act directly on uterine muscle. Conversely, synthetic oxytocin and prostaglandins can be used to induce labor when this is desired.

Once labor begins, the fetus can be monitored by electrocardiogram and through fetal scalp blood samples to detect distress and acidosis. If the fetus is found to be at risk in the womb it can be delivered promptly, often by cesarean section.

All these advances in the monitoring and control of labor and delivery have greatly improved the odds for the healthy delivery and survival of the infant. With these improvements, however, has come the risk that they will be overused. In developed countries throughout the world, the incidence of cesarean section has increased to a level that is almost certainly excessive. Aside from some preliminary impressions that the rate of cerebral palsy may have gone down as the rate of cesarean section has increased, there is no evidence that the increased use of this form of delivery has led to an overall improvement in the health of the infant population (although the procedure has certainly been lifesaving in those cases where it was truly necessary). The present challenge is not only to improve the techniques for prenatal and perinatal surveillance and care but to distinguish those cases where such techniques are really needed from those in which the infant could quite safely be delivered by a midwife. The present trend to natural childbirth and home delivery should help bring this issue into focus in the years ahead.

Medical intervention in pregnancy may not only be unnecessary but may actually be harmful. All too often drugs used to interfere with the reproductive process have been employed before their effectiveness was demonstrated and before the risks involved in their use were adequately assessed. The use of diethylstilbestrol (DES) is a dramatic example. This synthetic estrogen was given to women for decades for the purpose of maintaining pregnancy and preventing miscarriages, in spite of the fact that there were doubts as to its effectiveness. When DES was first introduced no harmful effects were known, and it was widely prescribed. In the past decade, however, it has been clearly demonstrated that the daughters of women given DES during pregnancy run an increased (but still low) risk of developing vaginal cancer. Recently the possibility of physiological abnormalities in sexual development of the sons of women given this drug have also been of concern.

The risks and benefits of interfering with hormonal levels must be considered in all areas of reproductive medicine. Side effects of DES and the birth control pill were discovered after these agents had been in use for some time, and have received considerable publicity. Very recently, the effects of hormonal intervention have been studied in another area: the use of estrogens to treat postmenopausal women.

The Menopausal State and Hormonal Intervention

The hormonal changes that occur with the onset of menopause are complex and poorly understood. Menopausal changes, which now affect nearly 30 million American women, can have major physiological consequences. Besides the discomfort of hot flashes, menopause and aging are associated with osteoporosis (softening of the bones), atrophy of the reproductive organs, and an increased risk for carcinoma of the breast and of the endometrium (the inner lining of the uterus). While the biological reason for these changes remained unclear, the idea arose some years ago that they might be treated by hormone replacement.

There were some problems with this approach. First, it may be unrealistic to expect hormonal replacement to be a panacea for the problems of menopause, since the menopausal state involves many physiological aging changes besides the most obvious hormonal ones. And second, there was never any evidence that synthetic estrogens given to postmenopausal women could actually have all the beneficial effects that were attributed to them. There still is no real evidence, for example, that these agents are effective in preventing osteoporosis. But in spite of these objections, a great many women were given estrogens, largely because these substances are effective in prolonging active sexual life and because (like DES) when they were first introduced they had no demonstrable bad effects. Although it was well known that giving estrogens to experimental animals could induce cancer, there was some confusion as to whether or not the induction of cancer was a direct or a secondary response to the estrogens. The applicability of these findings to human patients was also unclear. In any event, the risks were not considered major, and a large number of postmenopausal women began to use estrogens.

The overall wisdom of this trend is now being severely questioned. Since their use began, estrogens have been found to be associated with an increased risk of coronary disease, stroke, and thromboembolism. They have also been linked recently to cancer of the breast and endometrium. At the same time, many of the claims that were made for the beneficial effects of these substances remain unproven.

In principle, there is nothing wrong with the idea of hormone replacement for postmenopausal women. It is not unreasonable to expect that accurately mimicking the hormonal balance the woman experiences in reproductive life would effectively treat some of the problems of menopause. The major obstacle to doing this is that the changes women undergo with aging are very complex and are just beginning to be understood. Yet they must be understood before accurate hormonal control can take place.

Much work remains to be done, for example, to clarify the role of fat tissue in the synthesis of estrogen. The function of estrogen synthesized in such peripheral tissue is unclear; but some researchers have suggested that these hormones, which may differ from the estrogens synthesized at other sites during normal reproductive life, may be linked to the development of endometrial carcinoma in postmenopausal women. Very obese women are known to develop endometrial cancer after menopause nine times more frequently than their thinner contemporaries; this difference could conceivably be due to the greater production of peripheral estrogen in obese women. This speculation is still totally hypothetical. It is clear, however, that the interaction of peripheral estrogens, estrogens formed at other sites in the body, estrogen administered from outside the body, and cancer is very complex in women past the age of menopause. Our understanding of these areas has increased tremendously in the past two decades; virtually nothing at all was known about the biological synthesis of the estrogens before the 1950s. But much more basic research needs to be done before the hormonal changes of menopause can be effectively and safely controlled.

Future Research Needs

The need for basic research in reproductive medicine is clearly evident. Unfortunately, there are some very difficult problems that face the physician or biologist doing basic research in this area. The problem of extrapolating from animal studies to human problems is probably greater than in any other field of medicine (with the possible exception of neurological research); the differences between the reproductive systems of lower animals and those of human beings are especially great. For example, there are only a few animal species in which females menstruate, the higher apes and *Homo sapiens;* and human beings are essentially the only animals that cannot tell by sense perception or behavior when the female is fertile. The fact that reproduction is controlled by the brain puts the researcher in another double bind: one can perform only very limited studies of the human brain, yet the human brain is so highly evolved that brain studies of lower animals have questionable applicability to human medicine. The best that one can do is to study the higher primates and to extrapolate one's findings to people with caution.

In the realm of human research, epidemiologic studies will probably play an increasingly important role in reproductive medicine. The possible benefits and risks of different drugs and synthetic hormones can only be determined through long-term, well-organized studies of the effects of these agents on human populations. This has been demonstrated in the past; English physicians were able to gather information on the effects of the birth control pill much faster than were researchers in the United States, because England's national health insurance program and record keeping facilitated the collection of the necessary information. At present, much more research is devoted to getting a drug on the market than to following the effects of that drug once it enters public use. This unbalanced situation must certainly change.

Finally, research is turning increasingly to the study of the psychological and social factors that may affect the reproductive process. It is a measure of our ignorance that we have no idea what determines whether an individual becomes homosexual or heterosexual; the relative importance of such diverse factors as hormones and parental upbringing remain unclear. The physiological symptoms of the psychiatric condition anorexia nervosa are also under study; adult women who suffer from this disorder (in which the patient essentially refuses to eat) actually stop menstruating and undergo the same pattern of hormonal release as is seen in prepubescent girls. Nutritional and socioeconomic variables play an important role in prenatal care, and the effects of these factors are worthy of much further study.

The reproductive process is important at one time or another to all human beings; people's lives are deeply affected by their personal sexuality, the birth of a child, and the population problem. Modern science and research has done a great deal to improve our understanding and control of the reproductive process. But much more work must be done to make that understanding more complete, and that control safe and effective.

The Skin

RICHARD A. JOHNSON
THOMAS B. FITZPATRICK

19

The skin is unique among the body's organ systems; it is the only system which is readily visible. For this reason, the diseases which afflict the skin have been observed and recorded from prehistoric times. Scientific dermatology began in 1776 when Joseph Jacob Plenck of Vienna proposed a system for the classification and diagnosis of skin disorders by visible lesions. Personal experiences treating skin disorders were first recorded in book form by the British physician Robert Wilans about a quarter of a century later. Since that time, careful clinical observation has always been the essential first step in the description and treatment of skin disease. New environmental stresses and types of treatment have brought with them new disorders of the skin, all of which were first identified through primarily visual criteria. Today most dermatologic diagnoses are made through educated observation of the disease-induced changes in the normal structure of the skin and, when indicated, by a skin biopsy (removal and examination of living tissue).

Advances in Visual Diagnosis

Studies of symptomatology and improved microscopic technology have greatly facilitated the diagnosis of skin disorders. This has probably been most important in the treatment of skin cancer, where early detection is crucial to a successful cure.

Straightforward clinical observation has become central to the diagnosis and treatment of malignant melanoma. This serious form of skin cancer is a malignant transformation of the melanocyte, or pigment cell, that often arises in preexisting moles; it occurs most commonly during a patient's most productive years (the 30s and 40s) and kills one third of its victims. By the time melanomas become very noticeable through bleeding or ulceration, the cancer has likely invaded deeply and spread to the internal organs; at this later stage, there is no definite cure. Early detection is thus of the utmost importance in the treatment of this disease. Recently, criteria for the early detection of malignant melanoma were developed through a broad clinical study comparing photographs and case histories of over three hundred patients with this disorder. Moles with areas of blue-to-gray pigmentation and brown flat-to-raised skin lesions are now known to characterize malignant melanoma in its early, curable stages; moles present from birth are also known to be especially likely sites for the development of this type of cancer. Lesions can be cured in over 90 percent of all cases if they are brought to a physician's attention when color, border, or surface changes have been relatively recent. Visual diagnostic techniques have been essential in making the early detection and cure of this disease possible.

During the past decade, several new techniques have been developed for the microscopic examination of skin disorders. The electron microscope, which uses an electron beam rather than a visible light, gives much higher magnification than the light microscope and has been an invaluable research tool in revealing the structure, function, and interactions of single cells and small groups of cells. It has proved especially useful in the study of melanin granules, the units of brown pigment in the epidermis that give the skin a characteristic color.

In the innovative one micron section technique, tissue is prepared as if for use in the electron microscope, but the section of tissue is examined with a light microscope. A large field can be examined by this method. Alterations of all skin layers and appendages as well as of blood vessels and nerves can be observed with finely preserved cellular detail. This procedure has been especially useful in studying immunological reactions mediated by type T lymphocytes (see Chapter 7). The subtle difference between the healthy reaction of T lymphocytes to the tuberculosis bacillus and the allergic reaction seen when the epidermis is exposed to poison ivy can be distinguished by this thick-section technique. Vasculitis (inflammation of the blood vessels) mediated by T and B lymphocytes can also be diagnosed by this method.

Abnormal T lymphocytes seem to be the causative agents of the skin cancer mycosis fungoides. Many investigators believe that these malignant T lymphocytes are produced outside the skin but have a unique ability to congregate in the skin and form tumor masses there. While the site of their production remains the subject of some debate, there is no doubt as to the importance of early detection of malignant T lymphocytes in the treatment of this disease. It is here that thick-section technique may have its most important application, as it can be used to identify mycosis fungoides cells long before the characteristic tissue changes seen in this illness can be detected by other methods.

Another recent innovation has been the use of the scanning electron microscope to examine the surface of both normal and diseased skin. This instrument produces pictures of very high magnification with three-dimensional perspective, comparable to satellite photographs of the earth's surface. (Regular electron micrographs, in contrast, give a cross-sectional and flat perspective.) This new method of visualization should make possible even more sophisticated study and diagnosis of skin disorders.

Structure of the Skin and the Barrier Layer

The use of the microscope to study skin tissue is not new. As early as a century ago, investigators were able to use the light microscope to identify four functional subdivisions of the skin: the epidermis, the outer layer of the skin; the dermis, the "leather" layer with nerve and blood vessels which gives girdle-like support to the underlying muscles, joints, and internal organs; the subcutaneous fat, which acts as a bumper against mechanical injuries, and also a store of reserve energy; and the skin appendages, such as the sweat glands, oil glands, hair, and nails. In spite of this early understanding of the anatomy of the skin, many aspects of its structure and function remained a mystery until the past few decades. Especially puzzling was the barrier function of the skin. While the thickness of the epidermis and dermis varies from site to site within the body, the skin is nowhere more than a few millimeters thick; yet somewhere in these few millimeters is a physical barrier which not only prevents loss of the body's water, salt, and protein, but which simultaneously protects the body from microbial agents, chemicals, and harmful solar radiation. It has only been during the past thirty years that researchers have located this barrier in the stratum corneum or scale layer, which is formed in the last stages of epidermal growth (Figure 19-1).

The stratum corneum, which looks and feels like a semi-opaque plastic film, is composed primarily of nonliving membranes from skin cells

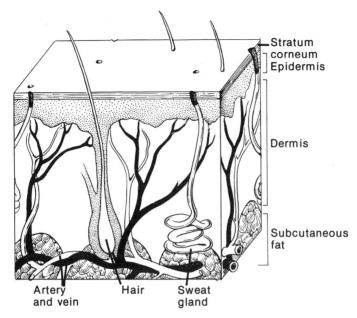

Figure 19–1. A three-dimensional cross-section of the skin. The three basic levels of the skin are shown, in addition to the skin appendages and the stratum (or scale layer).

whose cytoplasms and nuclei have been digested by enzymes within the cells. It is continually regenerated from below at the same rate that the outer position scales off. While membranes composed of living cells (such as those of the intestine and kidney tubules) can use energy to transport salt and water actively, these substances diffuse passively across the stratum corneum. The rate at which this passive transport occurs is determined by the protein-lipid composition of the scale layer.

Knowledge of the rate at which a substance passes through the stratum corneum and of the changes in this rate seen in altered states of the membrane (such as hydration) allows the pharmacologist to compound medications which react with the stratum corneum in different ways. Medications to be used as sun screens, for example, must deposit on this membrane, while a cortisone preparation used to reduce inflammation in the skin must be able to pass through the membrane into the dermis. Substances applied to the skin may have uses beyond the local treatment of skin disorders. Medication intended for systemic use may be able to be applied to the skin, pass through the stratum corneum into the blood vessels, and reach the appropriate organ. This is essentially the same principle that has been employed for centuries in the oral administration of pills and liquids, which relies on absorption through the intestinal membrane. There are many factors which make intestinal absorption erratic and undesirable, so that administration through the skin (percutaneous absorption) would often be preferable. Nitroglycerin, the agent used in angina pectoris to open the blood vessels supplying the heart muscles, is already available as a cream which can be rubbed into the skin. This substance passes through the scale layer into the dermal blood vessels and is in the heart within seconds of application; the patient can control the dose. Other agents do not pass through the stratum corneum by themselves but pass through readily when dissolved with a chemical known as DMSO. With further understanding of the scale layer and its barrier function, many other agents may be given systemically by this method of percutaneous absorption.

Methods of Treatment

While improved methods of visualization and anatomical studies have made much better diagnosis of dermatological disease possible, great strides have also been made in the treatment of these disorders. In the past few decades, increasingly safe and effective methods have been found for treating skin diseases through drug therapy and radiation.

Until the late 1930s dermatology wards at the major medical centers had two types of patient at high risk: those suffering from cellulitis, an infection of the dermis and subcutaneous tissues caused by the streptococcus bacterium; and those with pemphigus vulgaris, a blistering disease resulting in ulcer formation both on the skin and in the mouth. Lifesaving treatment for cellulitis came with advances in the development and availability of sulfonamides and later of antibiotics; penicillin drastically reduced the death rate for this disease. And pemphigus vulgaris, which once killed 95 percent of its victims within one or two years, was effectively treated with corticosteroid drugs after these agents became available in the early 1950s. Pemphigus vulgaris is a disease characterized by inflammation that the corticosteroids, which are similar to the cortisone normally produced in the adrenal glands, act to suppress. Their antiinflammatory action has made the corticosteroids useful in the treatment of many other dermatological diseases as well.

Although early victories in the treatment of pemphigus were extremely encouraging, serious drawbacks to these methods of drug therapy became evident almost as soon as they were instituted. Corticosteroid preparations must often be given in large doses and over long periods of time in order to be effective. For this reason, significant long-term side effects are common. Alternate drugs, such as the antimetabolites metho-trexate and azathioprine, are often prescribed instead. These agents were first used in cancer therapy and act by "poisoning" pathways of cellular metabolism. But unfortunately, these drugs, too, often have toxic effects.

Some success has been achieved in developing effective but harmless drugs to combat dermatological disorders. The tetracyclines, as well as certain other relatively inexpensive antibiotics, have proven very useful in the treatment of inflammatory pustular acne and do not have significant side effects. But in the treatment of other, more serious skin diseases, the use of powerful but toxic drugs (such as the coricosteroids and anti-metabolites) is being largely abandoned in favor of the rapidly develop-ing techniques of therapeutic radiation.

X-ray treatment of skin diseases was the earliest form of radiation therapy. When first introduced seven decades ago, X irradiation was used in the treatment of many common types of skin disorders. After this technique had been in use for several decades, however, a serious prob-lem was encountered: many patients who had undergone long-term X-ray treatment began to experience chronic X-ray burns (radiodermatitis). This serious effect makes X-ray therapy inadvisable except in the treat-ment of skin cancer patients over the age of forty-five; for these individ-uals, the expected therapeutic benefits outweigh the dangers of long-term damage. (Radiodermatitis usually does not occur to a significant degree until twenty years after X-ray treatment.) Even for these individuals, X irradiation could hardly be considered an ideal treatment. It is a danger-ous form of therapy that may have harmful effects besides radioderma-titis.

More recently safer yet equally effective forms of radiation therapy have been developed. Electron beam irradiation has been used as therapy for skin lymphomas, which involve extensive areas of skin. With this technique, the entire skin surface can be treated but only to a depth of several millimeters. This avoids the problem of toxic irradiation to the bone marrow and gastrointestinal tract, a major drawback of X-ray ther-apy. In the past few years, promising developments in phototherapy have also occurred. A high-intensity ultraviolet light source used in combina-tion with oral administration of psoralens (a naturally occurring group of plant photosensitizers) can now be used successfully to clear and main-tain patients with extensive disabling psoriasis, a hereditary disorder of rapid proliferation of the epidermis. The patient with psoriasis can be maintained on weekly to monthly therapy, as a diabetic is controlled on insulin. Before the advent of phototherapy, these patients had used the antimetabolites methotrexate, hydroxyurea, or azarabine, which are effective but frequently have to be discontinued because of their toxicity. Phototherapy appears to have no such serious side effects; it has been used for many years in the treatment of vitiligo, a depigmenting disorder, with no long-term adverse reactions.

These new types of radiation therapy should not be seen as replacements for drug therapy but rather as very useful additional methods for combating skin disorders. Treatment programs combining drug and radiation therapy have already been developed and appear to be safe and effective. Photochemotherapy in particular has been used very successfully in both the United States and Europe during the past years.

Epidemiology

As methods of treating dermatological disorders have improved, increasing attention has focused on the epidemiology of skin diseases. Paradoxically, some diseases have actually increased in prevalence at the same time that methods for treating them have improved. In these cases, treatment advances have simply been outweighed by epidemiologic factors that have increased the rate at which new cases of these disorders arise.

This effect has been especially marked in the case of syphilis. (Since this venereal disease manifests itself in the skin, diagnosis and treatment is usually carried out by the dermatologist.) Penicillin was first used in the treatment of syphilis about thirty-five years ago and proved to be highly effective; by 1956 it appeared from the yearly decrease in case reports that syphilis would soon be totally extinct. However, in 1957 syphilis began to spread again, and now the incidence of this disease is increasing by about 7 percent annually. Probably the major reason for this increase has been the change in sexual practices. Penicillin has remained curative in diagnosed cases of syphilis; the spiral bacterium that causes the disease has shown no signs of developing resistance to this antibiotic. But increased sexual promiscuity has placed so many more individuals at risk of infection that the disease remains a major public health problem. There is no naturally developed immunity to reinfection following syphilitic infection, and there are no signs of a breakthrough in the near future in developing syphilis immunization. Thus the tedious process of seeking out, interviewing, and treating contacts of active syphilis remains our only method of combating this illness. (One intriguing proposal for future investigation is the selective breeding of a harmless spiral bacterium which would have the ability to survive and reproduce in the body for the life of the patient. This bacterium would cause no disease itself but would be capable of maintaining persistent immunity against the pathogenic syphilis bacterium by its close similarity to it.)

In the past few years, epidemiologic studies have demonstrated a definite link between exposure to sunlight and skin cancer. Ultraviolet solar radiation of certain frequencies has long been known to have cumulative effects on the skin. High-frequency ultraviolet light, known as UVC, never reaches the surface of the earth; it is completely filtered out by the protective layer of ozone (O_3) in the stratosphere. Low-frequency ultraviolet light (UVA) reaches the earth unfiltered but does not appear to have significant medical effects. But UVB, ultraviolet light which is intermediate in frequency, presents a real problem. This type of radiation is only partially screened by the ozone layer and is of a high enough frequency to be a potential medical hazard. To UVB has been assigned the major responsibility for the irreversible damage to the skin which we appreciate as aging, namely wrinkling, dryness, old age spots, and localized areas of scaling. The more important, UVB is now being found to play a key role in the etiology of skin cancer.

Population studies of the incidence of skin cancer have shown that the people most likely to suffer from these cancers are those who have been bombarded by the most UVB radiation. Fair-skinned individuals are highly susceptible. Melanin (the brown pigment in the epidermis) functions as a highly effective sunscreen, so that blacks are nearly completely protected from UVB, but people of Celtic origin have very little natural protection against this radiation. Individuals whose work or recreational activities entail spending a great deal of time in the sunlight are also prone to skin cancer, as are those living near the equator where UVB radiation is greatest. Because the elderly may suffer from cumulative UVB damage, the incidence of skin cancer increases with age. (For reasons that remain unclear, patients receiving phototherapy with ultraviolet light show no increased tendency to develop skin cancer, even though phototherapy may often include exposure to UVB in the carcinogenic range. These patients are probably just not receiving enough ultraviolet light from these treatments to do any damage, or perhaps the brevity of sunlamp treatments and the time between treatments allow DNA repair to be carried out, minimizing the risk of mutational changes that could lead to cancer.) The link between sunlight exposure and less serious types of epidermal cancer, particularly basal and squamous cell carcinoma, has been well established for some time. But it is only recently that UVB has also been demonstrated to be a primary cause of malignant melanoma, a form of skin cancer which has a high mortality rate.

Recognition of the strong link between UVB radiation and the deadly forms of skin cancer has led investigators to study potential hazards to the stratospheric ozone layer. Since the ozone layer does screen out some UVB radiation, any damage to it would increase the amount of UVB radiation reaching the earth's surface, with potentially dangerous results. A recent report by the Climatic Impact Committee of the National Academy of Sciences, entitled "Environmental Impact of Stratospheric Flight," stressed the potential hazard to the ozone layer posed by emission pollutants from high-altitude jet flights. (It is known that these pollutants, particularly nitric oxide, can alter the molecular form of ozone.) According to this report, a 10 percent decrease in stratospheric ozone could be expected to result in about a 20 percent increase in melanoma mortality and a 20 to 30 percent increase in the incidence of basal and squamous cell carcinomas. Jet pollutants are not the only cause for concern; the inert fluorocarbon propellants used in aerosol cans have also been shown to destroy ozone. The hazard posed by these fluorocarbons has now become the subject of extensive debate, although no effective action has yet been taken to limit their use.

Research in dermatologic disease is still in its infancy. The clinical appearance and behavior of most dermatologic disorders have already been carefully observed. Many basic facts have been discovered about the pathophysiology of such common disorders as acne and psoriasis and such rare but deadly illnesses as malignant melanoma; yet the basic processes that cause and govern these diseases remain largely unknown. The deeper etiologic understanding that is now essential should come with a continuing dialogue between dermatologists, basic scientists, and other related specialists.

The Teeth
and Gums

PAUL GOLDHABER　　　　　　　　　　　　20

Dental disease is widespread and costly in the United States. In 1970 the total amount spent on dental disease in this country was 4.4 billion dollars, approximately 50 dollars for each person in the 42 percent of the population who saw a dentist at least once during that year. Even with this large expenditure, the dental health of the nation remains far from good. American children usually begin to get cavities at a very early age, and older people suffer from the added problem of periodontal disease, which leads to the destruction of the bone around the teeth and the subsequent loosening and loss of the teeth (Figure 20-1). Dental caries and periodontal disease account for the large number of Americans who have lost all their natural teeth. Tooth loss increases with age; three out of ten people past age 35, four of ten people past age 45, and five of ten people past age 55 have lost all their natural teeth. Particularly frustrating is the fact that the annual increase in dental decay matches the amount of dental services available each year, making it impossible to narrow the gap between needs and services without a significant increase in the dental workforce and the expenditure of enormous sums of money. At present, the backlog of accumulated untreated dental disease may include as many as one billion unfilled cavities.

It is obvious that dental caries and periodontal disease cannot be effectively controlled by present methods. New preventive and therapeutic measures must be developed and applied. In recent years, a great deal of research has been done to begin to make the development of such new approaches possible.

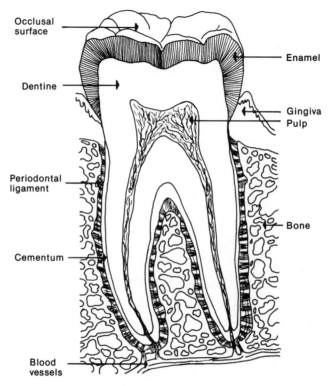

Occlusal surface

Enamel

Dentine

Gingiva
Pulp

Periodontal
ligament

Bone

Cementum

Blood
vessels

Figure 20–1. A lower molar tooth and surrounding tissues, in cross-section. From Jean Mayer, *Health* (Princeton, N.J.: D. Van Nostrand Co., 1974). Courtesy of D. Van Nostrand Co.

Dental Caries

Dental caries is a localized and progressive destruction of the hard tissue of the teeth, usually starting on the biting surfaces of the back teeth, the areas of contact between adjacent teeth, or along the gum line. Demineralization of the tooth substance results from acid production by bacteria on the teeth. Continued bacterial action, including the production of protein-destroying enzymes, leads to the formation of a cavity that will continue to expand unless checked by a dentist. The treatment of early or moderately advanced caries consists of cutting out the diseased portion of the tooth with a high-speed drill and rebuilding the missing portion with an artificial substance such as amalgam (an alloy containing several metals, primarily silver), gold, silicates, or plastics. If left untreated, the infection will eventually engulf the entire pulp, affect the tissues around the end of the root, and result in an abscess; the untreated abscess will expand, penetrate through the jawbone, and cause swelling in the surrounding soft tissue where it erupts. At this stage, the infection may spread through the tissue spaces and affect vital processes such as respiration, even endangering the life of the individual.

Once the pulpal tissue has died, the only two possible methods of treatment are root canal therapy or extraction. Unfortunately, extraction of the teeth, while solving the immediate problem of pain and infection, may create other long-term problems. For example, if a primary molar is prematurely lost, other teeth near the new space may shift position and prevent a permanent tooth from erupting into its proper position. This causes malocclusion, a condition in which the teeth are badly aligned and fail to interlock properly when the jaws are closed. Tooth loss may also encourage entrapment of food between the shifting teeth, increasing the risk of dental caries and periodontal disease in those areas. It is preferable to avoid extractions; where there is no alternative, the missing tooth or teeth should be replaced by a prosthetic appliance, preferably a fixed bridge, to minimize the risk of oral disease.

The best approach to the problem of dental caries is not through treatment after the fact but through programs aimed at prevention. Several methods of prevention have been tried and have met with various degrees of success.

Much attention has been given to the relationship of diet to caries. The most important dietary factor contributing to the development of dental caries is sucrose (sugar), which in this country is consumed at a per capita rate of 1 kilogram (2.2 pounds) per week, primarily in canned foods, baked food, soft drinks, ice cream, and snacks. The caries-producing effect of sucrose can be overcome by eliminating sugar-containing foods from the diet, substituting other sweetening agents, or attempting to block the bacterial production of acid. Unfortunately, there are problems with all these approaches. Modification of dietary habits, while possible in individual cases, is difficult if not impossible on a large scale. Many sweetening agents look promising as substitutes for sugar but as yet there are no data to prove that they inhibit caries formation in human teeth (except for the sweetener sorbitol, which has been shown to produce fewer caries than sucrose in chewing gum). The addition of organic or inorganic phosphates to the diet seems promising; glycerol phosphate has been shown to offer protection against caries in monkeys, while dibasic calcium phosphate added to sugar and flour has reduced the number of caries in Swedish children. But attempts to get large segments of the public to accept a dicalcium-phosphate-containing biscuit have not been successful. In general, the phosphates paradoxically seem to meet with the greatest acceptance when incorporated into caries-producing items like sugar lozenges and chewing gum.

Professionally supervised programs of oral hygiene can effectively prevent dental caries but only when such programs are carried out more intensively than may be generally practical. Swedish investigators have demonstrated that professional tooth cleaning by a dental nurse—repeated once every two weeks for two years and once every four weeks during a third year—resulted in excellent oral hygiene in a group of schoolchildren when combined with fluoride applications and toothbrushing instructions. The children of a control group, who only employed monthly supervised toothbrushing with a 0.2 percent sodium fluoride solution, developed about three carious lesions per child per year—20 times as many as the professionally cleaned group. The investigators concluded that substantial prevention of dental caries cannot be achieved simply by prophylactic treatment as infrequently as five to eight times a year.

The most effective and efficient means of preventing dental caries found so far is the fluoridation of drinking water. Extensive epidemiologic studies have clearly shown that the ingestion of one part per million of fluoride in the drinking water, if it begins in early childhood during the years of tooth development, will prevent the onset of dental caries by 60 percent. Controlled studies started 30 years ago have revealed that this approach is safe and that its cost-benefit ratio makes it an ideal public health measure; for each dollar expended on fluoridation, about thirty-five dollars' worth of dental care is prevented.

It is rather disappointing that despite the overwhelming evidence of fluoride's efficacy, safety, and economy only about 90 million Americans now drink artificially fluoridated water. (More than 163 million are on public water supplies that could potentially be fluoridated.) Exactly why water fluoridation continues to be one of the most controversial community health issues remains a mystery, even to anthropologists, sociologists, political scientists, and psychologists. The major arguments of the anti-fluoridationists appear to focus on three issues: the uncertainty of benefits, the possibility of injurious consequences, and the violation of individual rights. The first two objections have been answered by a mass of scientific data accumulated over the past 30 years; and the third point is one that could be raised about many of our city, state, and federal rules and regulations. What is urgently needed now is strong federal legislation to fluoridate community water supplies, instead of local referenda which can be repeatedly challenged even after fluoridation is voted in. Mandatory water fluoridation would put an additional 67 million people under the "fluoride-protection umbrella." Future dental manpower and economic savings would be enormous; eventually, this one step would totally arrest decay in an additional 20 percent of the population. For the 50 million people who live in areas that do not have central water supply systems and for whom community water fluoridation is therefore impossible, other solutions are feasible, primarily the fluoridation of school water supplies. Although this latter approach does not inhibit dental caries to the same extent as is possible with continuous ingestion of fluoride from a central community water supply, the protection afforded is significant.

Effective though it is, fluoride administered in the drinking water or through toothbrushing prevents caries primarily on the smooth surfaces between the teeth and along the gum margin; it is relatively ineffective on the biting surfaces (pits and fissures) of the back teeth, where almost half the total cavities experienced by elementary school children develop. During the past decade, a number of adhesive resins have been designed to seal the pits and fissures from direct contact with the major factors responsible for the production of dental caries: the caries-causing bacteria and fermentable carbohydrates found in the oral environment. Several types of sealant material have been developed and were used clinically as early as 1966. Despite the fact that early sealants were difficult to handle and usually needed to be reapplied at six-month intervals, the clinical findings were very encouraging; most studies after six months to two years demonstrated caries reductions of approximately 70 to 90 percent compared to a control group's teeth. A more effective liquid sealant system, introduced in 1968 and subsequently modified, can be applied to the biting surfaces of the back teeth with a thin brush and hardened in a few seconds by exposure to ultraviolet light. This procedure results in better adhesion to the teeth and better protection against dental disease; some investigators have found a 99 percent reduction in pit and fissure caries of permanent teeth two years after a single application of this sealant system. Less impressive caries reduction and sealant retention have been reported by others, but these poorer results can be ascribed to improper technique in etching the enamel surface, removing the conditioning solution, or in drying and cleaning the tooth enamel surface, or using ultraviolet light of improper intensity.

Concern has been expressed about the possibility that small carious lesions may be inadvertently covered with sealant and may worsen as a result. To date, however, the evidence suggests not only that these cavities do not progress rapidly but that in fact they are probably arrested, since the sealant keeps nutrients from reaching tooth bacteria.

The search for new and better sealants continues, for if the sealant approach is to have any appeal as a public health measure it must prove to have a favorable cost-benefit ratio. The ideal sealant must be easy to apply so that dental auxiliaries may perform this service where feasible; it must be retained for at least several years; it must prevent pit and fissure caries; and it must be inexpensive. Pit and fissure sealants are not a substitute for water fluoridation but should be considered an important part of the armamentarium available to the dental profession for the prevention of dental caries. Indeed, these sealants may well have the potential to complete the equation: water fluoridation plus pit and fissure sealants equals 100 percent prevention of dental caries.

In recent years, investigators have been taking a new look at the possible use of antibiotics to control dental caries. Although this concept was studied as early as three decades ago when penicillin was reported to inhibit dental caries in rats, it was not followed up in people except for one study which reported inhibition of caries in schoolchildren using a penicillin dentifrice under supervision. Because of concern about possible side effects from the use of antibiotics, the dental profession avoided investigating this means of combating dental decay and concentrated instead on the therapeutic use of fluorides and the regulation of diet. Since those early days, the caries-producing properties of dental plaque have been ascribed to a specific organism, *Streptococcus mutans*. The eradication of this bacterium should prevent dental caries from forming. At present, however, the problem of finding an antibiotic ideally suited to the destruction of *Streptococcus mutans* in dental plaque without unwanted side effects remains unsolved.

Finally, it is possible that the ultimate solution to the problem of dental caries may be a program of immunization. It has been shown recently that rabbits and rats immunized against a strain of *Streptococcus mutans* isolated from human subjects produced antibodies to the bacteria and had a lower rate of caries formation. The antibodies may protect against caries by interfering with the adherence of *Streptococcus mutans* to the tooth surface; another possibility is that antibodies interfere with the bacterial production of lactic acid. More work will have to be done to determine how anticaries immunization works and how effective it is before this approach can be used as a major means of preventing human dental caries.

Periodontal Disease

There are several types of periodontal disease—disease of the tissues surrounding the teeth, including the gums and the supporting bone to which each tooth is attached. Gingivitis, the most common periodontal disease, is characterized by redness, swelling, and bleeding of the margins of the gums. About half of all school-age children in the United States have gingivitis, which, like dental caries, seems to be caused largely by oral bacteria in the dental plaque. (This soft, adherent deposit, composed primarily of bacteria, their extracellular products, and salivary proteins, accumulates especially on tooth surfaces near the margins of the gums.) If ignored, gingival inflammation will eventually extend to the deeper periodontal tissues and will slowly destroy the underlying bone and ligament around the affected teeth, giving rise to chronic destructive periodontal disease. As the inflammation progresses, the gums become detached from the root surface and pockets form. Pus may form in the inflamed tissue. As a significant amount of the bony socket is destroyed and the periodontal ligament fibers lose their attachment to the bone, the affected teeth loosen. If this process is not arrested by therapy, the bone loss and tooth mobility will continue and will be accompanied by periodic episodes of periodontal abscess formation with pain and swelling, until the tooth must be extracted or is lost spontaneously.

While it is not clear how bacteria initiate inflammation of the gums, it is known that a number of bacterial products have the potential to damage gum tissue. The correlation of gingivitis with poor oral hygiene is striking. Experiments have shown that the cessation of hygiene procedures by students with healthy gums led to the accumulation of soft deposits of bacterial plaque around the gum margins and the development of gingivitis within several weeks. These changes were completely reversed when supervised oral hygiene procedures were reintroduced. Clinical observations also show that gingivitis in children or adults is usually reversible by proper treatment and the institution of a rigid regimen of oral hygiene. Unfortunately, the personal effort involved in carrying out the mechanical removal of plaque is too much for most individuals, despite the introduction of power-driven brushes and water irrigation devices. In order to have a real impact on the average standard of oral hygiene, a simple, inexpensive, and relatively effortless method of eliminating bacterial plaque is needed.

One such approach could be the use of an antiseptic agent. Studies have shown that two daily mouth rinsings with 0.2 percent chlorhexidine gluconate completely inhibits the development of plaque and gingivitis without any form of mechanical plaque removal. Furthermore, this procedure by itself causes heavy plaque accumulations to disappear and the inflamed gum tissue to revert to a healthy state. Longer-term studies of antiseptic agents used for up to two years continue to be promising and give no evidence of bacterial overgrowth or toxic reaction. Chlorhexidine may prove especially effective because it is selectively absorbed onto the tooth surface and slowly released; it thus prevents bacterial retention and growth between rinses. This compound has some negative features; it stains the teeth and may form harmful breakdown products, such as parachloraniline. However, this approach to plaque removal clearly is feasible and effective.

In recent years, attention has focused on the possible role of immunological processes in periodontal destruction. Although gum inflammation may serve as a key defense against bacterial invasion from the dental plaque, it may also lead to the subsequent destruction of the ligaments and bone attached to the teeth by activating several components of the immune system. The gums of patients with chronic destructive periodontal disease show an accumulation of white blood cells that is characteristic of a cellular immune response (see Chapter 7). It has also been shown that lymphocytes taken from patients with periodontal disease proliferate when exposed experimentally to plaque antigens. Initial gum inflammation may result from the activation of the complement system by bacterial toxins and protein—degrading enzymes in the plaque and from the accumulation in the gum tissue of bacterial substances that attract certain kinds of white cells. As the process of gum inflammation becomes better understood, it should become easier to prevent the pathological consequences of gingivitis.

Recently, researchers have begun to investigate the biochemical basis of the bone destruction that can occur in periodontal disease. Several years ago it was demonstrated that fragments of human gum tissue grown in combined culture with bone from the top of mouse skulls (calvaria) stimulated the dissolution of the calvaria both around the gum fragments and at some distance away. Subsequently, it was found that similar effects could be obtained with extracts from human gum tissue, suggesting that this tissue contains a factor capable of dissolving bone and that it is stored and need not be synthesized continuously; when gum fragments are grown in culture, they release this factor into the surrounding growth medium. Some recent results suggest that the factor acts on bone through a mechanism that may involve the production and release of prostaglandin (a special kind of biologically active lipid) by bone cells. Small concentrations of the aspirin-like drug indomethacin, a potent inhibitor of prostaglandin synthesis, will significantly inhibit bone dissolution due to gum fragment media. Levels of one type of prostaglandin in inflamed gum tissue are twice as high as levels seen in normal tissue and are high enough to stimulate bone dissolution in tissue culture. Perhaps the most intriguing aspect of prostaglandin studies is the possibility that aspirin or some other inhibitor of prostaglandin synthesis may be found to be effective in the treatment of chronic, destructive periodontal disease in conjunction with other types of treatment. Long-term studies with animals and human subjects are needed to determine the efficacy of such an approach to periodontal therapy.

Tooth Implants

In 1969, 15 percent of all dental visits in the United States involved tooth extractions; approximately 56 million teeth were removed. During that same year 14 million prosthetic appliances were fabricated: 4 million removable partial dentures, 4 million fixed partial dentures, and 6 million full dentures to replace all the teeth in the upper or lower jaw. Artificial replacement of missing permanent teeth is usually necessary for functional and esthetic reasons and to prevent the shifting or extrusion of teeth adjacent to or opposite the newly created space. (Teeth near these spaces have an increased risk for dental caries and chronic destructive periodontal disease.) Unfortunately, these protheses are not without their problems. Fixed partial bridges require solid teeth to act as abutments on both sides of the space; periodontally diseased teeth may not offer enough support for the bridge, and several teeth may have to be used on each side of the space. Frequently, healthy teeth may have to be cut down to construct crowns. Finally, the techniques used to construct these prostheses are complex and time-consuming, and great skill is required to provide a perfect fit, proper occlusion, strength, pleasing appearance, and the opportunity for good oral hygiene. For all these reasons, artificial teeth are extremely expensive; depending on the number of teeth involved, these appliances can cost as much as several thousand dollars. Removable partial prostheses are usually less expensive, since they generally require less complicated procedures to install and less time to prepare. They are bulky, however, and their usual attachment by clasps around the abutment teeth creates additional problems. The repeated insertion of the appliance and its removal for cleaning tend to put an untoward stress upon these teeth, which, together with the difficulty of cleaning the abutment teeth, may gradually lead to loss of bone support and to loosening and eventual loss of the abutment teeth. The complete full denture is the least stable prosthesis, since it does not use any teeth for support or attachment and must depend on a good fit and peripheral seal with the gums for its retention. Continued dissolution of the bone of the jaw even after the teeth have been extracted leads to the shrinkage of tissues under the denture and its subsequent loosening; in some instances, particularly in the lower jaw, the bone may have dissolved to such an extent that it is virtually impossible to fabricate a full denture that will have any retention.

Dental clinicians and researchers have been investigating the use of dental implants as a new approach to the replacement of extracted teeth. Metal implants have been designed that can be firmly retained even when massive dissolution of the lower jawbone has occurred. Other devices, known as endosseous implants, have screws or blades that are inserted directly into the body of the upper or lower jaw and acquire stability through the mechanical interlocking of bone and fibrous tissue with the implant. Despite their advantages, it appears that endosseous implants eventually fail because of progressive bone dissolution around the implant. Recently, researchers have been concentrating on the development of new materials and designs to improve the success rate of implants. Substances with microscopic pores have attracted much interest, since it is thought that tissue ingrowth into such pores may reduce the stress on the surrounding bone and decrease the rate of bone dissolution. Among the materials used or under review for endosseous implants are certain metals (like the chrome-cobalt alloys and titanium alloys), polymers, silicones, nylon, teflon, dacron, and the ceramics, such as alumina, spinel, calcium aluminate, and the carbons.

The use of acrylic tooth replicas to replace extracted teeth almost immediately is most intriguing. In this procedure, the extracted tooth is immediately duplicated in methylmethacrylate mixed with an agent that provides a porous surface to the plastic. The replica can be made and inserted into the extraction socket before the patient leaves the office. Animal and human studies indicate that such a plastic tooth is generally well tolerated by the surrounding tissues and that subsequent tissue growth around the implant root contributes to its stability and retention without subsequent bone dissolution and loosening. If these findings are substantiated by other investigators, the plastic-replica method will certainly be widely used; it offers a simple, quick, and inexpensive approach to the replacement of extracted teeth and does not require the cutting down of adjacent teeth for abutments, nor the use of removable prosthetic devices that depend on continuous clasping of adjacent teeth for retention.

We now have available to us many methods in various stages of development for the prevention and treatment of dental caries and periodontal disease. Some of these approaches, like the use of drugs that block prostaglandin synthesis to prevent jawbone dissolution, will require much more theoretical and experimental work before they can be put into practice. Other methods already seem to be feasible in theory, but technical problems remain in their application; much research will have to be done, for example, before immunization against caries becomes a reality. And still other preventive oral health measures, like the fluoridation of community water supplies, are blocked in their effectiveness only by the public's reluctance to accept them. With further research and better health education, these diverse approaches should yield the tools necessary to lower the national prevalence of oral disease to a level where it can more readily be treated at a reasonable cost.

Vision

W. MORTON GRANT

21

Various forms of blindness constitute a major health problem in the United States. It has been estimated that between 350,000 and 500,000 Americans are legally blind, meaning that they have distance vision that cannot be made better than 20/200 with glasses, or that they have a visual field of 20 degrees or less. Less serious visual impairments handicap many more, ranking third (after heart disease and arthritis) among the chronic diseases that prevent people from leading normal productive lives in this country. The annual income loss due to blindness in the United States is from 600 million to 1 billion dollars and the cost to public welfare agencies more than half a billion dollars.

Of the principal categories of eye disease responsible for blindness in the United States, glaucoma is the cause in 49,000 people, corneal disease in 21,000, cataract in 45,000, and diseases of the retina and choroid in 147,000. These numbers do not tell the whole story, for there are differences in the types of blindness within these groups. The last category includes both totally blind people and a number who are blind only in a central spot in the field of vision; in contrast, practically all those who are blind from glaucoma are severely disabled by permanent constriction of their visual fields. Some of those who suffer from corneal disease or cataract may be able to recover their vision through surgery.

Research into the mechanisms and diseases of the eye began over a hundred years ago. A large part of the research done at that time utilized eyes that had been removed surgically, because of disease or after death (Figure 21-1). A great deal was learned from these investigations concerning the physical abnormalities associated with cataract, inflammation,

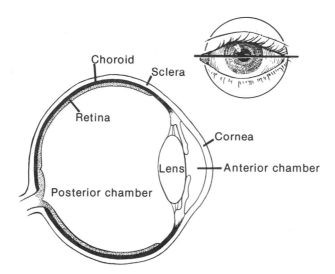

Figure 21–1. The anatomy of the normal eye, as revealed by dissection. The insert shows the line along which the eye has been dissected to obtain this cross-section.

tumors, and glaucoma. However, research was then limited to what one could learn by looking at tissue specimens with a microscope or by injecting fluid into the eye to imitate the circulation occurring in life. It has been less than fifty years since the beginning of biochemical, electrophysiological, and other truly biological studies on the eye and its connections to the brain. For abnormal circumstances in which some of the normally clear portions of the eye have become opaque and visual examination is prevented, it has become possible to study much that goes on within the eye by means of ultrasound, X rays, and radioisotopes. There are instruments for measuring the pressure within the eye and the pressure within the blood vessels of the eye; the circulation of the eye's fluids can also be gauged. Apparatus has vastly multiplied for evaluating all aspects of the visual process: the optical, the electrophysiological, and the psychophysical. Specialized instruments and methods have developed into clinical tools of great usefulness in diagnosing eye disorders and managing their medical and surgical treatment.

Glaucoma

Glaucoma was one of the first diseases to stimulate research on the eye. In the middle of the nineteenth century an acutely painful and rapidly blinding form of glaucoma, usually affecting one eye at a time, was recognized by its invariable association with a high pressure in the affected eye. We now know that there are other forms of glaucoma, at least 20 times as common, in which the pressure in the eye is only slightly elevated above the normal level and in which there is no pain; these forms of the disease have a much more gradual effect on vision, sometimes taking many years to cause significant loss of sight.

The first effective treatment for glaucoma came with the introduction of two drugs of botanical origin, pilocarpine and physostigmine. The acute, rapidly blinding form of the disease was commonly found to be accompanied by dilation of the pupils; pilocarpine and physostigmine were known to cause pupils to constrict and proved highly successful in the treatment of acute glaucoma as well. Pilocarpine is still the most frequently used drug in the treatment of glaucoma today, and there must now be hundreds of thousands of patients who owe the preservation of their vision to this drug and to drugs having a similar action.

The major breakthrough in the understanding of the nature of the various forms of glaucoma came through the use of gonioscopy to study the eyes of patients. Gonioscopy, basically a very simple procedure, consists of applying a type of contact lens to the patient's eye so that the investigator can look with a microscope at a small region that is otherwise hidden from view within the eye. This tiny area was named the filtration area more than a hundred years ago. At that time it was first hypothesized that clear, watery fluid (aqueous humor) was constantly being secreted into the eye and circulating through it, finally leaving the eye through a very small, highly specialized region composed of a fine meshwork of tissue (Figure 21-2). Clearly, anything that obstructs the escape of aqueous humor through this filtration area will cause the pressure in the eye to rise. Eyes that were removed surgically because of blindness and pain from acute glaucoma were dissected so that one could look directly at the filtration area, and causes of obstruction were almost always evident. The great advantage provided by gonioscopy was that it made possible the completely harmless and painless examination of the filtration area of a patient's eye, so that the nature of the obstruction and the cause of the glaucoma could be determined. Together with clinical means for examining the composition of the aqueous humor and for measuring resistance to its outflow, gonioscopy has led to the recognition of several dozen different causes of obstruction. This has made the choice of treatment for glaucoma more specific and efficient than was ever before possible. Perhaps the most significant distinction established through

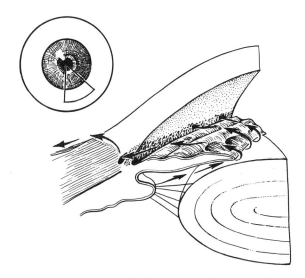

Figure 21–2. The filtration area. Fluid circulates between the iris and the lens into the anterior chamber; the fluid then filters out of the eye through the filtration area. The insert gives the orientation of this cross-section with reference to the rest of the eye; if one took a pie-shaped slice of the eye (as shown in the insert), the cross-section would be the view from one of the straight sides of the slice. (The outer circular rim of the pie slice is on the left in this cross-section.)

gonioscopy was between the two most common forms of glaucoma: the so-called angle-closure glaucoma, which can be completely cured by surgical removal of part of the iris (a safe and reliable operation), and open-angle glaucoma, which requires quite different types of medical and surgical treatment (Figure 21-3).

Biochemical research which has resulted in major progress in the treatment of glaucoma had its beginnings in the 1930s and 1940s and has been concentrated primarily on understanding the secretion of fluid into the eye. Jonas Friedenwald theorized that the process was probably helped by an enzyme, carbonic anhydrase, that was already known to aid the movement of carbon dioxide from the blood to other body fluids (such as cerebrospinal fluid and urine). His hypothesis seemed so logical that researchers sought and tested substances that might stop carbonic anhydrase from working, in the hopes of slowing down secretion of fluid into the eye and thereby reducing intraocular pressure in glaucoma.

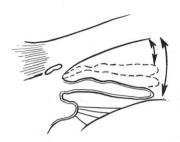

Figure 21–3. Different types of glaucoma. In open-angle glaucoma, the iris remains in its normal position near the lens (solid line). In angle-closure glaucoma, the iris and lens are closer to the cornea, and the iris blocks the filtration of fluid (dotted lines). The orientation for this cross-section is the same as for Figure 21–2.

Sulfanilamide was tried for this purpose by Everett Kinsey in the 1940s, but it was too weak and ineffectual. Finally, in the 1950s, pharmacologic research produced acetazolamide; this drug was able to reduce the rate of secretion of aqueous humor into the eye by about half, as determined in animals and patients by Bernard Becker, myself, and others. Acetazolamide and several closely related drugs have provided a very valuable means of reducing the intraocular pressure in both acute and chronic glaucoma, although their use may be limited by unpleasant side effects in some patients.

Today, glaucoma can usually be effectively treated if it is discovered reasonably early, before much damage has been done to the optic nerve head. Unfortunately, many patients still do not realize they have this disease until they have reached a desperate stage where blindness is very difficult or impossible to prevent. Greater awareness and better means of detection are improving the situation. Although some of the causes of glaucoma are still unclear, hereditary factors do seem to be important in most common forms of the disease. This makes it advisable for blood relatives of glaucoma patients to be examined regularly.

In this connection, an intriguing and practical discovery was made in the 1950s, when cortisone and related hormones were being widely used to treat various kinds of inflammation of the eye. Becker, Mansour Armaly, and others found that close relatives of patients with spontaneous open-angle glaucoma ran a high risk of developing high intraocular pressure upon using these drugs. The obvious practical implication seemed to be that if a simple means were devised of testing for this special responsiveness to these hormones, one might be able to identify very early those people who were likely to develop glaucoma. One of the most interesting investigations going on at present is the study of a peculiar laboratory reaction of certain blood cells to these hormones; the behavior of a patient's cells seems to be related in an important way to inheritance of the tendency for the intraocular pressure to rise. This opens up possibilities for the development of a blood test for the open-angle glaucoma trait.

In less common forms of glaucoma, major practical advances have also been made through clinical research and experimentation. The treatment of congenital glaucoma was vastly improved by Otto Barkan in the 1930s through careful clinical evaluation of an operation called goniotomy, which is performed (with the aid of considerable optical magnification) upon the tiny filtration area in the eyes of infants with this disease. This method has proven successful in a large majority of cases. Another form of glaucoma, known as malignant glaucoma, was virtually untreatable until new effective medical and surgical procedures were developed in the 1950s and 1960s.

In addition to continuing research on the system of fluid circulation in the eye, great attention is now being given to the structure and the blood supply of the optic nerve in the hopes of understanding how that nerve is damaged in glaucoma. It is well known that some people suffer rapidly blinding damage to their optic nerves with a given degree of elevation of intraocular pressure, whereas other people tolerate the same amount of pressure for years without perceptible damage. Evidently there is wide variation in the vulnerability of the optic nerve. The ultimate goal of research in this area is to explain this variation and to use that knowledge to develop some way of treating or altering the weak optic nerve heads to make them strong and better able to withstand pressure. This could be extremely valuable in the treatment of those patients in whom it is difficult to reduce intraocular pressure.

Cornea and External Diseases

The external surface of the eye consists of the conjunctiva, a loose and vascular tissue which overlies the sclera (the white of the eye), and the cornea, a transparent membrane which covers the pupil and iris much as the crystal of a watch covers its hands and face. The cornea is essential to vision; it is an important element of the optical system that focuses an image of the outside world on the retina in the back of the eye. Any irregularity of its outer surface, or any clouding, can cause visual impairment ranging from a slight blurring to near-total blindness. Besides causing loss of vision, corneal disorders may be extremely painful. Because of constant exposure to the outside world (except for the occasional protection provided by closure of the eyelids), the cornea and conjunctiva are subject to a great variety of injuries and infections. They are also prone to a variety of systemic diseases and inherited conditions.

Research has developed several antibacterial, antiviral, and antifungal agents that have proven effective in the prevention and treatment of infectious diseases of the cornea. Gonorrheal ophthalmia in infants has been nearly eliminated by the routine application of silver nitrate eye drops at birth; and new cases of syphilitic interstitial keratitis in young people have become practically unknown since the initiation of testing and treatment of pregnant women to prevent congenital syphilis in their children. In the less developed parts of the world the infectious eye disease trachoma remains an important problem, causing widespread blindness in some regions. This disease has gradually been yielding to research on its causes and treatment and has practically been eliminated from the more prosperous parts of the world; it could presumably be controlled worldwide with increased availability of preventive and therapeutic techniques. The first viral disease of the cornea to yield to drug treatment has been herpes simplex keratitis, also known as dendritic keratitis, a recurring condition caused by the herpes simplex virus which tended to leave varying degrees of scarring and interference with vision. The effective therapeutic agent, idoxuridine, evolved from the basic virologic research that was done by Herbert Kaufman while he was still a hospital resident in ophthalmology. Success with dendritic keratitis has encouraged the effort to develop antiviral agents to combat other viral corneal diseases.

Many diseases and injuries unfortunately produce opacity of the cornea that is unresponsive to any known medical treatment. In such cases, the only real chance for improvement of vision lies in the surgical transplantation of a clear cornea from another eye, usually donated at death through an eye bank. A long series of laboratory and clinical studies has vastly improved both the meticulous surgical procedures—performed under a microscope with sutures finer than a hair—and the means for maintaining the viability of the normal cornea after its excision from the deceased donor. Reasons for earlier failures have become better understood, including the immunological aspects of the problem; with technical improvements, the success rate of restoration of vision through corneal transplantation has improved considerably. Further research will almost certainly overcome some of the complications that still remain.

Cataract

The crystalline lens, situated in the pupils, is normally crystal clear. The properly functioning lens responds to a small ring of muscle within which it is suspended; this muscle can make the lens change shape to focus images of objects at varying distances from the viewer on the retina at the back of the eye. Under abnormal circumstances the lens may become cataractous and lose its transparency, or it may become detached and dislocated from the ring of suspending muscle. Even if one has a clear and normally focusing lens when young, it inevitably changes with age. From middle age onward the lens becomes hardened and less responsive to muscular control and gradually loses its ability to change focus back and forth from far to near. Many people then have to wear glasses for reading. Later in life, the nucleus of the lens not only becomes more hardened but also gradually becomes yellow. Everyone who lives long enough experiences the changes of so-called nuclear sclerosis; in many people, portions of the lens turn milky white. As such a cataract develops, vision is gradually reduced. Naturally one would like to know how to stop or at least slow down this process; otherwise, one would like to know how to make surgical removal of cataracts as easy, safe, and successful as possible. Research on the lens and on the development of cataract has produced some important and practical advances in both prevention and treatment.

One impressive example of the prevention of cataract in infants has been the near-elimination of rubella cataract by successful prevention of rubella (German measles) in the mother during the first three months of pregnancy. More recently, encouraging progress has been made by Jin Kinoshita and his associates in understanding the biochemical aspects of another type of cataract known as sugar cataract. These researchers have shown that under certain conditions in experimental animals (and also in human beings), sugar alcohols can be formed from sugars within the lens faster than they can be metabolized or escape from the lens. When these sugar alcohols accumulate, they cause the lens to swell and cloud. This condition can be reversed if treated early but develops in time into an irreversible cataract. Kinoshita and his associates have taken the logical step of seeking and testing substances that would slow down the formation of sugar alcohols within the lens in experimental animals and have demonstrated that such substances actually do retard the development of this special type of cataract. Eventually this type of treatment may become possible in human beings as well.

Efforts are constantly being made to improve surgical techniques for the removal of cataracts. Innovations are frequent, and they require much careful clinical appraisal. Some changes in surgical procedures appear to offer a real advantage in increased safety for the patient and more rapid return to a normal style of life, whereas others are still in a period of evaluation. One recent innovation that has proven particularly useful has been the introduction of an enzyme, alpha-chymotrypsin, to weaken the fine strands of protein that normally hold the lens in the eye and thus to permit easier surgical extraction of the lens. Advances have also been made through the development of low-temperature probes that grasp the lens by freezing to it, providing a safer and more secure hold than was obtained formerly with forceps or suction devices and reducing the risk of rupturing the lens. In young people, the lens may be so firmly anchored within the eye that removal as a whole is less practical; in these cases it is now possible to aspirate the contents of the lens by means of a slender needle and irrigating system introduced through a small opening, thus improving safety and reducing complications. Other recently proposed surgical procedures, however, need further clinical study before they can be applied on a widespread basis. For example, the use of high-frequency vibrations to fragment the lens and facilitate its removal from the eye, and the implantation of artificial plastic lenses in place of the original lens, entail definite risks that may or may not be outweighed by their merits.

Retina and Choroid

Disorders of the retina and the choroid (the middle coating of the eye lying between the retina and sclera) comprise numerous and widely varied causes of loss of vision. These include retinal detachment, diabetic changes in the retinal blood vessels, degenerative diseases of the retina, various types of intraocular inflammation, intraocular tumors, and many manifestations of systemic diseases and poisoning on the retina and choroid.

One of the most impressive practical results of research in this area has been accomplished in the case of retrolental fibroplasia. This is a disorder in the development of the blood vessels of the retina which mysteriously began to appear in large numbers of prematurely born infants in the late 1930s. After lengthy investigation, the cause of this disease was traced to an increase in the use of oxygen in the incubators for premature babies. This excess of oxygen had actually been responsible for causing the developing retinal vessels to constrict abnormally and then later to dilate, proliferate, and leak; the accompanying abnormal contraction of membranes caused blindness by distorting or detaching the retina. While the incidence of blindness from retrolental fibroplasia has dropped dramatically with the reduction of oxygen levels in incubators, the problem of how to provide just enough oxygen for the premature baby's survival, without the slight excess that can result in severe abnormality of the eye, remains a subject of very active concern and study.

Treatment of retinal detachment has changed greatly and has become increasingly successful during the last 25 years, thanks both to technical advances in methods of examining and evaluating the retina and to innovations in surgical procedures for reattaching the retina. Careful clinical research using improved instruments and technology has provided the understanding necessary to the development of appropriate treatments. One novel approach entails indenting the sclera (scleral buckling) to push the wall of the eye into contact with the detached retina, rather than trying to force the delicate, easily torn retina out into contact with the walls of the eye. This technique has given superior results in many cases of retinal detachment.

Diabetic retinopathy, unknown a hundred years ago, has become a very serious, blinding complication of diabetes today. Only since the advent of insulin have diabetics been able to live long enough to develop the severe degenerative changes in the small blood vessels that have especially serious consequences in the eye. Distorted and leaking vessels in the retina give rise to hemorrhages into the normally clear, jelly-like vitreous humor that fills the center of the eye, and thus severely reduce the patient's vision. Blood from hemorrhages in this area characteristically persists, and the hemorrhages may recur repeatedly. Diabetic retinopathy has been such a growing and widespread problem and has become such an important cause of blindness that it is now the subject of much clinical and experimental research. Clinicians have developed several different treatment approaches, including the use of intense focused light (photocoagulation or laser treatment) in an apparently promising attempt to prevent progression of the disease. Another approach has been the use of special miniature instruments equipped with high-speed rotating blades and a circulating system designed to remove persistent blood and produce a tunnel through the vitreous hemorrhage to permit vision. So far, some of these procedures have seemed to give immediate dramatic results; but their long-term value has yet to be determined and is presently the subject of worldwide clinical evaluation. An additional problem affecting many individuals with diabetic retinopathy is the development of a very severe form of glaucoma due to growth of blood vessels over the filtration area, preventing intraocular fluid from escaping from the eye. This form of glaucoma is extremely difficult to treat in such a way as to preserve vision and is another subject of current research.

Another visual problem that worsens with age is the degeneration of the macula, the central focus of the retina at the back of the eye responsible for the keenest central vision (such as is used in reading). In the elderly, and particularly in those who have undergone cataract operations, the macula commonly deteriorates and this central vision is lost. The patient has no trouble walking about unaided, since the rest of the retina is functioning and gives a broad field of vision, but he is greatly handicapped by not being able to read signs, recognize the faces of friends as they approach, or pass the visual acuity test for a drivers license. This is a problem of ever increasing frequency and importance and is receiving a great deal of attention in clinical and experimental research, but like diabetic retinopathy it remains a great challenge to solve.

Intraocular inflammation involving the retina and choroid in the back of the eye goes under the general name of uveitis. This is a less common cause of blindness than those already mentioned, but nevertheless it constitutes a frequent and serious problem that continues to challenge researchers. Actually, a great improvement in treatment has come about through clinical experimentation with the same corticosteroid hormones that were mentioned previously in conjunction with genetic characteristics of glaucoma. The first of this group of hormones, cortisone, has proven invaluable in the relief of the general inflammatory signs and symptoms of uveitis. One of the problems with uveitis is that it is not a single disease but actually a large family of similar diseases, presumably with many different causes. The effort to differentiate these diseases by etiology has been partially successful; research on uveitis has already arrived at the stage of devising specific treatments for types of uveitis with specific causes.

A whole family of substances which go under the name prostaglandins are formed and released within the eye in certain types of inflammation, including some types of uveitis. The properties of many of these substances have been studied, and it appears that they actually contribute to the inflammation. Drugs to counteract the prostaglandins are being sought and tested in the hope that they may be helpful in the treatment of uveitis as well as in treatment of other inflammatory diseases such as arthritis and gum disease (see Chapter 20). Some practical results have been obtained, but this problem is still in an early stage of study.

Advances have also been made in the treatment of certain types of blindness resulting from the action of toxic agents on the retina. Methyl alcohol poisoning, although rare, has been notorious for causing blindness through poisoning of the retina and optic nerve. Clinical research, largely stimulated by the astute observations and investigations of Oluf Røe in Scandinavia has made possible great improvements in emergency treatment; the administration of certain chemicals is now known to optimize the patient's chances for a healthy recovery.

Probable Future Developments

Great strides have been made in the past fifty years in the understanding and treatment of disorders of the eye. However, it is clear that extensive laboratory and clinical research is still needed in several areas.

The primary goal of eye research is the prevention of blindness. To prevent serious eye disorders, one must first understand them on a level that makes therapeutic intervention possible. The biochemical understanding of sugar cataracts and of the role of prostaglandins in uveitis has already given direction to the search for effective agents to combat these problems; and an increasing number of eye diseases should begin to come under control as we understand them biochemically.

One of the central questions of glaucoma research now is whether some metabolic or toxic factors control the processes by which aqueous humor normally is secreted into the eye and drains through the filtration area. Once these two complementary processes are understood, it should become possible to develop new drugs to correct them in glaucoma and to prevent the buildup of excessive pressure within the eye. Specific chemical substances may also be identified as causative agents of some of the more severe types of glaucoma, such as neovascular glaucoma (in which new blood vessels and fibrous tissues grow over the filtration area and obstruct it) and glaucoma that occurs following cataract extraction.

Cataracts may themselves become preventable through a combination of biochemical and structural research. Different kinds of cataract should be associated with different changes in the molecular structure of the proteins of the lens; these molecular changes may be identified and studied through electron microscopy and analytic methods that make use of laser technology. Some types of cataract may be traceable to abnormalities in metabolism and in the enzymes within the lens; others may be caused by the presence of toxic or injurious agents.

Finally, biochemical research is essential to further progress in the prevention and treatment of disorders of the cornea and retina. We need to learn much more about the cellular mechanisms that prevent the accumulation of fluid in the cornea, that keep the cornea from being overgrown by blood vessels and scar tissue, and that promote healing of the cornea after bacterial or viral attack. Pharmacologic research should help us develop better agents to combat infections of the cornea and conjunctiva and should also be useful in identifying those drugs and chemicals that may actually injure these parts of the eye (which are especially vulnerable to injury because of their contact with the environment). And diabetic retinopathy, probably the greatest current problem in retinal disease, cannot be effectively prevented or cured until we have a considerably better understanding of the fundamental biochemical abnormalities underlying this condition.

Targeted research into specific diseases is clearly important; but very basic research may also result in major improvements in the treatment and prevention of eye disorders. Recently, the rods and cones of the retina, which detect light and convert it into nerve impulses that are sent to the brain, have been discovered to be more complex structures than was originally thought. We now know that rods and cones are comprised of stacks of little discs essential to the detection of light; new discs are always being formed, while old ones are cast off the rods and cones to be devoured by the immediately adjacent pigment cells of the retina. It now appears that a failure in any part of this remarkable mechanism—whether caused by genetic factors, the toxic action of drugs, or other causes that have not yet been determined—can give rise to visual disturbances at the clinical level. Research into abnormalities of the retinal pigment cells and their interaction with the rods and cones should improve the understanding and treatment of different types of retinal degeneration, including the degeneration of the macula often seen in adults and the night blindness and gradual constriction of the visual field that characterizes the retinal disease retinitis pigmentosa in young people.

Fundamental research areas that may not even appear to impinge on the eye disorders may in fact be very relevant to the treatment and prevention of diseases of the eye. Very basic research on the healing of

wounds is badly needed to improve the chances for success of antiglau-
coma surgery in young people, who often cannot be treated for glaucoma
by other medical means. Drainage channels can be created surgically to
relieve the pressure within the eye. But young people have a special
ability to heal and form scar tissue easily; and tragically, they tend to
form scar tissue that blocks the drainage channels created to cure their
glaucoma. We still need to determine what biochemical or physiological
mechanisms may underlie this unwanted tendency to heal and scar and
we need to discover ways to overcome this problem with new drugs or
surgical techniques.

While many researchers have concentrated on the biochemical aspects of eye disorders in the hope of developing new methods of drug
therapy, others have worked to develop new technological methods for
correcting visual abnormalities. The progress that has already been made
in this area promises to continue in the future.

A great deal of inventive genius is now being devoted to the problem
of improving reduced vision. Optical aids for low vision and television
magnifiers to help people read in spite of degeneration of the macula are
already realities. Portable radar, sonar, and optical devices have also been
developed to make it easier for the visually impaired to walk around.
These new inventions are now in various stages of development and
experimental evaluation.

New technology has also been applied to major problems in eye
surgery. Many attempts have been made to replace the central portion of
opaque corneas with clear substances other than a transplanted natural
cornea, including glass and many types of plastic. A major obstacle to
these artificial corneal implants is the difficulty of maintaining a reliable
seal between the implant and the natural cornea; such a seal must be
maintained both to keep fluid within the eye and to keep infectious
agents out. No artificial corneal implant has yet had lasting success; often
a layer of opaque tissue grows over the inside surface and obstructs
vision. But the advantages of the artificial cornea—including the fact that
plastic does not cause the same immune reaction as living tissue—make
these implants worthy of further investigation.

Plastic lenses have been somewhat more successful to date and are
coming into increasing clinical use as replacements for lenses that have
become cataractous. After years spent perfecting these devices, it is now
possible to replace the opaque part of the cataract with a plastic lens that
enables the patient to see without the contact lenses or heavy spectacles
usually required after cataract extraction. Many patients are pleased with

the immediate visual results, but most ophthalmologists continue to be cautious in deciding who may best benefit by the implantation of a lens. Experience with the most modern lenses has been too brief to know how well or how poorly they may be tolerated by the patient after a number of years; the process is still not as successful or safe as standard cataract extraction. Nevertheless, the development of lens implants has been a major step, and it is to be hoped that their use will become increasingly safe and have fewer complications.

The ultimate goal of being able to replace a blinded eye by actually transplanting a whole eye from a human donor is still far beyond the grasp of available knowledge and technology. Unlike the relatively simple corneal transplants, the transplantation of a whole eye involves very difficult problems of blood supply, survival of the optic nerve, and the connection of the optic nerve with the brain. These problems seem virtually insurmountable; but nevertheless, they are the subject of active investigation. Even the prospects for developing an artificial eye are being examined hopefully.

At present, the outlook for different types of eye research is somewhat mixed. Some eye disorders, especially the progressive conditions like diabetic retinopathy and degeneration of the macula, remain baffling clinical problems. But current research in other areas has been very encouraging; and there is every reason to expect that continued study of the biochemistry and physiology of the eye will lead to the understanding of many causes of blindness, including glaucoma, cataract, and diseases of the cornea, retina, choroid, and optic nerve. As our understanding of these disorders improves, so should our ability to treat them with effective drugs or surgical procedures. Eye research already has a fine record of success, and its future promises to bring even more important results.

Hearing

HAROLD F. SCHUKNECHT

22

Hearing loss is the most important cause of impaired capability for communication. Many kinds of developmental defects, diseases, injuries, and other malfunctions cause impairment of hearing (and consequently of speech), which disrupts personal maturation and delays social development in the child and interferes with well-adjusted and productive living in the adult. Auditory communication is basic to our world; it is the cohesive force in every human culture and the dominant influence in the personal lives of all of us. It is simultaneously the mechanism for influencing the masses, the foundation for social organization, the vehicle for our intellectual heritage, and the medium whereby each individual adjusts to his fellow man. Disorders of hearing may handicap the individual at any of several levels: severe loss of acuity (inability to hear, deafness); partial loss of acuity (hard of hearing); and dysacusic disturbances (garbled hearing of sounds and speech).

A 1971 survey by the Public Health Service indicates that there are over 13 million Americans who suffer from impaired hearing, and that two to three million of these cannot hear or understand normal speech. A health problem of this magnitude cannot be taken lightly. The national expenditure made necessary by disorders of hearing, while difficult to estimate precisely, is definitely quite sizable. A Subcommittee on Human Communication and Its Disorders of the National Institutes for Neurological Diseases and Stroke estimated the annual direct costs to the nation for the education, management, and compensation of the hearing-impaired to be over 400 million dollars. No monetary value can be placed on the personal tragedies and social misunderstandings which result from hearing loss.

In the broad sense, auditory communicative disorders are divided into three categories: disorders of the receptor system (the ear); disorders of the central processing mechanism (the brain); and disorders of the effector system (primarily the muscular system). In this chapter the discussion will be limited to disorders of the first category.

The Anatomy and Physiology of the Ear

On the basis of anatomical, physiological, and clinical features, the ear can be divided into three principal parts (Figure 22-1). The first part

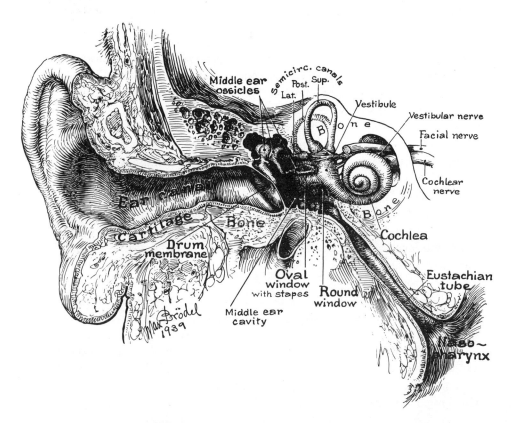

Figure 22–1. The human ear seen in cross-section. From Max Brödel, *The Anatomy of the Human Ear* (Philadelphia: W. B. Saunders Co., 1946). Reproduced by permission.

is the external ear, which consists of the auricle and ear canal, and has the purpose of funneling sound to the eardrum. The second part, the middle ear, transmits the physical stimulus, sound, to the fluids of the inner ear. The major structures of the middle ear are the tympanic membrane (the eardrum) and the malleus, incus, and stapes (the ossicles), a sequence of three tiny bones connected to the tympanic membrane. Sound stimulates the tympanic membrane to vibrate; these vibrations are transmitted through the malleus and incus to the stapes, which in turn applies pressure to the fluids of the inner ear through the oval window. Defects which impair the function of the external and middle parts (the sound-conducting system) cause conductive deafness, which is characterized by an elevation of the threshold of hearing. It is for disorders of this part of the ear that surgical correction is most successful.

The third part of the auditory system, the inner ear, consists primarily of a snail-shaped structure called the cochlea. Its function is to code the sound stimulus into patterns of nerve impulses in the auditory nerve. Other inner-ear structures, the three semicircular canals and vestibule, contain sense organs of balance and may be affected by some of the diseases the inner ear is subject to; this is why vertigo accompanies certain types of deafness. Lesions affecting the inner ear often cause distorted or garbled hearing as well as elevation of the threshold of hearing; such hearing problems are types of sensorineural deafness. Conductive and sensorineural deafness can usually be differentiated by tests that measure the ability to hear pure tones and speech.

The mechanical aspects of sound conduction in the external and middle ear have been studied extensively over the past hundred years and are now quite well understood; but the translation of the mechanical stimulus of sound into patterns of neural excitation remains a somewhat mysterious process of great interest to current researchers. By opening the cochlea and observing its delicate membranes under high magnification, George von Békésy was able to describe the mechanical events occurring in the coiled cochlear duct at the moment of nerve excitation. It is known that the excitatory event is mediated by a group of 12,000 sensory cells (also known as hair cells) which are located along the cochlear duct. In some way that is not yet clearly understood, hair cells respond to the mechanical vibrations they receive and initiate patterns of impulses in the 30,000 auditory nerve fibers, which are then conducted to the brain for neural integration and decoding. In 1936 Glen Wever and C. W. Bray discovered that the cochlea when stimulated by sound generated an electrical response. Subsequently, several additional types of electrical response have been discovered and are now measured and used to study auditory function. Much recent research has been directed toward determining the exact relationship between the original stimulus of sound and its neural encoding in the cochlea. The code for simple stimuli has been determined in some detail through the use of microelectrodes (which can be inserted into single nerve fibers), the development of electronic control of stimuli, and computers, which can handle vast amounts of data quickly. With the aid of computers it is now possible to examine cochlear and auditory nerve responses, as well as brainstem activity, in human individuals with hearing defects. These techniques show promise of becoming an important diagnostic tool in determining the site and nature of auditory lesions.

The Pathology of the Auditory System

Many studies of the auditory system in humans and animals have been performed to determine the causes and mechanism of pathological changes in the ear, their resulting dysfunctions, and possible methods of repair. Great emphasis has been placed upon studying the microscopic appearance, normal and abnormal, of the structures comprising the ear, the bone that encases it (the temporal bone), and the surrounding tissues; these studies have markedly improved our understanding of several types of hearing disorder. Light microscopic studies on human and animal specimens have been conducted using procedures fundamentally unchanged for a century: fixation of tissue, decalcification, embedding, sectioning, staining, and mounting. Simple light microscopy is now being supplemented by electron microscopy, histochemistry, phase-contrast microscopy, and scanning-electron microscopy to provide new dimensions for the acquisition of pathological data. Selected examples will illustrate how pathological studies have provided a basis for improved understanding of several types of hearing disorder.

Before the Second World War, the most widespread causes of hearing loss were infections and their complications. Recent advances in the use of antibiotics have virtually eliminated deafness resulting from acute bacterial infection. Chronic infections, however, are still common and continue to be an important cause of conductive hearing loss. The soft-tissue and bony alterations occurring in chronic bacterial infections are being carefully studied; when combined with astute clinical observations, such information provides the otologic surgeon with a clearer concept of the indications for surgery, as well as of the surgical techniques most suitable for the elimination of disease and improvement of hearing. Pathological studies, too, have pinpointed an unexpected way in which bacterial infections may indirectly lead to deafness: the antibiotics used to combat infection may themselves be harmful to the ear. It has been demonstrated that one class of antibiotic drugs, the aminoglycosides, are toxic to the inner ear; a study of the effects of streptomycin, for example, has demonstrated that repeated injections result in an accumulation of the drug within the inner-ear fluids. Similar behavior has been demonstrated for neomycin and kanamycin; these two drugs as well as dihydro-streptomycin frequently cause deafness due to an irreversible loss of cochlear sensory cells when given in therapeutic dosages. Other commonly used drugs have also been found to be ototoxic: gentamicin, quinine, chloroquine, ethacrynic acid, thalidomide, nitrogen mustard, and tetanus antitoxin. The use of all of these substances must be effectively regulated to prevent their potentially harmful effects.

With the elimination of acute bacterial infection as a cause of hearing loss, the most common type of deafness has become presbycusis, or deafness of aging. Presbycusis is in fact not only a disorder of the elderly but may have its onset at any age; it affects the ears symmetrically and is slowly progressive. It appears to be genetically determined and, at present, there are no therapeutic measures which alter the course of this disorder. However, histological studies have provided the basis for identifying several types of presbycusis based on the selective atrophy of different structures within the cochlea. These structures may be involved individually or in combination. When occurring separately, each type of structural degeneration is manifested by a characteristic pattern of functional disturbance that can be identified by medical history, otologic examination, and auditory testing.

Pathological studies have also been useful in determining the origins of sudden deafness in individual cases. There are many known causes for sudden deafness; these include inner ear infections, ototoxic drugs, fracture of the base of the skull, inner ear hemorrhage, multiple sclerosis, and leukemia. But there are also many cases of sudden deafness in which the etiology is not so obvious. Some occur in association with mild upper-respiratory infections or pneumonia, others in patients complaining only of mild lethargy or headache. Although pathological studies are not entirely conclusive, the weight of evidence favors viral labyrinthitis (viral infection of the inner ear) as the cause for the majority of cases of sudden deafness.

Another common cause of hearing loss is otosclerosis, a disorder of the bone surrounding the inner ear that causes deafness by fixing the stapes so that it can no longer vibrate. A very large literature exists on the pathology of otosclerosis, including possible etiologies, hereditary factors, results of surgery, and effects of the disease on the inner ear. The impact of ostosclerosis on the cochlea has not yet been established. However, increasing numbers of temporal bones from individuals who have had surgery for otosclerosis, particularly removal of the stapes, are becoming available for study. In general, it now appears that careful surgery can effectively reestablish sound transmission through the oval window area without causing inner-ear injury and can be expected to result in long-term hearing improvements.

Ménière's disease is a prevalent inner-ear disorder characterized by attacks of severe vertigo and progressive hearing loss; in about 20 percent of cases both ears are involved. This disease results from imbalances in the two fluid systems of the inner ear, which have distinctly different chemical compositions and functions. The endolymphatic system is located within the membranous labyrinth, the membrane-walled tube running throughout the inner ear. Endolymph has a high potassium and low sodium concentration. The perilymphatic system is located outside the membranous labyrinth; perilymph has a low potassium and high sodium concentration. Numerous studies of temporal bones from individuals with classic symptoms of Ménière's disease have confirmed endolymphatic hydrops (distension of the endolymphatic system) as the most spectacular underlying pathological lesion. Endolymphatic hydrops can be produced experimentally in animals through surgical removal of the endolymphatic sac; the inner-ear changes found in these animal studies are similar to those seen in human individuals with Ménière's disease and include occasional atrophy of the sensorineural structures in the innermost region of the cochlea. Ruptures of the endolymphatic system are also a common pathological finding in Ménière's disease. In these cases the cochlear and vestibular nerve fibers, which appear to be bathed in perilymph, may be adversely affected by the potassium of the endolymph spilling episodically into the perilymph through these ruptures. Such a picture would provide an explanation for the episodic vertigo and hearing loss that occur in this disease.

Finally, much recent pathological research has been directed to the widespread problem of noise deafness. Studies on human subjects and animals have shown that moderate intensities of acoustic stimulation may induce temporary hearing loss accompanied by depletion of cochlear enzymes and stores of the carbohydrate glycogen and by reversible alterations in the cochlear sensory cells and nerve endings. More intense stimulation results in irreversible structural damage and permanent hearing loss. These studies have led to the establishment of damage-risk criteria, that is, maximum levels and durations of sound of different spectra to which the ear can safely be exposed. Such criteria provide the basis for noise-control programs which attempt either to reduce noise at its source or to provide the worker with noise protection devices.

The Prevention and Treatment of Hearing Loss

The most effective approach to the problem of hearing loss, or any disease for that matter, is to prevent it from happening in the first place. This is particularly true for most neurological and sensory disorders, in which the loss of tissue substance through disease or injury is not followed by regeneration but results in permanent loss of function. In the past three decades, considerable attention has been paid to the problem of the prevention of deafness.

One of the most obvious and most important aspects of this problem has been the prevention of exposure to noise. Although it had been known for a century that high-intensity noise exposure could impair hearing, this danger was considered in years past to be one of the unavoidable hazards to be endured and suffered by those engaged in certain occupations and in the military. With the technological explosion came even noisier environments; hundreds of thousands of people suffered hearing losses through exposure to noise generated by machinery, vehicles, firearms, and explosive devices. Many individuals who suffered mild losses could function quite adequately through most of their adult lives but began to exhibit real disability with the added losses caused by aging. In recent years, however, awareness of this problem has led to extensive programs for noise abatement, ear protection, and education of the public. Data acquired through hearing surveys on noise-exposed populations and through controlled animal studies have led to legislation (Occupational Safety and Health Act of 1970) that should alleviate the industrial noise-deafness problem; similar standards are being adopted by the military as well.

Health surveys have also been instrumental in identifying ototoxic drugs and limiting their use. Dihydrostreptomycin was widely used therapeutically until 1959, when George Shambaugh, Jr., and coworkers described deafness of delayed onset in thirty-two patients receiving this drug, mostly in combination with penicillin. On the basis of this study, the Food and Drug Administration forbade the manufacture and sale of antibiotic preparations combining dihydrostreptomycin with other antibiotics. Today, such drugs as dihydrostreptomycin, kanamycin, and neomycin, because of their known ototoxic effects, are used only in exceptional circumstances.

Another key area in the prevention of deafness is the control and prevention of diseases that can lead indirectly to hearing loss. The incidence of conductive and sensorineural deafness occurring as a complication of contagious disease has been greatly reduced through immunizations and prophylactic antibiotic therapy. Smallpox, typhus, typhoid, tuberculosis, diphtheria, tetanus, and measles (morbilli) have ceased to be significant causes of deafness. In the early part of this century, about 20 percent of deaf institutionalized children had lost their hearing through aural complications of meningococcal meningitis; today, improved health standards have virtually eliminated this disease in America. Rubella (German measles) occurring in the early part of pregnancy frequently causes multiple anomalies in the offspring, with deafness occurring in about 15 percent of such infants; but the development of a rubella virus vaccine promises control of this disease in the near future. Erythroblastosis fetalis, another disease of pregnancy, has also been associated with infant deafness. This disease, usually caused by Rh incompatibility between the mother and the fetus, often results in deafness in the newborn. But this type of deafness has been almost eliminated, thanks to improved methods in the treatment of Rh incompatibility; these include the administration of immunoglobulin G antibodies and exchange transfusions for the newborn infant (see Chapter 15). Finally, the prevention of acute ear infections through improved health standards and early treatment of upper-respiratory infections has greatly reduced the incidence of middle-ear and mastoid complications. Mastoidectomy for acute infection, which entails the removal of a portion of the temporal bone, was a frequently performed surgical procedure just four decades ago. It is a rare operation today.

Unfortunately, it is still far from possible to control all forms of deafness through preventive measures alone. However, the alleviation of deafness through treatment has also been successful in many cases. The prompt treatment of acute ear infections with appropriate antibiotic drugs (penicillin, tetracycline, and so on) usually arrests the process before destruction of the tympanic membrane and ossicles can occur and prevents the infection from becoming chronic. Additionally, antibiotic drugs are now used effectively to control certain forms of meningitis, which when untreated result in a high incidence of profound deafness in survivors.

Surgical correction can effectively remedy many types of conductive hearing loss. Advances in this area must be attributed to knowledge gained in laboratory and clinical research, to improvements in surgical equipment, and to the design and manufacture of prosthetic middle-ear devices. The success of middle-ear surgery depends largely on favorable reparative reactions to surgical trauma; consequently, these reactions have been studied extensively in the normal animal ear. The adaptation of the stereoscopic microscope to surgical use has allowed the otologic surgeon not only to remove disease but also to undertake reconstructive procedures to improve hearing. The use of tissue grafts and prostheses has been most successful in restoring hearing in patients with congenital anomalies, otosclerosis, or chronic ear infection. The most spectacular example of success is in otosclerosis, where the fixed stapes can be replaced with a steel or plastic one. Given a normal inner ear, hearing can be restored in such cases.

In cases of hearing loss which cannot be treated by drug therapy or by surgery, the use of amplifying devices is often helpful. With the advent of the transistor, microcircuitry, and improved power packs, the hearing aid has rendered convenient, indispensable aid to millions of Americans. Almost all individuals with hearing problems, whether they be conductive or sensorineural in type, will be benefited to some extent by amplification.

Fruitful Areas for Future Research

It is obvious that there are many areas in which well-conceived and carefully executed research on the mechanisms of hearing can provide needed information; there is still a great deal to be learned. The investigation of the anatomy, physiology, and chemistry of the inner ear is of primary importance. A detailed knowledge of the normal cochlea is fundamental to understanding the causes of inner-ear deafness. We must know the mechanics of the cochlea, how it initiates nerve excitation, and how the stimulus is coded into patterns of nervous activity. More information on the chemistry of the inner-ear fluids in health and disease is also needed. At least one type of deafness, strial atrophy, occurs with no obvious structural changes in the sensory cells or neurons of the cochlea; thus it is likely that this common form of deafness of aging may be caused by a chemical deficit. Studies of inner-ear fluid chemistry could clarify the etiology of this disease.

A knowledge of pathology is basic to progress in any field of medicine, and studies of temporal bone pathology are vital to the understanding of diseases of the ear. To understand deafness, we must determine the structural changes occurring in the middle and inner ears and correlate these with the functional deficits resulting from such changes. This knowledge is essential if one is to dignify a clinical study with an intelligent diagnosis and logical management.

Much work is still needed to determine the behavioral correlates of lesions in the auditory system (the middle ear, cochlea, cochlear nerve, brainstem, and cortex). It is already quite clear that most of these lesions are expressed by characteristic abnormalities in psychoacoustic behavior and electrical response. Further research on such functions as speech discrimination, loudness sensation, and sound localization holds promise of providing new, useful tests for determining the site of a lesion through behavioral criteria. Another attractive approach to the problem is through the further development of electrical recordings from the ear and brain. At the very least, it seems probable that refinement of these methods will facilitate the diagnosis of hearing loss in infants and children and will permit the earliest possible initiation of educational and rehabilitative procedures.

In the realm of treatment, much progress can be made through the development of technological devices to aid the profoundly deaf. A rough estimate places the number of profoundly deaf persons (those who cannot hear or understand speech) at between two and three million in the United States alone. In addition to acquiring lip-reading skills, these individuals would be aided by some form of sensory experience resulting from sound stimulation. Under investigation (and needing much more development and study in the laboratory before clinical application) are methods of direct electrical stimulation of the auditory nerve by cochlear implants. The development of an implant that will convey speech understanding will not be a simple task; such a device will require a multiple-electrode system, spatially distributed so as to selectively excite populations of auditory nerve fibers with electrical discharges accurately simulating those given out by the cochlea. Other areas which deserve further study are the investigation of high-gain hearing aids, which may function through a combination of auditory and tactile stimuli, and the development of devices to convert sound energy into vibratory stimuli to be applied to the skin.

Finally, improvements are needed in the educational and rehabilitative management of auditory disorders. The question of how deprivation of auditory experience in early life modifies and interferes with the acquisition of communicative skills is of importance. Improved methods of teaching the deaf to communicate can be expected to result from laboratory studies of the fundamental speech process. Other areas worthy of study include the special problems of the doubly handicapped (auditory and visual), the training methods to be used for children with different degrees of deafness, the most effective methods of maintaining and improving the communicative skills of the hearing-handicapped adult, and vocational training and placement for individuals with hearing problems. Finally, we must have more carefully designed epidemiological studies to define the prevalence, incidence, and etiology of each type of hearing impairment, those that occur in combination with other disorders as well as those that occur alone.

New Techniques of
Diagnosis and Intervention

PART FIVE

Orthopedics

HENRY J. MANKIN

23

Man's curiosity about the workings of his musculoskeletal system dates back to antiquity. Since the early periods of recorded history investigators have examined the mechanisms of limb function, spinal support, joints, and muscular attachment and function. The pathological processes of the musculoskeletal system have been similarly studied; early writings of ancient Egyptian, Greek, and Roman physicians display a fairly sophisticated knowledge of dislocations, osteomyelitis, muscle paralysis, and arthritis. The path followed by orthopedic research over the centuries has been long and arduous, characterized by false starts, blind alleys, and the inevitable perpetuation of ancient misconceptions. The earliest modern investigators used crude tools and were primarily dependent on anatomical observation and the interpretation of microscopic preparations. With the advent of the twentieth century, however, the newer techniques of biochemistry and physiology have been applied to the study of the musculoskeletal system, and slowly the ancient mysteries have yielded to the tireless efforts of the research scientist. In the last two decades there has been a remarkable surge of interest in the disorders of locomotion, culminating in some spectacular advances in clinical care. Orthopedics today is riding a crest of enthusiastic research and development, thanks largely to the growing participation of engineers and research biochemists. Judicious application of recent advances in chemistry, materials science, and mechanical and electrical engineering has enormously speeded the progress of orthopedic research in the seventies and promises to continue to do so in the decades to follow.

The Problems

Disorders of the musculoskeletal system exact an enormous toll in the United States today, in terms of both disability and financial cost. It has been estimated that over 20 percent of the complaints for which patients in the United States seek health care fall within the category of problems of the musculoskeletal system; patients with such disorders approximate 18 percent of the total hospitalized population in America today. At least 20 million Americans require medical care for arthritis. The cost in terms of the reduction of the labor force can be estimated from the fact that approximately 20 percent of these individuals are significantly disabled; 8 percent are restricted to bed for varying periods of time, 4 percent for 8 or more days per year. Trauma constitutes another major health problem. Accidental injury represents the third ranking cause of death in adults and the first in children; but this fact alone does not tell the full story of the impact of such injuries on our society. It is estimated that of the over 10.5 million accidental injuries occurring each year, there are more than 2 million fractures of the extremities, and 400,000 injuries which result in permanent disability. Major trauma to the limbs or spine remains the most devastating of the nonfatal illnesses in terms of the total number of individuals affected and economic impact. Fracture of an extremity, even when optimally treated and with no apparent complications, can easily result in 12 months or more of total disability, followed by a permanent impairment which limits the individual's earning power and his ability to function normally in work in leisure activities. Abnormalities in the extremities in children are another frequent sources of serious disability. Club foot occurs in one out of every two hundred live births; a dislocated hip, in approximately the same percentage; and scoliosis (curvature of the spine) in one child out of a hundred. Rarer lesions such as meningomyelocele, Perthes disease of the hip, and a variety of genetically determined disorders of the entire skeleton (including dwarfism, rickets, and fragile bones) cause untold hardship for the afflicted individual and his family. Bone tumors, although rare, occur most frequently in children; they are often extremely malignant and prove fatal in more than 75 percent of all cases, despite amputation, radiation therapy, and drug therapy. Osteoporosis (an increased porousness of the bone resulting from calcium deficiency) produces significant musculoskeletal problems, particularly in relation to fractures of the vertebrae, hips, and upper extremities in the elderly population. It is estimated that there are over 8 million postmenopausal women in this country who suffer from advanced degrees of this disorder and that 75 percent of the female and 40 percent of the male population over the age of 60 experience some such diminution in mineral content of the bones. Most fractures in patients over the age of 60 are "pathological" in the sense that they occur in bones already weakened by osteoporosis; and fractures of the hip in the elderly are a major cause of permanent disability, loss of independence, and even death.

It is apparent from this small sampling of health data that orthopedic problems represent a major segment of the spectrum of disorders that affect the American people and that they have a vast impact on the health pattern and economics of this country. If even some of these problems could be solved, the resultant gains in alleviation of suffering, restoration of disability, and reduction of the cost of health care would be enormous. The major research activities in orthopedics in the United States today fall into eight broad categories, discussed below. It should be emphasized that a rank order of importance is not implied by the presentation of these areas here; researchers in all these areas are making contributions of vital importance to individuals affected by orthopedic disorders.

Bone Formation

Throughout medical history, scientists have been puzzled by the phenomenon of bone formation. No other of the body's tissues appear to have quite the capacity for self-renewal that the bones do, and the nature of the process by which this occurs remains obscure. Studies have progressed, however, and considerable information is now available regarding the complex process of bone formation by the cell. Bone formation begins with the production of an organic framework consisting of a specialized protein known as collagen, which is characterized by a triple helix of repeating units extended into very long strands. Tiny crystals of a calcium- and phosphorus-containing mineral known as hydroxyapatite are deposited on the collagen. The organic and mineral phases are then combined in a highly organized framework which assumes the structure of the specific bone according to a variety of complex factors. The osteoblast (a bone-forming cell) is central to this entire system; it synthesizes the collagen and dictates the alignment of the collagen fibers by controlling chemical cross-linking between them. The hydroxyapatite crystals are also produced by the cell, in apparent defiance of the relative insolubility of the component ions in water, by an elaborate and as yet poorly defined intracellular mechanism. These crystals are then deposited at specific sites on the collagen fiber, where they grow (like rock salt) by precipitation from a supersaturated solution. The control mechanisms of this process are not fully understood, but investigation proceeds at a rapid pace toward their elucidation. Over recent years, the nature of the collagen fiber and the interrelationship of its various regions with the crystallite have been the subjects of intensive study. The mechanism by which the cell is able to concentrate the component calcium and phosphorus ions has been partially determined, and the control systems of this process are now under further investigation.

Numerous outgrowths of this research are of great importance in such areas as fracture healing, bone growth, and metabolic bone disease. Of special importance is the potential for controlling the process of bone formation by chemical or hormonal agents, such as magnesium, pyrophosphates, diphosphonates, parathormone, Vitamin D or calcitonin. Present studies are certain to lead to a better understanding of the abnormalities of bone structure which accompany certain genetic disorders of collagen or mineral metabolism. It is hoped that over the next decade or so, further information will solve the final mysteries of the complicated process of bone formation and will lead to important developments in many of the other fields discussed in this chapter.

Growth Disturbances

There is probably no more distressing problem in all of orthopedics than that of the child in whom an injury to one or several growth plates of the long bones has altered the growth of the segment, leading to eventual shortening of an extremity. If the disorder is systemically widespread, as occurs in certain genetic abnormalities, the child may be dwarfed and show bizarre deformities related to disturbances in the pattern of growth and in the rate of new bone formation. If the disturbance is localized, as may occur in trauma, there is considerable shortening of the affected part, and sometimes a disturbance in alignment, resulting in grotesque deformity.

The hope of developing effective treatments for systemic disorders (with generalized disturbances) has been encouraged by research suggesting that these disorders are caused by specific metabolic abnormalities. Specific enzyme defects are known to occur in Gaucher's disease, and are strongly suspected to play a role in Morquio's and Hurler's syndromes. Electron microscope studies of patients with a variety of other growth disorders have demonstrated abnormalities in the endoplasmic reticulum of the cell (that portion of the cell where protein synthesis is thought to occur); this suggests that some form of enzyme defect may be involved in these disorders as well. Continued work in this area may lead to the development of some forms of replacement therapy similar to that now employed for Gaucher's disease. (In this systemic lipid storage disease, the patient's condition may be improved by administration of the specific enzyme in which he is deficient.)

New treatments are already available for those children in whom Vitamin D resistant rickets limits the growth of the epiphysis (the spongy, cartilage-covered bone process that forms the joints). This type of rickets usually results from a genetic abnormality in the kidney's handling of phosphorus or in the production of important metabolic products of Vitamin D. Patients with this disease respond well either to oral administration of neutral phosphate, or in some cases to administration of a new and very potent Vitamin D analog, 1-alpha, 25-dihydroxy Vitamin D. This synthetic material closely resembles the natural active principle of Vitamin D—1,25-dihydroxy Vitamin D—which is a product of the metabolism of Vitamin D by enzyme action in the liver and kidney. In some patients with Vitamin D resistant rickets, the kidney enzyme appears to be either absent or defective, resulting in an inadequate supply of this very important metabolic product. Introduction of the snythetic material has greatly enhanced the pediatrician's and orthopedist's ability to deal with problems of Vitamin D resistant rickets, in which dwarfism and skeletal deformity are the usual consequences.

For patients with localized injuries to the growth plate, numerous methods have been used to stimulate the epiphyseal plate in order to achieve a limb length reasonably close to that of the opposite member. Some of these techniques includes interruption of the arterial supply of the affected bone, arteriovenous anastamosis (dilation of small arteries and veins achieved by the blocking of large ones), and heating of the extremity; none of these have been found to be very effective, however. Recent studies have indicated that venous blockade may enhance epiphyseal growth and that periodic applications of tourniquets can gradually increase the rate of growth of the limb. This method is unfortunately limited in its usefulness, particularly if there has been significant damage to the plate. With better understanding of epiphyseal cartilage physiology, it may become possible to stimulate epiphyseal plates locally, perhaps using electrical fields, in order to equalize limb lengths. This is an area of important research for the future, and additional time will be required to assess the value of current research programs.

Fracture Healing

Of all the disorders of the musculoskeletal system, none produces more suffering than fractures. A fracture of the bone is a major medical event that can result in prolonged hospitalization and treatment, loss of earnings, and often permanent disability. Despite the attention paid to this area by orthopedists since antiquity, little is known about the process of fracture healing; numerous investigators are currently attempting to understand the normal process of fracture repair and to find means of enhancing it. This area of investigation, although embryonic in its current state, may lead in the next two or three decades to the development of substances which when locally or systemically introduced could improve the quality and rapidity of fracture repair.

A development of more immediate practical significance has been the introduction of superbly designed metallic implants for the purpose of compression and rigid immobilization of fractures (Figure 23-1). Following the pioneering work in this area performed by Swiss orthopedists and engineers, clinicians throughout the United States and abroad have put these devices to widespread use. These implants have markedly altered the orthopedist's approach to the treatment of fractures; early operative procedures now make prolonged immobilization unnecessary and result in predictable healing of the fracture with solid union occur-

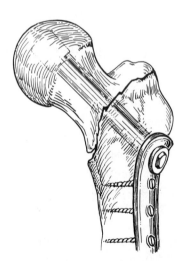

Figure 23–1. A metal implant for a fracture of the femur (thigh bone).

ring in a relatively short period of time. There are still, however, numerous problems with the introduction of these metallic compression fixation devices. The designs, although excellent, still require improvement, and techniques for their use must be simplified. Infection rates for some implant procedures are still too high. Furthermore, the basic problem remains that the devices by their very nature limit the normal function of the bone in terms of turnover and remodeling and occasionally cause weakening of the bony structure adjacent to the hardware or even remote from it. These are problems under study, and new designs for plates are currently in progress. An example of such an effort is the production of plates made of materials with elastic properties more closely resembling those of bone, thus decreasing the interference with the normal resonance of the limb and bony structure. Such materials include pyrolytic carbon and titanium, both of which are lighter in weight and have mechanical characteristics more like those of bone than the currently used stainless steel and cobalt-chrome alloys.

Of perhaps equal interest and potential value are the exciting investigations into the effect of electrical currents and fields on fracture healing. In the 1950s, several investigators demonstrated that bone, when stressed, produced tiny currents of electricity (piezo-electricity). It was thought that these micro-amperage levels of current might serve as a stimulus to normal remodeling and day-to-day repair, which are important processes in maintaining the resistance of bone structure to stress failure and fracture. Experimental studies clearly demonstrated that new bone formation could in fact be invoked by the appropriate application of direct current; although this effect was observed only through a limited range of current intensity, it was a predictable result. Armed with this information, scientists performed animal studies which demonstrated that electrical currents and fields delivered through implanted electrodes connected to battery packs appeared to enhance the rate of repair of long bone fractures. Preliminary studies have now been extended to people; in a small series of patients, fractures which ordinarily would be somewhat delayed in healing or characterized by unstable repair have healed much more effectively under the application of an appropriate electrical field. The devices are still somewhat crude, but with the continued participation of electrical engineers and orthopedists, research directed to improvements in electrode design and the development of better calibrated and smaller battery packs is likely to yield a more reliable instrument. Over the next few years, these devices will probably play an important role in the orthopedist's daily struggle with complicated and disabling fractures.

Prosthetic Replacement of Joints

In the course of the twentieth century, the replacement of damaged joints with prosthetic implants has been first a dream, then a research goal, and now, in the last two decades, a practical realization. Experience gained during the 1930s and 1940s with the use of hemi-joint replacements for fractures of the hip and knee has in the last two decades been applied by ingenious investigators and engineers to the design of metal and plastic replacement parts for many of the body's joints. The hip device, originally developed by John Charnley and subsequently modified by a number of investigators, was the first such artificial joint; it now represents an extraordinarily effective means of dealing with a very serious problem. The device in its current form consists of a highly polished metal head fixed into the femur by a stem and articulating with a polyethylene socket contained within the pelvis. Both components are firmly fixed to the bones of the femur and pelvis respectively by methylmethacrylate, another plastic which serves as a "cement" (Figure 23-2). With well over fifteen years of experience and some 150,000 cases in the United States alone, it is apparent that this device is far superior to any prior approach to problems like osteoarthritis and rheumatoid arthritis of the hip, the "failed" hip fracture, and fractures of the acetabulum (the pelvic socket in which the head of the femur rests). Nevertheless, problems still exist in the use of these hip replacements, and considerable research is devoted to their further development. Current research efforts are seeking improvements in many aspects of the procedure: improved tissue acceptance of the implants, more secure methods of anchoring the metal and plastic components to the bone, plastic socket materials with reduced rates of wear, modifications in the design of the femoral component to decrease the likelihood of stress fractures, and improved instrumentation for easier insertion of the devices. The formerly formidable and hazardous operative procedure required to introduce the total hip replacement has already been made relatively safe by such innovations as hypotensive anesthesia, clean air systems, prophylactic antibiotics, and antithromboembolic measures; in the hands of qualified and experienced orthopedists, the procedure now has a relatively low morbidity and mortality rate.

Encouraged by the results of replacement surgery for the hip, surgeons and engineers have now turned to other joints of the body; there are currently over three hundred and fifty designs for knee prostheses using essentially the same materials as are used for the hip. These include

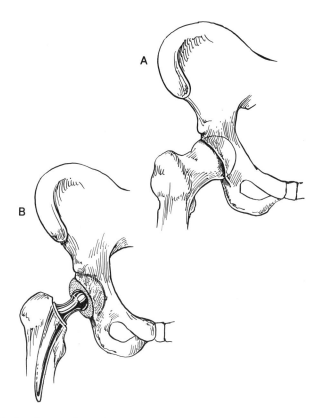

Figure 23–2. The artificial hip. A shows a normal hip. In B, a polyethylene socket has been "cemented" to the pelvis; a metal prosthesis at the head of the femur fits into this socket.

hinge joints, "sleds on runners" joints, and polycentric devices, all of which attempt to meet the requirements dictated by the complex functional anatomy of the knee joint. As yet none of these designs is completely satisfactory, and considerably more investigation will certainly be required to perfect them. Progress is being made through animal research, design analysis, and human trials to improve knee implants.

Perhaps the best of the prosthetic devices currently in use are those pioneered by Alfred Swanson for the replacement of damaged small joints of the fingers and hand. The principles and materials for these tiny implants are considerably different than those for the larger joints, in that no cement is used; the entire device is made of a solid piece of inert silastic rubber. The value of such devices in the treatment of the patient whose hands have been destroyed by rheumatoid arthritis is obvious, and many patients have been restored to useful function by this means. Work continues in this area toward improvement of both the design and materials to eliminate such complications as breakage or limitation of the range of motion.

Inspired by all these successes with joint replacement, the interest of investigators has extended to the ankle, elbow, and shoulder, and in a limited way to the wrist. Each of these joints has served as the focus of attention for several groups of investigators who have proposed theoretical solutions and who, in some cases, have actually fabricated devices which have been successfully implanted into patients suffering with arthritis or trauma to these joints. It is too soon to analyze the data obtained by studying these patients, but it is hoped that the years to come will bring further improvements in design and methods of implantation.

Cartilage Metabolism and Osteoarthritis

In a sense, joint replacement is a defeatist approach, since it is useful only when the anatomical structure of the joint has been irreparably damaged to a degree that necessitates the removal of the original joint and the substitution of a prosthetic device. For this reason, many orthopedists have chosen to study joint physiology and mechanics, focusing especially on the articular cartilages; if these tissues can be saved from the ravages of disease, restoration of function can be accomplished without joint replacement. The articular cartilages are a complex connective tissue structure which serve as the gliding surfaces of the joints and ordinarily move in relationship to each other with considerably less friction than ice against ice. This smooth glistening white material, familiar to all as the "gristle" covering the ends of the long bones, has been of considerable interest to investigators for over a hundred years. Most recently, studies have illuminated the biochemical and metabolic characteristics of this tissue; once thought to be an inert type of shock absorber, articular cartilage is now considered to be an active participant in the complex biochemistry of the joint. Considerable work has been done to analyze the components of the cartilage cell, which include collagen and proteoglycan, and the metabolic activity associated with the production of these materials by the cell. Especially important is the analytic work that has carefully detailed the changes undergone by normal tissue under the stress of trauma or osteoarthritis. In trauma, repair of the articular surfaces is limited and incomplete; several studies have attempted to discover why the reparative response fails in this way. It is hoped that further study will lead to techniques or chemical methods for enhancing the reparative ability of this tissue and thus decrease the likelihood of the development of arthritis following joint injury. Osteoarthritis has appeared in recent studies to be accompanied by specific chemical changes in the cartilage. One of the most important of these changes is a depletion of proteoglycan by locally produced enzyme complexes which can alter the biochemistry of the cell in such a way that proteoglycan is solubilized and more readily lost from the tissue. Methods for enhancing cartilage repair and for diminishing the enzymatic degradation of intracellular substance are currently under study; if these methods prove successful, it is possible that chemical agents may also be utilized to ameliorate osteoarthritis of joints. This would indeed be a major breakthrough, and it is anticipated that, with continued research in this area, such approaches may be introduced into clinical trial within the next decade.

Spinal Surgery

Some of the most significant problems facing the orthopedist are those encountered in scoliosis (curvature of the spine) and in congenital malformation of the spinal column and its underlying neural contents. In the past, the treatment of these problems was uniformly difficult, time-consuming, and extremely distressing to the patient (who frequently was bedridden for months). Surgery often consisted of the removal of a deforming structure, correction of the curve by traction or other means, and an arthrodesis (surgical bony fusion) of the involved segments to prevent recurrent or advancing deformity. Such operative procedures were massive and complicated and often failed because of the inability to properly immobilize the operative site long enough for bone to grow across the fused segments.

A major breakthrough occurred in the latter part of the 1950s, when Paul Harrington introduced the use of posteriorly applied rigid rods equipped with jacks, compression devices, and hooks at both ends to anchor to the vertebral processes. These enabled the surgeon to correct the deformity by jacking up one side of the spinal column or compressing the other, while at the same time fusing across the spinal segments involved. The jacks and compression rods were left in place after the fusion and served as an internal form of immobilization. These techniques, along with better means of external immobilization, have revolutionized the treatment of scoliosis and complicated malformations of the spine. How-

ever, they are inapplicable to certain types of deformities, particularly
those in which the posterior elements of the spinal column are not strong
enough to withstand the forces generated by the jacks and compression
devices. More recently, careful experimental work has produced a new
technique. Utilizing the anterior approach, eye hooks are drilled into
the bodies of the vertebra on the convex side of the curve and a cable
passed through the eyes; the cable is then pulled taut to correct the curve,
and is held by affixing a bead at the proper location in the cable. This
method has introduced a broad new dimension to scoliosis surgery and
has increased the ability of surgeons to deal with very complicated problems (Figure 23–3).

Scoliosis surgeons have also studied various aspects of spinal deformity from the standpoint of epidemiology, biochemical abnormalities in

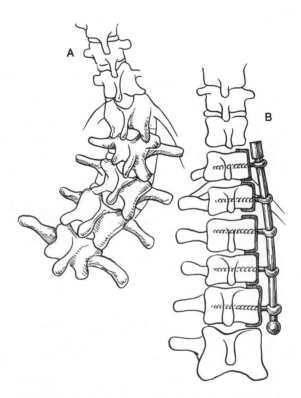

Figure 23–3. Surgical correction of scoliosis (curvature of the spine). A shows
the spine of a patient with scoliosis. B shows the condition corrected; the spine
is held straight by a cable pulled through eye-hooks that have been affixed to
the vertebrae.

disc and adjacent structures, and chemical aberrations suggestive of systemic disorders. There is some evidence that the disorder may be a partially hereditary one of polygenic origin. More research is definitely required, however, before this observation can be of clinical value.

Tumors of the Bone

Perhaps the most discouraging aspect of orthopedic management over the past hundred years has been in the field of the malignant tumors of bone. The first fifty years of this century were devoted to identification and study of the various types of tumors which occur in the skeletal system. These lesions are rare and principally occur in young people. When they do occur, the malignant tumors are very aggressive, with spread of tumors to the lungs occurring in most patients despite mutilating operative procedures. Up until recently, the rate of salvage for chondrosarcoma (tumor of the cartilage) was less than 40 percent; for osteosarcoma (bone sarcoma), less than 25 percent; for Ewing's tumor, less than 15 percent; and for other bone tumors, equally dismal prognoses.

Over the past fifteen years, increasing knowledge of these tumors has provided some clues as to methods of therapy. Osteosarcoma is now treated much more effectively than was previously possible through the combination of radical surgery, radiation therapy, and chemotherapy using such drugs as adriamycin and methotrexate (highly potent antibiotics which selectively kill tumor cells). Ewing's tumor appears to respond well to X-ray therapy coupled with a combination of several potent drugs; the rate of survival on a three-year basis is now as high as 60 percent. Several of the tumors have shown characteristic immunologic responses which suggest that immunotherapy may hold great promise for the future development of methods of treatment. The tumors appear to be potent antigens which cause the development of specific cell-killing antibodies; these antibodies could theoretically be used to control the growth of the tumor and perhaps to eradicate small foci of tumor spread. This area of research is just beginning to blossom, and several laboratories are deeply involved in antigen-antibody studies of the malignant tumors of childhood.

Another recent development of some interest has been the demonstration that human osteosarcoma can be transferred from man to experimental animals and retains its potential as a malignant tumor over several such passages. This suggests a viral cause for this disorder, and the finding of small particles within the cell on electron microscopy supports this speculation. If further work confirms this, osteosarcoma will be the first of the connective tumors with a virus demonstrated to be an etiologic agent.

Although the traditional method of surgical management for malignant tumors has been amputation of the affected limb, the recent advent of newer methods of systemic treatment and more refined surgical procedures has made it possible to devise techniques which spare the limb. One such method consists of the introduction of a metallic implant after wide surgical removal of sections of bone. Another technique, perhaps more exciting, is the use of transplants taken from cadavers for replacement of large bone segments after massive surgery. Such experimental transplants have now been successfully performed in patients with a variety of malignant tumors. Follow-up suggests that replacement of the entire tibia, or of half a femur or humerus, can be performed with relative ease; moreover, the patients do retain reasonable function of the part. The problems associated with transplantation of bone and cartilage are somewhat different from those involved in kidney transplants in that a standard form of rejection is not clearly noted in massive bone transplants. The principal problems that are associated with such bone surgery are maintenance of joint function and reattachment of ligaments and tendons to the cadaver bone. If these can be overcome, this type of procedure may become an important method of dealing with many types of disorder.

Sports Medicine

In the last two decades, it has become apparent to orthopedists throughout this country and abroad that many of the injuries associated with trauma sustained during sporting events are avoidable and can be eliminated by better protective devices and improved physical conditioning. Properly designed and fitted headgear, improved padding for contact sports, better knee braces, and other advances will clearly decrease the morbidity and mortality associated with amateur and professional athletics in the United States. Improved training and physical conditioning may be critical in preventing an injury or reducing the likelihood of serious consequences.

The physicians who deal with sports medicine have also recognized the need to improve current techniques for the repair of injuries that do occur, with particular emphasis on major tears of ligaments around the knee and ankle. Over the past decade, numerous new surgical techniques have been devised, including the use of artificial tendons and ligaments. These can help restore a badly damaged knee to reasonable function and in some cases can enable a player who years ago might have been totally disabled to return to the athletic field.

Other Areas

The items listed in the eight sections above only include those areas of orthopedic research that are currently the focus of major efforts in many of the laboratory and clinical research units in this country. But there are numerous other areas in which research—performed not only by orthopedists but also by such specialists as rheumatologists, endocrinologists, and pediatricians—will clearly have major effects on the practice of orthopedics in the future. Many of these are detailed elsewhere in this volume; suffice it to say that the orthopedist shares the interest of scientists in other disciplines in such conditions as osteoporosis, rheumatoid arthritis, meningomyelocele, disproportionately short stature, and organ transplantation. There are also some areas within the field of orthopedics proper in which smaller groups of investigators have generated considerable enthusiasm and are now providing interesting data. These areas encompass research programs of great diversity: the use of sound and light absorption for the determination of bone mineral content and for the healing of fractures; prevention of excessive scar tissue formation in hand and nerve injuries by administration of collagen inhibitors; studies of the effects of corticosteroid hormones, vitamins, and other materials on bone and cartilage formation; studies of gait disturbances using instrumented walkways, cameras, and computerized data analysis; analyses of the effects of trace elements derived from metallic implants on physiological systems; theortical muscle force analyses of the lumbar and cervical spines; studies of the biochemical aspects of bone tumors; development of new designs for limb prostheses and their control mechanisms; and many, many more.

It is difficult to measure research progress in a field like orthopedics, partly because advances occur rather slowly and partly because orthopedics is a "practical" specialty in which the physician traditionally remains heavily involved in the clinical care of the patient. Nevertheless, it is apparent to those who are familiar with the annals of the past that the quality of orthopedic care enjoyed by patients today is vastly superior to that available to their forbears. These advances are primarily the result of competent, clinically directed investigation of patient problems for which previous methods of treatment were inadequate or unsatisfactory. In the last decade there have been great strides made in relieving suffering and improving the quality of life for patients with crippling musculoskeletal disorders. It is hoped that the decades that follow will show similar advances; and considering the promise shown by current research in progress, this is likely to occur.

Surgical Care

FRANCIS D. MOORE

24

The word surgery is related to the French *chirurgie,* which in turn derives from Greek and means "doing with the hands." Surgery is the active practical intervention in the progress of bodily disease through removal of disease or rearrangement of anatomy. Over the past century, such intervention has been carried out through the technique of anesthetized sterile tissue dissection.

A great many diseases are best treated by direct repair or removal of parts of the anatomy. Treatment of trauma, burns, and fractures, removal of solid tumors, repair of congenital defects, restoration of vision in cataract disease, drainage of abcesses, repair of the interior of the heart, restoration of blood flow to limbs—all are examples of modern applications of this ancient and once-simple science of "doing with the hands."

Basic medical advances in the eighteenth and nineteenth centuries were instrumental in bringing surgery to its present level of effectiveness; these included the development of pathology (the study of disease processes themselves), control of infection, and the introduction of anesthetic drugs. In all these areas surgeons such as John Hunter, Joseph Lister, and John Collins Warren played a major role. These men were effective clinicians who also maintained contact with the basic science of their age; they were in a sense the conduit bringing advances in biological knowledge to the bedside of the surgical patient. In the past 50 years, surgery has continued to advance through the specific research activities of surgeons and through studies conducted in surgical wards and laboratories. This chapter will focus on six areas that have seen especially dramatic progress: treatment of burns and shock, metabolic management of patients, and the surgical treatment of cancer, heart disease, and kidney disease.

Burns

The skin injury of a burn results from the heat-induced coagulation of protein in the deeper layers of the skin with destruction, death, and shedding off of the burned skin. But the medical problem of burn goes beyond the immediate destruction of skin itself. The area of the burned skin becomes a dead "pablum" or culture medium in which bacteria grow luxuriantly; the properties of the skin which help control temperature and water loss are destroyed; and blood circulating through the skin at the time of the burn is destroyed by the heat and releases hemoglobin pigments that damage the kidney. Until the early years of this century, death from extensive burns generally occurred within two to four days.

A major problem was the loss of fluid from the circulation. Starting at the time of the Second World War, research began to demonstrate that much of this fluid was not lost outside the body but was instead redistributed within the body, in a large area immediately beneath the burn. We now know that this lost fluid can be reabsorbed if the patient survives the early days after his injury. Once the watery tissue fluid disappears, the patient and surgeon can begin the long task of resurfacing the burned area by skin grafts. The discoveries that lead to the early improvements in burn management were related to a better understanding of body composition, fluid balance, and the metabolism of water, minerals, and protein. The standard treatment of burns is now largely based on one general principle: provide to the patient's bloodstream those components that have been lost.

Replacing the surface of burned skin is still a severe problem but one that may have many possible solutions. The use of dog skin, pigskin, placental membranes, and artificial skin has been explored for several decades; skin grafted from a living or dead donor has also often been employed, with varying success. With persistent effort and the avoidance of lethal infection, skin replacement can finally be achieved even in remarkably extensive burns.

The problem of infection has yet to be solved; it remains the largest obstacle to the safe and effective treatment of burns. Despite antibiotics, germ-free isolation chambers, and ultraviolet light screens, infection remains the leading cause of death in burn patients. Antibiotics, while they can be effective, are also dangerous; the overuse of these drugs, which can lead to the induction of resistant strains and abolition of the patient's own immune processes, has been part of the problem in the treatment of burns in the last 20 years. In the past decade, however, the national mortality figures for various types of burns have begun to fall for the first time since the Second World War. This recent advance in burn treatment has resulted from the use of various types of therapeutic baths, improved grafting in the early days after the burn, and, above all, better local use of antibiotics and avoidance of their overuse.

Shock

Although the term shock was first used about 1915, the clinical picture of shock has been known since the middle of the nineteenth century. Surgeons in the American Civil War described soldiers heavily injured in combat who suffered tissue destruction, blood loss, pain, and anxiety. Within a few minutes or hours, such a victim of shock develops a very rapid, thready pulse and a very low blood pressure, becomes "hungry for air," and feels thirsty; without therapy, the patient dies within a few hours.

Walter Cannon, a physiologist at the Harvard Medical School, began to study shock intensively at the time of the First World War. He and several other investigators in the Allied cause soon demonstrated that time factors were of the greatest importance in the treatment of shock. A brief period of reduced blood flow (which occurs in shock) can be well tolerated, especially by young people in good condition. But as time passes the devastating effects of this low-flow state become more marked, until finally even a modest reduction in blood flow over the course of a day or two may result in irreversible damage to the kidneys, the heart, and the brain. (In older patients, these effects may occur after a much shorter time interval.) If blood flow to the brain and heart is reduced sharply enough, death immediately results. To restore blood pressure and flow to normal, the restoration of blood volume is the first priority.

The great advances in the treatment of shock in this century have been drawn from other medical fields, mainly immunology. The description about 1915 of the immunologically different blood types (A, B, and O) made possible the modern use of blood transfusion to support patients in traumatic shock. Despite the advances in hematology and immunology, however, it was not until the end of the First World War that transfusion of large amounts of blood was widely practicable, and it became possible to revitalize patients suffering such devastating injury as direct wounds of the heart and the aorta with massive losses of blood.

The effects of shock on the kidney have been clarified in the past 25 years. Eric Bywaters in London first described the "crush syndrome," or traumatic nephrosis, in air-raid casualties. This temporary shutdown of kidney function is a by-product of shock that occurs especially when abnormal pigments have been circulated to the kidneys. Chapter 14 describes the development of dialysis by Willem Kolff in Holland during the war; the first application of the artificial kidney in this country, and perhaps its primary use until the advent of kidney transplantation, was to tide over patients with temporary kidney failure resulting from shock. This clinical problem was not restricted to combat injuries. It could also occur in pregnancy following a hemorrhage at the time of delivery, in the young woman with a ruptured ectopic pregnancy, in the athlete with a ruptured spleen, or in the patient with a severe burn.

In the treatment of shock, as with burn treatment, the problem of infection remains paramount. Jacob Fine of Boston demonstrated around 1940 that some of the endotoxins produced by the bacteria in the normal human colon (*E. coli*) produce a shocklike state. All the clinical signs of surgical shock can be produced by such infection alone, without any actual loss of blood or plasma. Infection with shock-producing bacteria markedly reduces the chance for survival of patients in shock with kidney failure, especially those who also suffer lung damage. The control of these infections remains one of the many unsolved problems in the treatment of individuals suffering from shock.

Metabolic Care

One of the most thoroughly modern branches of surgical research has involved the application of chemistry to surgical problems. The advances of the nineteenth century widened the scope of surgery to the point where the chemical problems in the field could be clearly defined; and surgery has advanced in the twentieth century largely through the use of biochemical techniques. Biochemists in the first half of the century—especially John Peters of Yale, Donald van Slyke of New York, and James Gamble of Boston—described alterations in extracellular fluid chemistry that were rapidly assimilated by surgeons. Over the past 25 years these have been incorporated into a new body of knowledge regarding what might be called the metabolic response to surgery.

After severe injury the normal human body goes through an integrated set of orderly changes, beginning with the loss of lean muscular tissue. This process is essential to the healing of the wound; the breakdown of muscle protein provides substances used by the body to make collagen, the body's major connective protein and an essential material in wound healing. Fat is burned up to provide the body's energy needs, while extracellular fluid is jealously saved; kidney mechanisms conserve water and sodium salts. There are evolutionary reasons for these metabolic processes. Think of the primitive vertebrate, wounded or injured, crawling under cover to heal his wounds. He must have sources of energy within himself and synthesize collagen, and must save fluids and minerals from which his plasma was made. The similar metabolic response to surgery probably evolved from such survival mechanisms.

The early breakdown of lean tissue is followed by a dramatic turning point that has been recognized by surgeons and patients for many centuries. This feeling of suddenly getting well after a severe injury is associated with the cessation of lean tissue destruction, increased excretion of water and salt in the urine, and a restoration of appetite and intestinal function. There follows a phase of reconstruction of body tissues during which the patient returns home and gradually regains a normal level of activity.

Many surgical patients suffer from disorders of this remarkable chemical sequence. These may be associated with obstruction or leakage in the gastrointestinal tract, failure of the kidney or lungs, or the accumulation of fluid in the lungs or brain. The chemical understanding of these disorders and their treatment through special feedings and intravenous administration of fluids have been major advances of surgery in the past 50 years. Many surgical laboratories have become concerned with improving the metabolic management of patients. The so-called isotope dilution methods for studying body composition have grown up in surgical laboratories; by injecting a few radioactive and stable isotopes at very low and safe dosages and sampling the blood a few hours later, the physician can now determine exactly how many quarts of blood a patient has, how many pounds of red cells and muscle tissue, and the total amount of extracellular fluid. These body compositional methods, originally developed to improve surgical care, have been used by surgeons and physicians all over the world to gain a better understanding of different diseases.

The intravenous provision of rich nutriments began many years ago with the development of glucose infusion, followed by the availability of fat and amino acids. At the present time it is possible to keep patients alive, gaining weight and making new tissue quite normally through intravenous nutrition (see Chapter 16). Unfortunately, it is still almost impossible to maintain patients on this basis for more than one or two years. Nearly all laboratories that have studied this problem find that difficulties (usually involving infection) eventually kill patients who are being maintained entirely by intravenous means.

The Removal of Cancer

It is a platitude to state that cancer is a systemic disease that cannot generally be solved by local means; once a cancer has spread beyond a localized area it cannot be cured by methods of irradiation, drug therapy, or surgery that focus on only one small part of the body. Despite these limitations, the fact remains that the great majority of former cancer patients who are healthy today have been cured by the surgical removal of cancer. To be effective, this approach requires the early diagnosis of cancer, usually by X ray.

The means to improve the surgical removal of cancer and to make such operations safe and effective have constituted one of the largest areas of surgical progress in the past century. Techniques for removing cancers of the bowel, developed as major research advances around 1900, are taken for granted today. Cancer of the left colon, including the rectum, is now one of the most favorable areas for radical surgical removal. If the cancer has not invaded blood vessels or spread to the lymph nodes, the patient has a 75 to 85 percent likelihood of being cured. The removal of cancer of the lung, first performed about 1930, involves a much bolder approach to cancer, since it entails the removal of a seemingly vital organ. Preliminary work carried out in laboratory animals provided the essential demonstration that it was possible to live without one lung; the operation was first performed successfully on dogs. (It should be noted that many surgical advances are based on expensive and demanding research carried out, as humanely as possible, in animals.)

Surgery is not always an appropriate treatment for cancer. The examination of a large number of cancer cases where surgery was employed has made it clear that the surgical operation should not be done at all when the cancer has advanced beyond a certain point. This is certainly true for cancer of the breast, the commonest cancer in American women. If breast cancer is small and localized, removal of the tumor is effective and high cure rates are achieved, with over three-quarters of patients remaining free of the disease for at least five years. When the tumor is larger, however, the patient's life may be shortened by an inadvisable surgical operation which may actually spread the cancer.

Surgical care of cancer is but one component of what must be a joint approach or team effort. In some cases operation should be followed by the use of anticancer drugs; radiation treatment may also have an important role after surgery if there is a suspicion that tumor cells have been left behind (see Chapter 3). Although the biology of cancer still escapes our understanding, the removal of early cancers remains the most effective treatment. An unsolved problem that remains for the future is to determine the optimal combination of surgical removal with other systemic means for combating the disease once it has become widespread.

The Repair of Heart Disease

The most dramatic advance to occur in the management of heart disease since 1930 has been the development of techniques for the direct surgical repair of the heart. Congenital heart diseases—those that are present in the heart when the child is born—were the first to be treated effectively by surgical intervention. One of these congenital disorders originates when a small blood vessel connecting the aorta to the pulmonary artery remains open. This little blood vessel (called the ductus arteriosus) is essential to the life of the baby in the mother's womb, when the lungs are not being ventilated with air; after birth, the duct closes. If it remains open, the baby will circulate nonoxygenated blood (causing a blueness of the skin) and will probably develop a lethal infection.

Surgeons who were considering surgical treatment of heart disease as early as 1930 thought that the open ductus might be surgically corrected. But it was not until 1938 that Robert Gross, working at the Children's Hospital, carried out the first such operation successfully. (Very careful anesthesia is required; and the anatomical dissection must be of the greatest elegance and accuracy, since even a small slip can release a massive hemorrhage.) Gross's success with this operation stimulated other surgeons to develop procedures for treating another congenital anomaly called coarctation (narrowing) of the aorta. Before effective surgery became possible, children born with this disorder could expect to live no longer than two or three decades; today, they can be cured surgically and live normal lives.

By 1950 it was clear that further advances in heart surgery would be impossible unless the circulation to the heart and lungs could be maintained by some sort of machinery so that the heart could lie quiet and open for the surgeon's dissection and treatment. Fortunately, one brilliant American surgeon, John Gibbon, had already been working on this problem for 17 years (first at the Massachusetts General Hospital with Edward Churchill, then at the Jefferson Medical College in Philadelphia). Gibbon gradually perfected a machine which made it possible to divert the entire blood supply of the heart and lungs in dogs and cats, enabling the surgeon to open the heart or close off the vessels to the heart temporarily without lowering the animal's chances for survival.

A major problem was to find a way of pumping the blood through plastic tubing without injuring the blood in the process. Michael de Bakey of Texas found the solution: an ingenious pumping mechanism that does not touch the blood at all, but which operates through a roller that impels blood along flexible tubing.

The problem of adding oxygen to the blood and removing carbon dioxide was much more difficult. When oxygen is administered through a membrane in contact with the blood, a "boundary layer" phenomenon occurs; the cells immediately next to the membrane become oxygenated very rapidly, but the oxygen does not penetrate deeper into the blood. Methods of producing turbulent blood flow without damaging the blood have therefore been essential. Gibbon's early device used a screen; some methods have used a rotating disc, while others have bubbled oxygen through the blood.

In 1953 the first operation using this new technology was carried out in a child with congenital heart disease; circulation was completely maintained by machine while the open heart was repaired. Over the past twenty years a variety of methods has become available to pump and oxygenate the blood with virtually no blood damage and with no danger of bubbles being injected into the patient's bloodstream. Open heart operations up to seven hours in length can now be carried out with safety.

Kidney Transplantation

Open-heart surgery was made possible through an impressive series of technical advances and mechanical improvements which could be successfully applied once they were theoretically perfected. The problems involved in organ transplantation are more complex. The anatomical problems of kidney transplantation, for example, have finally been solved satisfactorily; but the immunological problems involved still remain major obstacles to the success of this and other types of organ transplants.

The French surgeon Alexis Carrel, working first at the University of Chicago and later at the Rockefeller Institute in New York, became the first to accomplish the anatomical transplantation of kidneys. This operation involved the direct suture of blood vessels and necessitated an understanding of the healing of blood vessels after suture. Carrel's work broke new ground and eventually won him the Nobel Prize (he was the first surgeon in America to be so honored). But if Carrel's operations were technically successful, they were clinical failures; the kidneys that he transplanted were always rejected. Rejection could not be attributed to infection or to lack of blood flow. Carrel perceived that some other process must be at work, but he did not know what this process was or how to control it.

It remained for the surgeons of the 1930s, especially Emile Holman, to understand the phenomenon of immunologic rejection. Holman carried out and studied a number of skin grafts using skin taken from donors related to the patient; eventually he came to conceive of the rejection or casting off of this grafted skin as an immunologic process. His early speculation that this process might possibly be related to certain skin diseases was confirmed much later when researchers began to understand the autoimmune diseases (see Chapter 7).

After the Second World War, once dialysis and the artificial kidney had been developed, several laboratories used a standard animal model to study kidney rejection; in this model a dog's own kidneys were removed and one transplant sutured in place. These studies were a classic example of the value of animal experimentation; the experiments conducted in dogs made it possible to understand the nature of the process of rejection and to devise strategies for interfering with that process. In the early 1950s, a team of Boston doctors demonstrated the technical feasibility of human kidney transplantation (see Chapter 14); immunologic problems thus remained the last obstacle to the success of such an operation.

Initial attempts to block the rejection of grafted tissues involved radiation and other injurious methods. A major breakthrough came in 1960, when Robert Schwartz and William Dameshek of Boston described the immunologic effects of 6-mercaptopurine, a drug then being tested as an anticancer chemical. Their remarkable observation that this drug could block the immunologic response to foreign protein was immediately applied by a young surgeon in Great Britain, Roy Calne. Within a few months he had shown that kidney grafts in dogs could be greatly prolonged by the use of 6-mercaptopurine. Calne came to Boston, where he worked at the Peter Bent Brigham Hospital with Joseph Murray and George Hitchings; this team developed a new drug, azothioprine, which is still used throughout the world for suppression of the immune rejection of grafts. The first kidney transplant using immunosuppressive drug therapy was finally carried out in 1962.

Although the immunosuppressive drugs are a vast improvement over earlier methods of preventing tissue rejection, their use entails some very real problems. These agents act by interfering with essential cellular processes; they have specific effects on the synthesis of protein, and some of these chemicals also interfere with cell division. It is difficult to find agents that will effectively interfere with the immune process that leads to rejection of the kidneys and other organs and yet will allow protein synthesis to contrive so that the cells of the body are not seriously injured.

In spite of the problem of immunosuppression, kidney transplantation has been carried out on a wide scale; approximately 35,000 patients throughout the world have undergone kidney transplants in the past decade and a half. Many of these operations have not been totally successful; a large percentage of patients have died some months or years after receiving a transplanted kidney. But thousands of others have been effectively treated by this operation. As the immunologic problems associated with this procedure come under further study, the chances of success will certainly improve.

Surgery has always advanced through a combination of technical innovation and progress in basic science; the interaction between researchers in these complementary areas should continue to be productive in the future.

Technical advances on all levels may have important implications. Cardiac surgery and transplantation would have been impossible without the very basic development of plastic sutures that can hold tissues together firmly and permit very rapid healing without producing an adverse tissue reaction. Much more sophisticated technical research, also important in the past, will certainly continue to play a central role in the future. For example, research is still needed to perfect techniques for maintaining circulation outside the body for more than seven hours. The machine used for this purpose has sometimes been called the "artificial lung," and is being developed for the treatment of patients with reversible pneumonia.

The surgeon faces many problems that are biological rather than mechanical; safe anesthesia, metabolic management, and avoidance of excessive fluid and minerals have all been essential to surgical progress.

Yet, basic biological problems in surgery remain. Probably the biggest obstacle still to be overcome is the difficulty of controlling infection effectively. Infection remains the primary cause of death from burns and also is a major complication of shock and intravenous nutrition. Infection is also frequently an undesirable side effect of immunosuppressive therapy given to patients receiving organ transplants. The answer to the problem of infection—like the ability to prevent the rejection of organ transplants safely and effectively—will have to come from basic medical research. Only through a combination of basic biological studies and sophisticated technical improvements can surgery continue to move forward with the impressive speed seen in the last few decades.

Radiology

HERBERT L. ABRAMS 25

Radiology is the field of medicine in which radiant energy (X rays, gamma rays, ultrasound) is used to produce images of viscera, organs, and bones for diagnostic purposes. The image is stored on X-ray film, motion picture film, or photographic paper. The radiologist's role is to interpret the examination on the basis of his knowledge of normal anatomy and physiology and to inform the referring internist, pediatrician, or surgeon of the precise diagnosis, the location of disease, its extent, and its relationship to surrounding structures. Although X-ray films of the chest and bones are best known to the public, every organ can be visualized radiologically when required. Few patients requiring surgery of the heart, brain, lungs, kidney, stomach and colon, liver, or gallbladder reach the operating room before the radiologist has defined the diagnostic problem and provided a "road map" for the surgeon.

The Past

Radiology is a young field as branches of medicine go; its eightieth anniversary was celebrated as the new year of 1976 dawned. It was a moment to take stock, look back to the beginning, define the present, and speculate on the future.

It all began on November 8, 1895. William Conrad Roentgen, during an experiment with a device called the Hittorf-Crookes tube, observed a bright fluorescence of barium platinocyanide crystals. He assumed initially that the fluorescence might be caused by cathode (beta) rays. But when he removed a fluorescent screen beyond the range of cathode rays, the fluorescence persisted; and Roentgen became aware that the effect was produced by a new, more powerful kind of ray. Soon he replaced the fluorescent screen by a recording photographic plate, and made the first X-ray pictures. (One of the dramatic results of this experiment was a picture of his wife's hand.) On December 28, 1895, after eight weeks of intensive investigation, Roentgen delivered the manuscript reporting his discovery of X rays to the Physical Medical Society in Würzburg. Printed as a preliminary communication in the annals of the society, it was a remarkably succinct and careful description of the behavior of X rays. His two classic papers of March 1896 and May 1897 completed the recording of many fundamental observations to which little was added for many years.

By early January 1896, word of Roentgen's discovery and its import had spread around the world. Almost immediately the possibilities of applying the new "photography" to traumatic lesions of bone fired the imaginative, and within a month X rays of fractures had been obtained and published. Early in the year, Thomas Edison and many others began intensive work on the fluoroscope. By the end of March 1896, W. Becher had studied the stomach and intestines of a guinea pig with X rays; these organs were outlined with lead subacetate to delineate them more clearly. In the fall of 1896, the great Harvard physiologist Walter B. Cannon, who was then still a medical student, undertook a study of the gastrointestinal tract of cats. Mixing bismuth subnitrate with the cats' food, he observed the movements of the opaque mass in the stomach and subsequently described in detail the nature and site of peristaltic activity as he saw it on the fluoroscopic screen. He noted in particular the "extreme sensitiveness" of the cat stomach to anxiety or rage and the marked inhibition of peristalsis that resulted. The usefulness of contrast agents—substances like lead subacetate or bismuth subnitrate used to outline the organs under study—was already becoming apparent. Such agents were also used to visualize the blood vessels in man early in 1896; the month after the announcement of Roentgen's discovery, E. Haschek and O. T. Lindenthal injected an opaque mixture into the blood vessels of an amputated hand, which they then x-rayed.

The first textbook on radiology was published by the end of 1896. W. G. Morton, "Professor of Diseases of the Mind and Nervous System" at the New York Post-Graduate Medical School, was fascinated by the new field of roentgenology. In collaboration with an electrical engineer named E. W. Hammer he wrote a text entitled *The X-Ray, or, Photography of the Invisible and Its Value in Surgery.* In it were not only chapters on normal anatomy, fractures, and dislocations, stiff joints, and foreign objects in the body but also a section on medicolegal applications of X rays. By 1900 an entire volume entitled *The Use of the Roentgen Ray by the Medical Department of the U.S. Army in the War with Spain* had been published. Gunshot fragments in the soft tissues and traumatic lesions of bone were illustrated in large plates in this volume. Soon a number of medical schools had organized departments of roentgenology, and exploration of the field grew rapidly. In M. K. Kassabian's voluminous textbook of 1907, *Roentgen Rays and Electro-therapeutics,* the chapters on diseases of the chest cavity and of the abdominal organs warranted sixty pages for adequate description.

Cannon's research interests in gastrointestinal physiology bore remarkable fruit within a decade after the discovery of X rays as clinical radiology of the gastrointestinal tract became a reality. By 1908 the radiographic appearance of gastric ulcer and gastric cancer had been fully described. The study of peristaltic activity in the gastrointestinal tract of man by fluoroscopy and films rapidly became as important as bone and joint radiology.

Important technical improvements early in the century made radiography safer and more effective and new areas became more accessible. In 1918 Walter E. Dandy of Johns Hopkins performed the first air ventriculogram, a type of brain X ray that Dandy used to visualize the brains of children with hydrocephalus (an excess of fluid in the ventricles of the brain). Soon afterwards, the discovery that intravenous sodium iodide was not only excreted by the kidneys but also made the urine opaque to X rays led to the description of clinical urography in 1923. About the same time, intravenous contrast agents were first injected in arteries and veins. E. Graham and L. G. Cole used their knowledge of physiology and chemistry to develop cholecystography—radiography of the gallbladder —by utilizing brominated phenophthalein, a substance excreted into the gallbladder that makes it opaque to X rays. A year later, Merrill Sosman of the Peter Bent Brigham Hospital observed that the gallbladder became opaque again three days after the Graham-Cole test. Realizing that the opaque salt must have been reabsorbed from the gastrointestinal tract, he pointed out the possibility of using an oral agent to render the gallbladder opaque; and the application of oral cholecystography to man was completed the same year. Radiography of the bronchi of the lungs (bronchography, introduced in 1922), of the arteries to the brain (1928), and of the chambers of the heart (1931) were other important milestones in the development of radiology.

The most important technical advance that followed was the development of image amplified fluoroscopy, initiated in the 1940s and completed in the 1950s. Fluoroscopy could previously be done only in a dark room at a high X-ray dose and yielded a relatively poor image. With image amplification, progressive improvements in the image became feasible and the versatility of the fluoroscopic method was remarkably increased.

The Present

Radiology in the mid-1970s represents the central method for delineating pathologic anatomy in sick patients, as well as one of the most important approaches to defining disordered physiology. It is literally the foundation of every creative new surgical therapeutic approach of the twentieth century. Without a sophisticated radiology, there could be no sophisticated surgery of the central nervous system, the lungs, the stomach, the duodenum, the large bowel, or the kidneys, and certainly not of the heart and circulatory system.

Radiology depicts the relationship of gross pathology to clinical signs and symptoms with a special kind of elegance. It reflects functional anatomy with clarity and with an unimpaired fidelity to fact; the structure of bones and joints can be examined or the position of calcified heart valves determined. Radiology can define many of the pathologic features of lung or kidney disease that permit a precise resolution of the underlying problem. As a physiologic tool, it has augmented our understanding of such diverse processes as gastrointestinal peristalsis, emptying of the bladder, and the mechanics of contraction of the heart. Pharmacologic effects have also been clarified, such as the effect of adrenaline on normal and tumor vessels in the kidney. Finally, radiologic techniques have been and remain essential elements in the entire gamut of differential diagnosis in medicine. The cause of such a common symptom as vomiting of blood—whether ulcer, cancer, distended esophageal veins, or acute gastritis—can usually be accurately detected by the radiologist.

The radiologist works as a consultant and teacher not only with the medical student or the resident; throughout his professional life, his teaching is directed as well at the internist, the pediatrician, the surgeon, indeed all the specialists in medicine (with the possible exception of the psychiatrist). He spends relatively less time with patients and a great deal more with physicians than most of his colleagues; and he must speak their language with lucidity and sophistication. His opinions are almost invariably subject to verification by the clinical course of the patient, the surgeon's knife, or the pathologist's microscope. Because he deals with gross disorders of visceral anatomy and physiology with a high degree of specificity, he and his colleagues may learn not only about the accuracy of diagnostic methods but equally about the chronology and biology of disease. In no other way can the sequence of the biological changes that occur in illness be mirrored with such precision over a period of many years, with the original data intact for all to see and the professional commitment available for all to evaluate.

Research in Radiology

Research in radiology until the last fifteen or twenty years was largely technical and reportorial. Clinical observation and analysis formed an important element in the scholarly activity of the radiologist, and for good reason; the field was still very young. A wealth of perceptive observations, correlations of radiography with other diagnostic methods, and astute interpretations amplified and deepened the whole framework of medical diagnosis in the years after Roentgen.

Techniques developed within the past fifteen years have concentrated on the circulation (arterial, venous, and lymphatic). These methods have added broad dimensions to our capacity to diagnose disease, to analyze the spread of cancer in the lymphatics, and to undertake fundamental cardiovascular investigations. As a clinical investigator, the radiologist has continuing opportunities to study blood flow and circulatory dynamics as a part of his examination.

In the modern era, research in diagnostic radiology finds its application in the study of function, normal and abnormal; the approach is uniquely capable of recording information of value and significance when correlated with other physiologic parameters. With the gastroenterologist, the radiologist may concentrate on the problems of the movement of the intestinal walls in man; with the urologist, on bladder and kidney function; with the neurologist, on cerebral blood flow. In the laboratory he may work in physiology, pharmacology, neuroanatomy, microradiography, biochemistry, and other areas.

But it is important to emphasize that the field of radiology goes far beyond the application of X rays from external sources to the diagnosis and characterization of human disease. Nuclear medicine—the diagnostic use of radioactive materials introduced into the body—has become an important segment of the field of radiology and has contributed to techniques for producing radiologic images and for collecting physiological data. Radioactive isotopes have been applied to the study of virtually every human organ and have made it possible to study many normal and abnormal physiologic processes without using more invasive techniques such as catheterization or surgery.

Another important and growing field of exploration in radiology is the use of diagnostic ultrasound, a technique rather like sonar that uses reflected sound waves to study physiologic structures. This method, which has been with us for decades, has suddenly become the center of an explosion in technology. The information derived from scanning of the abdomen as well as the valuable data attainable from cardiac ultrasound (see Chapter 12) have given a remarkable impetus to obtaining sharper and more dynamic images. One of the most important aspects of ultrasound is not only its noninvasive character but the fact that it has no demonstrated injurious effects, in contrast to X rays and gamma rays. Its harmlessness has made ultrasound an ideal method for prenatal diagnosis of the fetus (see Chapters 4 and 18).

Radiologic methods have become so integral to our approach to organic human disease that it seems highly likely that most of the conventional radiologic examinations now in use will continue to be applied for a long period of time. The special procedures are equally important in their yield of diagnostic and physiologic information. Although some may be modified or replaced within the coming years, this will occur only when major improvements in information-gathering techniques have become available.

Within the past ten years, the field of interventional (as opposed to diagnostic) radiology has become an important aspect of the radiologist's approach to patient care. The radiologist may now use a catheter not only to inject an opaque contrast agent and thus define the site of gastrointestinal bleeding but also to infuse pharmacologic agents which constrict the vessels and stop the bleeding. Similarly, he has become concerned with the technology of balloon catheters as a means of obstructing flow in circulatory beds in which uncontrolled hemorrhage is a threat to life. The characterization of intravascular materials that obstruct blood flow and the delivery of those materials to control local bleeding without decreasing blood flow to other segments has become both an art and a science.

Many other methods of therapeutic intervention have become routine radiologic procedures. Using ultrasound, the radiologist has become involved in obtaining tissue for examination from such organs as the liver, pancreas, lymph nodes, and kidney. He may now remove gallstones or intervene actively to correct special types of bowel obstruction or abnormal twisting of the colon. He may infuse antitumor drugs or materials to obstruct blood flow into cancerous areas. Removal of lung tissue for study, performed with the image-amplified fluoroscope, is now a standardized procedure. Blood sampling for parathyroid and adrenal tumors and for hypertension caused by narrowing of arteries to the kidney is an everyday occurrence in the radiology department; skilled radiologists know exactly how and where to place the sampling catheter so that specific sampling can be performed. In the patient threatened with pulmonary embolism (blocking of the lung arteries) from a clot formed in peripheral veins, the radiologist now may place a filter in the inferior vena cava (a large vein leading to the heart) to stop the progress of the clot toward the lung. When the intestine is deprived of adequate blood because of constriction of the blood vessels supplying it, the radiologist may infuse drugs to dilate those vessels. As a therapist, the diagnostic radiologist has even become involved in nonsurgical destruction of the adrenal gland and in the treatment of pancreatic cancer by catheter infusion of radioactive beads.

Most of these techniques have originated because of clinical need, have been developed in the experimental laboratory, and have subsequently been returned to the clinical setting and used in treatment. Problems that cannot be solved in clinical investigation, unanswered questions that relate ultimately to the diagnosis or treatment of human disease, are the stimuli that prompt animal experimentation in the radiology laboratory. Radiologists involved in the intra-arterial injection of the substance vasopressin to control intestinal bleeding have taken a new look at the effects of the drug on the vascular beds of other organs. Because they often deal with impairment of blood flow to the kidney and because the collateral (secondary) circulation of virtually all organ systems is very much a part of their examinations, radiologists have become interested in the stimulus for the collateral circulation. (In our own laboratory we are investigating a substance that stimulates blood vessel formation and is found in tissue with decreased blood flow.) Because they utilize the special drug responses of tumor vessels to enhance blood flow to tumors for diagnostic or therapeutic purposes, radiologists have naturally studied the nature of the blood vessels of tumors and the ways in which they differ from normal blood vessels. Because the patient in acute renal failure who excretes abnormally little or no urine is frequently studied by radiologic methods, the radiologist has developed and studied models of kidney failure in the animal laboratory. The architecture of the blood vessels supplying the lymph node during the immune response; the changes that occur in lymphatic tissue with the implantation and growth of tumor cells; the role of the hormone angiotensin in mediating constriction of blood vessels; the changes in the blood vessels of the kidney that accompany hypertension; the changes in blood flow to the aortic wall associated with the development of some types of aortic atherosclerosis; the development of new tissue-specific and tumor-specific radioactive drugs for diagnosis and treatment; the assessment of variations in the response of different tissues to ultrasound; and the capacity to distinguish between normal and cancerous tissue—these are but a few of the areas that radiologists are now exploring.

An important area of research in radiology concentrates in decreasing the radiation dose and increasing the information yield to make X-ray studies safer and more effective. This is a critical concern, because medical radiation is probably the most important single source of radiation to the human bone marrow and reproductive organs. Because radiology plays such a central role in clinical diagnosis, over 140 million X-ray examinations are performed in the United States each year. This means that every man, woman, and child, on the average, has a radiographic examination every other year. The problems of decreasing dose and improving the quality of data retrieval are obviously the central concern of a large and important sector of radiologic research, namely, equipment development and evaluation.

The Future

Radiology has recently experienced the most important single development in the field since image intensified fluoroscopy: computerized axial tomography, or CAT scanning. This new technique has become familiar to the biomedical community very recently indeed, but the principle behind it has been known for a long time. Different tissues are known to attenuate X-ray beams to different degrees; the attenuation or absorption coefficient varies significantly between tissues. Except when these differences are of great magnitude, however, conventional radiography cannot depict them; it thus has limited usefulness in distinguishing between tissues with relatively small differences in absorption coefficients. It was G. N. Hounsfield, an English physicist, who devised the first instrument to detect these relatively fine differences, which can be stored in a computer programmed to construct an image which reflects differing tissue densities. The basic principle of tomography—to eradicate the structural noise in all except a single plane so that only the information in that plane is conveyed with clarity—had been a part of radiology for many years. What the computerized tomograph did was to combine a sensitive detecting system that recorded the variations in absorption from multiple angles with a series of complex equations for reconstructing a useful image of a visual "slice" of tissue.

Because the scanning time was relatively long and demanded immobilization, the process was highly sensitive to blurring from motion. Consequently the initial application of computerized tomography was to the brain, because patients could lie with the skull immobilized for relatively long periods of time (Figure 25-1). Shortly after its first application, it became clear that computed tomography could detect intracranial tumors, specific disorders of cerebral circulation, and other abnormalities which previously had been definable only by relatively invasive approaches (Figures 25-2 and 25-3). Once the usefulness of cranial CAT scanning had been demonstrated, it was only a matter of time before application of the method to body scanning was realized. The differing

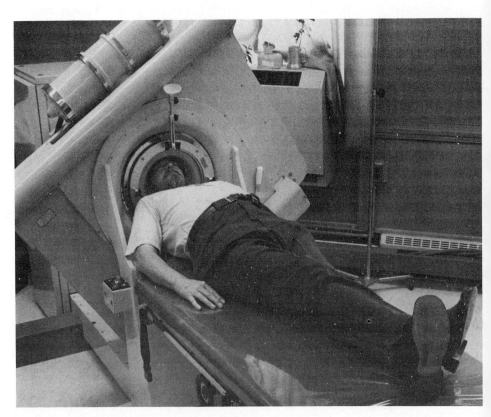

Figure 25–1. A patient with his skull in a CAT scanner.

attenuation coefficients of various organs permit identification of specific organs in the abdomen or chest cavity; the gallbladder, for example, is different in density from the surrounding liver. Types of gallstones not ordinarily visualized through standard X rays may now be detected through scanning. Since the scanner is exquisitely sensitive to small amounts of iodine-containing compounds, the ducts that carry liver bile may soon be visualized in jaundiced patients. (Today, these ducts can only be seen through direct puncture of the liver.)

Future improvements in scanning techniques can be expected to lead to breakthroughs in diagnostic methodology. Because the attenuation coefficient of cancerous tissue differs from that of normal tissue, it may become possible to detect tumors in areas in which they are not now presently definable; chemicals may also be given to make tumors more visible. The spread of tumor to the liver should be apparent on routine scan if the tumor is above a certain size. Techniques should also improve

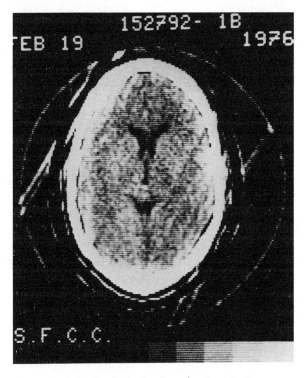

Figure 25–2. A normal CAT scan of a brain. The black areas in the center represent the cerebral ventricles in normal position.

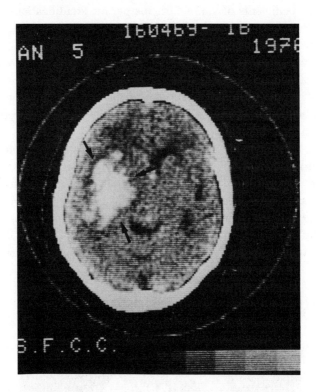

Figure 25–3. A CAT scan of another patient's brain showing a large collection of blood in the brain (arrows) after intracerebral hemorrhage.

for visualizing small lesions in the pancreas, an organ that at present can be evaluated only with great difficulty. Visualization of the pancreas, together with analysis of tissue samples taken with fine needles guided ultrasonically, will enable the physician to diagnose lesions that cannot be detected today except by far more complex procedures. Similar enhanced diagnostic capacities should be applicable to the adrenal gland, the bladder, the prostate, the uterus, the ovary, the spleen, and the kidneys.

In the chest cavity, the structures of the blood vessels of the lungs may become visible; perhaps more important, it may become possible to separate the esophagus, trachea, and the great vessels from each other on transverse images of the thorax. An entire new field of radiopharmacology—the use of drugs in radiology for diagnostic purposes—will concern itself with the enhancement of organ and lesion visualization.

CAT scanning will be highly effective in planning radiation therapy.

It represents an ideal tool for imaging tumor mass and the relationship to surrounding organs. The image can be put into digital form and fed into a computer, which can then calculate the best method for giving optimal dosages to the tumor and surrounding tissues. This may also represent an effective method of monitoring the results of tumor therapy.

Cardiac computerized tomography promises to make a major contribution to the diagnosis of heart disease. It has already been demonstrated that infarcted heart muscle (muscle that has died in a heart attack) has a different attenuation coefficient from that of normal heart muscle. As a consequence, the area of infarcted muscle is readily defined in animal models by CAT scanning. It seems highly likely that this will soon be applicable to humans, once the technology advances to the point where more rapid CAT scans synchronized to the events of the heart cycle are available. Similarly, when an agent that increases radiographic contrast is added to the blood, the blood pool within the heart's left ventricle is readily visualized in contrast to the wall of heart muscle. Thus, the internal anatomy of the ventricle may be defined, as well as the volume of blood contained at different points in the heart cycle.

With the new developments in computerized scanning, with three-dimensional reconstruction from ultrasound data on the horizon, and with the development of new radioactive substances which are taken up specifically by particular tumors or organs (and therefore enable further advances either in imaging or in therapy), the field of radiology is very much in the middle of a remarkable growth phase today.

The Implementation
of Research

PART SIX

Economics of
Health Research

RASHI FEIN

26

Had the chapters in this volume been written a decade ago, they would have been far different; if similar essays are written a decade hence, they will be more different still. Biomedical knowledge has grown and continues to grow. The increase in knowledge and understanding is not the product of a process in which individuals, marginally supported out of limited personal funds, labor in cold garrets or conceptualize on the banks of still rivers. Appealing as such romantic notions about the nature of research may be, they are not descriptive of reality. Modern research is an organized activity involving large numbers of people and significant sums of money. Modern research requires resources.

It is true, of course, that resources are needed to sustain any activity, even that of the legendary lonely scientist who improvised, patched his equipment together out of junk, and had sudden bursts of inspiration. The difference between the past and present does not lie in the fact that today's research, in contrast with yesterday's, requires support, but in the scale of support needed—in the resources required if research is to be sustained and in the resources allocated to the effort. Only 25 years ago, government, industry, and private nonprofit funding of health research and development totaled 161 million dollars. Today, expenditures total 4.3 billion dollars, 2.8 billion of which is contributed by the federal government. On a per capita basis, annual expenditures have increased from $1.16 to $20.05 per person.

Health research is a major economic activity. No longer an individual or marginal budget item, it now accounts for over 13 percent of national expenditures for all research and development and almost 10 percent of all federal health expenditures. Because it absorbs a sizable amount of public funds, medical research is the object of scrutiny and the subject of controversy. To grow to its present dimensions, medical research required federal support. But that support made it inevitable that sooner or later—and certainly in an era of tight budgets, a topsy-turvy economy, and an increased sensitivity to the evaluation of the impact of federal expenditures—medical research would face a set of hard questions. It is the purpose of this chapter to set forth some of these questions. Although they have occasionally been raised in a spirit of antagonism or anti-intellectualism, many of the questions asked are reasonable; they are the kinds of questions that can and should be asked of any economic activity supported with taxpayers' dollars.

The Rationale for Government Support

The classic argument in favor of government support for research—an argument that applies especially to basic research, in contrast to applied research and development—is that the private sector, applying private criteria, would engage in lower levels of research investment than would be socially optimal. The private sector can capture some but not all of the potential benefits of research findings. Public support of research is, therefore, warranted in order to supplement private efforts and to support research endeavors whose benefits cannot be fully translated into private profits.

In addition, government funding may be required to take advantage of the significant economies of scale that can exist in research. Individual firms may not be able fully to exploit existing economies of scale, and competitive factors may inhibit cooperative joint ventures in which costs or information would be shared. Furthermore, government may be able to mobilize the personnel required for research at lower monetary costs than might be incurred by a privately funded effort. This is partly because government funds can more readily be channeled to researchers in medical schools, where research activity yields multiple products (research, medical education, and service) and where opportunities for psychic income may be greater. These arguments are not purely theoretical; they are consistent with present patterns of government and private funding. Private funds, for example, play a larger role in pharmaceutical research than in research on psychological counseling or human development, and private money has gone primarily to developmental efforts rather than basic research.

An additional argument for government research support stems from the fact that government pays for a significant proportion of medical services. In fiscal year 1975, federal spending for health totaled 34 billion dollars out of a national health expenditure of 118 billion (and 29 billion dollars out of the 103 billion that represented personal health care expenditures). These sums and the proportion that is federally financed will grow. Aside from the benefits to the individual citizen of research that helps reduce sickness and the death rate and improve the quality of life, there is the additional argument (narrow but nonetheless persuasive) that today's federal investment in research may help contain tomorrow's federal bill for personal health care services. It is likely that the federal government will come to dominate the financing arrangements for medical care under national health insurance; the federal government therefore has a direct interest in minimizing the future cost of health care through successful research.

Finally, health research is already taking place in an established structure that has been fueled by government funds. Federal support has had both a direct impact on research and an indirect impact on the higher education institutions which house much of the research activity. Federal funds and university resources have created a set of structures that expresses a partnership. Medical education, medical care, and medical research are closely intertwined; the lines between these three activities are not drawn sharply. Often they all take place in the same institution, at the same time and with the same facilities and personnel. Significant changes in the level and structure of research support clearly would have implications not only for research but for other activities as well. As a consequence of years of federal funding for research—and the relative neglect of educational support—medical schools have come to rely on research funding as a mainstay of their total budget. If federal research support were to be altered without impairing medical education and research, account would have to be taken of the patterns that have developed and new sources of support would be necessary.

The importance of government funding for medical research is thus supported by theoretical arguments as well as by historical developments. Similar arguments can be advanced for medical research support by private philanthropy. It is of course the case that the funds available through private philanthropy are less than those available from government. This, however, does not deny their importance, since on occasion private philanthropic efforts may utilize their funds in a more flexible manner, designed to increase the diversity of research approaches and to support both fields and people who are not yet established. The importance of such "seed" money cannot be minimized. Even so, the scale of government support is such that there is little reason to believe that the private sector would or could compensate for major declines in federal funding.

Federal funding for medical research is clearly appropriate. What is at issue is how large this funding should be, what specific areas of research should receive priority, and who should make these decisions.

Determining the Level of Research Support

Let us begin by imagining that we live in a world in which those who construct budgets are called upon to make a decision regarding the total expenditure to be allocated for health research. Since research uses resources, important choices must be made. Shall available funds go to medical research or delivery of services, medical research or national parks, medical research or lower taxes? Similar questions of choice arise in the private financing of research whether at the individual, corporate, or philanthropic level. The difference lies in the scale of the decisions to be made and in the criteria to be used. The scientist of the past who supported himself out of his own funds and those of friends or family was engaged in a private matter, with financing made available to support private goals (perhaps as simple as maximizing the sheer enjoyment of the scientist or of the benefactor). The corporate funding of research is justified by the desire to maximize long-run profits. In both situations the criteria are private, and the range of choices—the things for which scarce dollars can be used—are limited by those criteria.

Government funding is qualitatively and quantitatively different from private funding. The various choices possible and the number of dollars available are much greater. In considering the possible choices, decision makers must ask how the benefits derived from the last dollar used for research compare with the benefits that might be derived from the various possible alternative uses of that incremental dollar. Marginal economic analysis teaches us that if the last or marginal dollar used for research would yield fewer benefits than in alternative uses, it should be shifted to those alternatives (and vice versa). Total benefits would be maximized when benefits are equated at the margin. The question posed, therefore, reminds us of a number of things: that our evaluation is of dollars at the margin, of increments to existing budgets; that it is crucial to specify the benefits to be gained from these marginal dollars; that the same benefit-cost question asked of those who advocate health research expenditures must be asked of the proponents of programs in other areas. The question establishes a general conceptual framework within which to consider budgetary decisions.

The first matter, the fact that we are dealing with the impact of the last dollar, with the impact "at the margin," tells us that our concern must be with marginal rather than with average rates of return to various government expenditures, including those for health research. Indeed, since this is the case, it becomes evident that we cannot speak of health research in general but must speak of specific projects. There is no reason, after all, to imagine that the health research dollar is equally productive in each and every health research area. Thus, analysis of the return on the marginal dollar in individual areas rather than the analysis of average returns to health research in the main is necessary.

In analyzing the appropriate level of health research funding in benefit-cost terms, it is first necessary to grapple with the very basic and difficult question of how a benefit in the field of health care should be measured. Government support is predicated on the assumption that the research funded will be productive in the sense that there will be scientific discoveries, that these discoveries will have relevance to health, and that they will be applied to improving the population's health. It could be argued that any research is valuable if it increases our store of knowledge, that a civilized society needs science as it needs art, music, and poetry. However, the level of support for health research and the legislative debate over appropriations indicate that the public's representatives believe—and have been led to believe—that they are buying more than an intellectual activity that provides enjoyment to those involved in it. This chapter cannot examine all the conceptual issues that are raised by the term benefit, used within a government perspective, or explore the inherent theoretical problems and measurement difficulties that analysts face in attempting to estimate benefits. But a few considerations can be discussed briefly to demonstrate the danger of a mechanistic or limited definition of benefit.

It is very convenient to emphasize those improvements in health care that reduce days lost from work through illness and death; those benefits can readily be translated into dollar values related to the gross national product. But an emphasis on productivity is narrow and may be misplaced. The alleviation of discomfort, pain, and concern is part of a broad definition of health. These are worthy goals even if they may have less impact on productivity and even though they cannot easily be quantitatively incorporated into economic benefit-cost calculations. Health researchers have often stressed the potential impact their discoveries might have in helping increase the GNP or in reducing the direct monetary costs of health care. While such arguments may be persuasive to some budget analysts and decision makers, there is a danger in this emphasis; it tends to narrow the focus of interest and to constrain the terms of debate. It may lead to allocations that are at variance with consumer preferences. Furthermore, accounting principles are not substitutes for ethical imperatives. It may be more socially useful to call upon the nobler motives of decency, humanity, compassion, and concern in an effort to bring forth the best in us.

The estimate of benefits is made more difficult by the question of the appropriate time horizon. Research is an investment that, at best, will lead to improved health at some point in the perhaps distant future and that is funded with money that might otherwise buy goods and services that increase satisfaction, perhaps even health, in the present. How, then, are the future and the present to be compared? How much are benefits that will accrue in the future to be discounted? What is the appropriate balance between consumption in the present and investment for the future?

Also related to the problem of defining health benefits is the question for whom. Diseases affect different population groups classified by age, sex, race, and socioeconomic status. Should calculations that determine research allocations only consider the total number of persons who might benefit and the degree of benefit, or are different groups of people to be weighted in some manner? Government, after all, is concerned not only with efficiency but also with distributive justice. But what are the principles of distribution that should guide the decision-making process? Furthermore, how can these principles be quantified?

If research is justified on the basis that research discoveries may promote the public's health, what consideration should be given to the various links in the chain required to translate these discoveries into better health care? Imagine that a research endeavor results in the acquisition of new knowledge but that this knowledge is not applied because of shortcomings and failures in the organization or financing of the health care delivery system. Should such a successful but unapplied research effort be viewed in the same way as a research endeavor that fails in the laboratory and that yields no applicable advances in knowledge? In both cases, but for different reasons, there is no improvement in health status; in the first case the delivery system fails to distribute the fruits of research, and in the second there are no fruits to distribute. Surely the research endeavor's potential must be considered in the light of existing constraints in the rest of the health care system, not to mention socioeconomic conditions (such as poor housing) that may limit the application, the impact, and thus the improvements in the public health. But these constraints will change over time; in fact, the fruits of research will themselves affect the speed with which constraints may change. Understandably, research scientists may feel a measure of resentment when their efforts are called into question, not because they have failed but because legislative and other governing bodies have not taken steps to ensure that the health care delivery system incorporates the products of the laboratory and distributes them to all the people.

In considering the health research budget, we must take note of the concept of a health dollar, a concept that has grown in importance in recent years and especially since the enactment of Medicare and Medicaid and the consequent expansion of federal financing of health care services. The attempt to constrain the expansion of total federal health expenditures, even while federal expenditures for personal health services (already mandated by law) increase, has inevitably put great pressure on the nonservice federal health programs. This has pitted the various parts of the health field against each other. Health research has been forced to compete for scarce resources against other health programs, not against all other federal and private expenditures. This is particularly the case with research programs whose effects will not be seen until some time in the future and which are often easily controlled by limiting expenditures (for example, through reduction of appropriations or impoundment of funds). Of course, all budget items are controllable, but new legislation or significantly tighter regulation would often be required if the expansion of health service costs were to be constrained. It is, therefore, easier to attempt to control research appropriations.

The difficulty of ensuring adequate federal health research appropriations stems not from the fact that they must compete for scarce resources but from the terms of the competition. To a significant extent, federal funds for research are put at jeopardy by the concept of the health dollar. That concept transforms research from a competitor with all other programs to a residual claimant for those resources available after the claims of other health programs have been satisfied.

Rather than being a cause for cutting research spending, the growth of service programs should provide an even greater incentive for investment in research, since such investments may reduce health care costs in the long run. In any case, the idea of controlling the total health budget by limiting research spending is highly questionable. Since health research represents only about 10 percent of all federal health expenditures, total health expenditures will not be substantially affected even by major changes in the budget for health research. Furthermore, the very concept of a health dollar appears at variance with the goal of designing the budget on the basis of benefit-cost considerations on a program-by-program basis. But these arguments have not been totally effective against the convenient (albeit simplistic) approach to health funding that has gained currency in the recent past.

Allocating the Research Budget

Let us suppose that a decision has been reached on an appropriate sum to be expended for health research. Whatever the basis on which that total sum has been determined, it must be allocated among the various competing areas and problems to be investigated. The considerations that would determine the allocation of the federal research dollar are similar to those that have already been examined in the discussion of the determination of the federal health research budget: the costs of various endeavors and their potential benefits. While the comparison of benefits of various alternatives may be easier when our focus is limited only to health research—we need not consider the satisfaction derived from less polio as compared with the satisfaction derived from less illiteracy or more national parkland—it still remains difficult. As already indicated, health is a multidimensional matter. It is impossible to bring precision to the comparison of different kinds of improvements in health appearing at different times in the future, affecting different population groups, and all subject to different probability estimates of the potential success of the various research efforts.

In judging where to place research emphasis it is not only important to know the significance of a disease in terms of the number (and characteristics) of people affected; it is also important to assess the probable fruitfulness of the research. Is there reason to believe that a breakthrough is at hand or is the probability of success, within a given time period or budget allocation, one half or one third or one fifth? It has often been argued that the bank which never has a loan default and the shortstop who never commits an error are both behaving in too conservative a fashion. Maximal success requires the taking of risk. So, too, with the world of research. Some proportion of the research activity should be expected to fail. If the budgeteer expects a 100 percent success ratio, he is likely to fund pedestrian research; there will be few failures, but there will also be few glowing successes. Yet even if one is aware of this situation, the pressures are likely to be toward conservatism and the avoidance of risk. Breakthroughs not achieved are harder to criticize than are visible failures. One of the powerful arguments for supplementary private funding of research efforts is that individual benefactors and foundations may often be readier to take risks in research funding, since the penalty associated with failure tends to be smaller.

Funding for specific research endeavors—and, ultimately, budget allocations must deal in specifics—must also consider the possible relationship between the specific endeavor and other important areas of knowledge. It is in the nature of research, particularly basic research, that boundaries between areas of investigation are sometimes blurred. That which at first appears to be important in understanding one disease may turn out to have considerable relevance to another; research that is stimulated by an interest in field X may yield knowledge about problem Y. Although obviously unpredictable, the possibilities of such spillovers cannot be ignored (or, for that matter, assumed).

The preceding observations make clear that the analysis of benefits and costs at the margin is difficult and complex. To imagine that such analysis can be undertaken for each and every health research area and project is clearly fallacious. Projects do compete against each other, but we do not live in a world in which each possible incremental federal research expenditure is evaluated on an individual basis against every alternative federal program. Were that the case, there would not be a decision on a total health research expenditure but a set of decisions on individual programs. One would arrive at the federal health research budget by totaling up the individual programs. In the real world, therefore, the budget process is one of interplay between an *ex ante* target total to be divided between various research endeavors and an *ex post* derivative total that represents the resultant of individual program decisions. We move back and forth—adjusting totals and programs.

Thus it is not surprising that the federal health research budget exhibits a significant degree of stability in real terms (adjusted for inflation) from year to year. Budget decisions in fact are made on an incremental basis—sums are added to or subtracted from the previous year's budget. Base-line expenditure figures are taken as given, and the analytic effort is devoted to analysis of the potential impact of changes at the margin. Such a procedure can be justified on various grounds: political and administrative feasibility or a belief that last year's budget was optimal in equating benefits at the margin (that is, that any shift of funds would have reduced total benefits) and, therefore, serves as a valid point of departure.

The Need for Balance

Decisions concerning research support and effort require a substantial degree of judgment. We do not know the "correct" answer or allocation and will never know it. Indeed, given the different views concerning trade-offs between present and future benefits, between improvement in the quality of life (alleviation of suffering) and extension of life, (reduction in mortality), there can be no correct answer. Thus, allocative decisions are not technical but are value or social decisions to be made by those who are society's representatives, though with as much advice as can be provided by professionals in medicine.

The setting of priorities and objectives is the responsibility of those who are empowered by the public to be its representatives. It is true that this responsibility to the taxpayers would not be fulfilled were public funds to be turned over to scientists to do with as they saw fit. Yet, it is important for the public's representatives to recognize the limits that are placed on government intervention by the very nature of scientific research and of the university, where much of the research is carried forward. It is one thing to set priorities. It is quite another to attempt to direct the nature of scientific inquiry or to select the particular research avenues to be followed. To do so is to change the nature of the fragile institution called the university—an institution which has served society well. The costs of such change may be high indeed. It is true that the preservation of freedom of inquiry in the scientific community is an expression of faith in that community and its processes; in fact, so is the support of research itself. But history vindicates these acts of faith; and while it is inappropriate to rely blindly on history, it is irresponsible to treat it lightly.

A balance is required, a balance between the need for scientific freedom and the requirements for social responsibility. To achieve that balance is vital, for much is at stake. Budget decisions require consideration of many alternatives: basic or applied and developmental research, medical care delivery or medical research, this area of investigation or that, support of general research programs or of specific research projects, institutions, or people. To decide wisely we need to know more than we now do about research itself. We need research on health research. What benefits has it brought? What processes, structures, and organizations enhance the probabilities of success? What increases the chances of spill-over effects? What speeds the diffusion of knowledge and the application of new insights? All these questions, and more, are themselves areas for study. We are dealing with large sums and complex organizations. Even if research support has been and will remain an "act of faith," we must increase our understanding of the way knowledge is acquired in order to allocate resources and organize activities more effectively.

The resources of the economy are limited; the needs are great. Resources must be used wisely and opportunities to advance the public welfare must be exploited. These challenges can be met but only if the issues are recognized and if all concerned with them attempt to solve them together.

Spreading the Medical Word

FRANZ J. INGELFINGER

27

Studies of the physical molecular mechanisms whereby soap facilitates the intermingling of grease and water seem to have few clinical uses except, perhaps, for sanitary purposes. Yet published reports of such studies, with descriptions of the methods used to analyze and measure the detergent properties of soap, led to the application of similar methods to assess the detergent effects of human bile. Once these methods became standardized and better known, they were seized upon by numerous clinical investigators, who confirmed what had been suspected on the basis of less sophisticated techniques: the detergent properties of bile are less than normal in persons with cholesterol gallstones, the most common type of gallstone among Western peoples. When such stones, moreover, were agitated in watery solutions containing bile salts and phospholipids (natural substances that confer upon human bile its detergent effects), the stones lost weight.

Such observations lent support to the hypothesis that gallstones form when the biliary concentrations of bile salts and phospholipids relative to that of the fatty substance cholesterol fall below a certain level. Actual measurement of these three substances in normal bile and in bile from patients with gallstones yielded further confirmatory evidence. The final step was now obvious: why not feed bile salts to such patients in the hope of dissolving the stones? Methods were therefore developed to prepare adequate quantities of a natural human bile salt, chenodeoxycholic acid, in a form that was about 98 percent pure. In numerous, but still preliminary, clinical tests that involved feeding the chenodeoxycholic acid to patients with gallstones that had not yet become calcified, about half such stones either disappeared or became smaller. The efficacy of the treatment, however, must be more sharply defined, and, even more important, its safety must be documented. Large doses of chenodeoxycholic acid, for example, might damage the liver. As of this writing, therefore, a multicenter clinical trial to evaluate the usefulness of chenodeoxycholic acid in the treatment of cholesterol gallstones is under way. If the results are satisfactory, the practitioner of the future will have the choice of treating his patients with gallstones medically or surgically.

The sequence leading from dissolution of grease by soap to the dissolution of gallstones, which required about 10 years, illustrates a common but far from invariable process whereby a notion is converted into something that may be medically useful. Clearly an elaborate structure of diverse professional activities is involved, including: basic scientists (physical chemists, physiologists, pharmacologists); developers (biochemists, pharmacists, entrepreneurs); clinical investigators; and practicing doctors (family physicians, emergency care physicians, internists, surgeons, pediatricians, and so on).

The lifeblood of this complex structure is communication, which must flow horizontally within a given level of peer investigators and also vertically from one level to another. Since the system of communication enabling the exchange of ideas and information among the first three levels—which may be subsumed under the heading research and development or R&D—differs from that connecting R&D with the practitioner, the two systems are described separately.

At R&D levels, the information exchange that keeps the cutting edge of experimentation well honed is primarily verbal. By telephone, by visits to colleagues, and at informal ad hoc meetings that convene experts to discuss a promising but sharply defined and limited topic, new ideas and observations are described and discussed. Collectively such verbal exchanges make up what have been called "invisible colleges." The advantages are clear. In view of academicians' penchant for travel, the technology of modern transportation, and the funds abundantly available—at least until recently—to support trips to exotic meeting places, invisible colleges have made possible a grass-fire propagation of new and worthwhile biomedical ideas. The informality permitted by the small and elite groups that usually make up invisible colleges fosters sharp exchange and criticism. Furthermore, since experts attending a given meeting may represent a variety of levels, a matrix of researchers and developers can gather to discuss a limited categorical subject—bile salts, for example. The invisible college system thus serves both vertical and horizontal communication at virtually all R&D steps.

The system also has its drawbacks. The person who might be able to contribute most to a certain topic might not be invited to participate at a given meeting. Conversely, the elitist nature of invisible colleges tends to exclude the young investigator, who could benefit from the stimulus of attending. These, however, are relatively minor problems: invisible colleges facilitate rapid dissemination of a large volume of research results.

The R&D community is also served by formal meetings. When the Federation of American Societies of Experimental Biology convene, some 20,000 attend to select what they want to hear from some 450 brief (10 minutes) presentations. (These 450 presentations are selected from several thousand abstracts submitted.) Clinical investigators and specialists hold similar if smaller meetings, primarily to hear what peer investigators at various R&D levels have to say. To the co-expert, however, the reports usually comes as no surprise; he has been alerted by the invisible college system.

Except as they are used to supplement both formal and informal verbal presentations, communication at R&D levels makes little use of audiovisual aids. The principal communication step that supplements verbal presentation is the printed page. Although a few rapid publication services are available, including the dissemination of abstracts of papers presented at meetings, the speed of such services cannot compare with that of the invisible colleges. Their content, moreover, is so abbreviated that they serve no more than an alerting function. Sooner or later, all biomedical research of any consequence is printed with considerable detail and care in appropriate and conventional biomedical journals.

Conventional and standard biomedical journals are as a rule tortoise-paced: months, a year, or even more may pass between submission of an article and its publication. A common complaint, therefore, is that R&D is delayed because of the lethargic pace of most medical publications. At one time the charge may have been in order, but today the invisible college system has made the complaint irrelevant. Printed records of research findings are nevertheless essential for purposes other than that of rapidly spreading the news. In the first place, most reputable and respected biomedical research publications—such as the *Journal of Experimental Medicine,* the *Journal of Clinical Investigation,* the *Journal of Biological Chemistry,* or the *American Journal of Physiology*—make use of referees in determining their content. A report usually is not published unless two or more peer experts as well as the editors are convinced that the article's substance is valid, reasonably original, and expressed with at least a modicum of clarity. Thus, reports of research appearing in most standard biomedical journals have received the Good Scientific House-keeping stamp of approval. Second, research reports in such journals tend to be detailed enough for co-experts to judge the methods of the investigation and, if they are so inclined, to repeat the experiment (or experiments) for confirmatory purposes. Third, a report published in the approved format in an established journal serves a valuable archival function: it is part of the record that makes up the body of biomedical knowledge. Even more important, at least from the author's point of view, is the fact that the report identifies his intellectual property. Priority for biomedical discovery is usually determined by the publication date of the journal issue in which the new research is described.

The system is not without its pitfalls. It is as rigid and ritualistic as academic protocol at graduation time. It is also dominated and shaped by the establishment. A radical idea that eventually may prove seminal may not be recognized as such by referees and editors, usually prime representatives of the establishment. Many published reports, moreover, reflect changes demanded by the editor and his consultants. The revised report may thus be shaped by their own notions. The long evaluative process, as well as a variety of organizational problems, accounts for the fact that the results of a research project may not be published for many months after its completion.

Claims of priority are also not without their quarrels. The report of a new phenomenon that is really second, as determined by the date of its submission, may appear in print before the actual first report if the latter is submitted to a journal with a longer lag period between receipt of a manuscript and its publication. Some journals try to correct for this possible source of injustice by printing the dates both of receipt of the manuscript and of its acceptance in its final and approved form. Even such stratagems, however, are not foolproof. Finally, the priority-establishing function of rapidly published items, such as letters to the editor or abstracts of material presented at meetings, is, in view of their brevity, a source of controversy. But the scientific community's reaction to a research report published in the lay press or in medical news journals that are entirely supported by advertising and whose contents are not refereed by co-experts is hard and fast. Material of this type, often selected because of its sensational qualities—that is, the much ballyhooed "break-through"—is not accepted as warranting the claim of having been first.

The mechanisms provided by the invisible colleges, formal meetings, and scientific journals provide a communication system that is on the whole very satisfactory. Communication is rapid and reasonably accurate. Moreover, these mechanisms are so abundantly available that there is no constraint on volume. On the other hand, the volume of the available media is so huge and their orientation so specialized that size of the communication system is an encumbrance as well as an advantage. A scientist may be unable to find the information he needs; he may, indeed, even be unaware of its existence. To mitigate this problem and to facilitate discovery, accessibility, and retrieval of available biomedical scientific information, a vast system of secondary services exists. The National Library of Medicine publishes the *Index Medicus*, which indexes and cross-indexes by title and author the contents of some 2,300 biomedical publications. But the size of the *Index Medicus* is itself forbidding—the 1973 edition comprises eight volumes totaling up to about 1,000 pages. To help scientists get at what they want more rapidly, the National Library of Medicine also publishes selected indices, often with abstracts, in certain categories—diabetes, for example. The library, moreover, offers on-line data bases such as Medline, Toxline, and Catline; in response to telephone requests, these computer-based systems will provide the inquirer with a list of sources that deal in one way or another with the topics about which the inquirer seeks information. (Medline provides the caller with citations from issues of some 3,000 biomedical journals published in the last few years; Catline is a computerized catalogue of serials and monographs; and Toxline provides information on known toxins, environmental pollutants, and drugs that may cause adverse reactions.) During July 1974 to May 1975 inclusive, the National Library of Medicine received 368,772 requests of this type, leading to 62,860 on-line (that is, immediately displayed on a computer terminal) titles that might help the requester and to 88,638 print-outs of such lists. The system is rapid, but it too suffers from excessive volume. Any list may contain many items known as "noise"—that is, titles that refer to the topic identified by the requester but in fact do not contain the specific information he is looking for.

The National Library of Medicine's efforts to organize biomedical information and make it more accessible are supplemented by numerous other services, some nonprofit, some commercial. Extensively used, for example, are *Biological* and *Chemical Abstracts*. A firm in Philadelphia issues a variety of reference publications. One, *Current Contents*, is a publication anxiously scanned by many investigators, for *Current Contents* reproduces the tables of contents of the better known biomedical journals. All such secondary publications serve an invaluable alerting function in keeping the investigator aware of what is going on, especially in fields not covered by the invisible colleges, formal meetings, and publications that serve his own special interests.

The entire communication system serving biomedical R&D is formidable. It is so massive as to be cumbersome. It is also far from perfect. The total system is punctured by many gaps, and needed information may not be caught in its nets. Yet, considering the intensity, explosiveness, variety, and volume of biomedical research, the means of communication that permits the research to grow rapidly (in fact, exponentially) is highly satisfactory. If an important discovery languishes unknown, the cause probably is not the inadequacy of the communication system but rather the failure of scientists to recognize the importance of the discovery.

The brisk and determined exchange of information that tends to keep the biomedical R&D contingent reasonably up to date unfortunately falters in its final task, that of linking biomedical science to medical practice. The communication stricture at this junction has been deplored by many. President Johnson chided the National Institutes of Health for their failure to promote the application of their research; Senator Edward Kennedy has charged that doctors are not adequately instructed about the use of new drugs; and some officials at the National Cancer Institute are forever complaining that practitioners are not sufficiently aware of the latest treatments for cancer.

Whatever the reasons for the slow and uncertain application of the results of R&D in medical practice, they do not include a dearth of the necessary instruments. In fact, the variety and number of the means of communication between the researcher and the practitioner are larger than those that serve R&D. The standard and traditional means is the medical journal. Some such journals are specially designed to acquaint the practitioner with new medical developments, but most of the best known and largest publications of this type are addressed to both town and gown. Thus, journals such as the *Lancet, Journal of the American Medical Association,* the *New England Journal of Medicine,* and many devoted to the broad specialties of internal medicine, surgery, and pediatrics feature sections devoted to original articles in which clinical investigators describe their experiments.

The relatively slow publication rate of practically all such journals—*Lancet* excepted—is often identified as a major cause of the unsatisfactory aspects of communication between scientist and practitioner. This criticism, however, is inappropriate. Many of the advances described have only a potential and indirect bearing on medical practice. Reports of the early stages in the development of chenodeoxycholic acid, for example, were of no immediate practical value. Even reports describing an actual clinical experience do not mean that the new diagnostic or therapeutic method is ready for general use. Additional testing and maturing experience are generally desirable. In addition, some new devices or drugs can be managed safely only by the expert. When the members of the National Cancer Institute complain that doctors are not sufficiently aware of new cancer therapies, they do not mean that the average practitioner should use the treatments himself. They merely wish to alert him to the availability of certain new methods at highly specialized institutions.

Even if a competent physician wishes to use a new drug, he cannot do so because the substance has not yet been cleared by the Food and Drug Administration (FDA) for general use. Today, all American physicians who open their medical journals or who attend major medical meetings know that cromolyn was used in England to treat asthma for six years before the FDA authorized use of the agent in the United States, and that carbenoxolone is given to the patient with gastric ulcer in Paris and London but is not available in New York. They also know that in 1967 in the *New England Journal of Medicine* George Cotzias described the remarkable relief that L-dopa brings to the parkinsonian patient but that the FDA did not authorize its widespread use until 1971.

The innovations of the laboratory and of the research ward are indeed slow to become part of the practitioner's therapeutic armamentarium, but the constraints are as a rule not those imposed by medical journals. New drugs are for the most part too toxic to permit their use by all physicians, and the FDA is properly cautious. Medical journals are frustratingly slow, but this characteristic rarely harms the patient by depriving him of new diagnostic and therapeutic modalities. If the slowness of medical journals does any harm, it is to medical egos. The doctor's ego and authority are at risk when patients ask him about this or that sensational breakthrough which they, but not the doctor, had seen on television the night before.

The principal difficulty accounting for the fact that the standard medical journal does not serve as an efficient means of communication between R&D and application is that the author of an original article in a medical journal sees his prime audience as his peers. After all, if his article is to be published it must first pass the muster of peer review, and even after its publication the author's ideas and research must meet with the favor of fellow experts before he is credited with expanding the vistas of biomedicine.

In an effort to present biomedical information in a manner that serves the readers' rather than the author's needs, a vast volume of so-called secondary literature is published. This consists of reviews that summarize, integrate, analyze, and restate material that has already been published. Many of these reviews appear in the same standard medical journals that present original articles; others make up journals devoted exclusively to recapitulation. In addition, there is a large variety of books and monographs published at periodic intervals and bearing titles such as *Progress in . . . , Yearbook of . . .* , or *Annual Review of . . .* The goals and quality of this secondary literature vary as much as its format. Reviews appearing in standard medical journals are at their best scholarly, exhaustive, and accurate. The same qualities, however, impair their comprehensibility and readability, at least as far as the practitioner is concerned. Too often, the scientist-author is still addressing his colleagues rather than the doctor caring for patients.

At the other end of the spectrum of biomedical review publications are what might be called rehash journals. At their worst, they are vulgarized, superficial, and inaccurate. They offer little that cannot be found in textbooks. Yet their style is popular and their illustrations often both attractive and useful. Perhaps their most serious fault is that they serve as information booths rather than colleges of medicine. They instruct the physician-reader in a "do this, do that" fashion—so-called algorithms or flow charts are popular—but they do little to promote the doctor's understanding of the why of his actions.

Between the extremes of heavy erudition and frothy shallowness there are, fortunately, reviews solid in substance and written with the practitioner in mind. Their number, however, is not large. In spite of good intentions, many a scientist-author is not innately a gifted writer, and his style tends to reflect his training to present material precisely and parsimoniously but not eloquently or appealingly. Furthermore, the motivation of the scientist who writes for the practitioner is limited. One good original contribution may lead to a professorship, but the impeccable review, particularly if written for the practitioner, will not enhance the author's academic status. Some publications therefore try to offer pecuniary rewards, but in these days of large incomes for the academic as well as practicing doctor, a 500 to 1,000 dollar stipend, half of which goes to the Internal Revenue Service, is meager compensation for the labor that a good review entails.

In spite of its deficiencies the secondary medical literature is so vast and redundant that it could give the practitioner all the information he needs to practice top-notch medicine—provided he could find the articles he needs and provided he could read them. The practitioner has to contend with the same problems of discovery and retrieval faced by the biomedical scientist, but the practitioner's difficulties in overcoming the problems are far greater, for he is much less adept than the scientist in using the library and the multiple indexing and abstracting services that are available. But even these barriers are only relative. I am convinced that a practitioner who assiduously scans five or so medical publications throughout the year and reads with care the items pertinent to his practice can keep up in a fashion that, though not ideal, is at least entirely adequate.

"Too busy to read" is the doctor's conventional excuse. A more accurate statement is that he is too busy to learn how to read. Although I am perhaps biased, my conviction is that about one third of practicing doctors reads frequently and effectively, but that another third never reads—or reads at least nothing more difficult than the sports page or the weekly news magazine. In between there is a group that reads once in a while. Those who never or rarely read either professional or serious nonmedical literature are handicapped for want of practice. The once-a-month golfer hooks and slices; the once-a-month reader is in the rough. The once-a-week reader is not much better off. Hence, for a large proportion of practicing physicians, the suggestion that they might keep up by reading about five medical journals is entirely impractical. They must rely on verbal communication.

Fortunately, such verbal means are abundantly available. Many formal medical meetings feature state-of-the-art lectures. Other meetings essentially consist of post-graduate teaching exercises, and most medical societies, teaching hospitals, and medical schools offer a wide spectrum of refresher courses. Audio-visual means of instruction have also been extensively developed. Television programs or cassettes serve admirably to demonstrate new techniques, but particularly popular are audiotapes, for they, as opposed to printed or audio-visual media, permit the busy practitioner to learn while he is doing something else—while driving from hospital to hospital, for example, or as he applies the morning razor. Finally, although he has no invisible colleges, informal communications such as conversation with colleagues, consultation with specialists, or—to many a pedagogue's distress—advice from the detail man (representative of a pharmaceutical company) play a large role in keeping the practitioner abreast of what is going on.

In spite of their abundance, the verbal means of communicating the results of biomedical investigation to the practitioner are relatively inefficient. The information so provided obviously lacks all semblance of organization. Hence, the learning experience tends to be fragmentary and haphazard. The doctor hears about new developments in fits and starts. Although his post-graduate education is continued, it is, alas, not continuous.

The inadequacy of communication between R&D on one hand and the practicing physician on the other is widely recognized. To counteract the deficiencies, major medical organizations engage in intensive publicity campaigns exhorting the doctor to keep up. The American College of Physicians has with considerable success encouraged internists to assess their knowledge by a carefully structured system of self-examination. The rules of many medical societies, moreover, require their members to take a certain number of post-graduate courses yearly. Finally, there is the threat of mandatory recertification imposed either by medical organizations or—to the dismay of many a doctor—by government.

In spite of such efforts, however, the results are disappointing. After thousands of original articles, hundreds of good reviews, and a plethora of post-graduate exercises, the use of antibiotics in 1974 and 1975 was apparently still so unsatisfactory that both the American Medical Association and the American College of Physicians undertook special measures to improve the situation. A tongue-in-cheek letter written by W. R. Lockwood to the *New England Journal of Medicine* proposes a solution that would not be necessary if communication between scientist and practitioner were better.

Antibiotics Anonymous

To the Editor: The syndrome of compulsive antibiotic prescribing (CAP), so widespread among physicians, is a serious affliction as attested to by the many learned articles on the subject itself and one of the consequences of CAP—namely, the appearance of antibiotic-resistant bacteria in hospitals.

Years of attempting to cure fellow physicians of CAP by sitting down and reasoning with them (Puzo M: The Godfather, New York, Putnam, 1969) has led us to the opinion that CAP is not inherited but is an acquired disease and should be treated as such. First-year medical students do not seem to have the disease, whereas nearly all interns and first-year residents are severely afflicted, only a few recovering by the time they reach staff status. Thus, it seems that CAP is acquired during the association with older physicians who are already hooked, and who seem to be possessed of a demon who not only refuses to allow them to break their own bad habits but insists that they inflict them on their colleagues.

Once such a chain of events is begun, it is very difficult to break, for not only are cures uncommon (there are none recorded at the Medical Center) but those who have the problem encourage others to acquire it too, perhaps in a subconscious effort to justify their own behavior. Furthermore, members of a well organized and aggressive group of pushers are ever present to encourage CAP for their own gain and that of the large syndicates with which they have close ties. Because the habit is a bad one, causing more harm than the little pleasure that it brings, and also because it is very expensive to support and, further, as traditional approaches to its cure have totally failed, we have decided that the best we can offer is help to physicians who wish to break the habit but find that they are incapable of doing so. Therefore, we have created a self-help organization for such physicians. We realize, of course, that few would wish to advertise their weakness and shortcomings, and, certainly no one wants them publicly displayed; accordingly, the organization membership will be kept strictly secret from nonmembers, no advertising will be allowed, and membership will be on a voluntary basis. The name of this new self-help organization is Antibiotics Anonymous (AA) . . .

New England Journal of Medicine 290 (1974), 465.

SUGGESTIONS FOR
FURTHER READING

INDEX

Suggestions for
Further Reading

Chapter 2

Clark, D. W., and B. MacMahon, eds. *Preventive Medicine.* Boston: Little, Brown & Co., 1967.

Erhardt, C. L., and J. Berlin, eds. *Mortality and Morbidity in the United States.* Cambridge: Harvard University Press, 1974.

Chapter 3

Baltimore, David. "Viruses, Polymerases, and Cancer." *Science* 192 (1976), 632–636.

Cairns, John. "The Cancer Problem." *Scientific American,* November 1975, pp. 64–78.

Dulbecco, Renato. "The Induction of Cancer by Viruses." *Scientific American,* April 1967, pp. 28–37.

Dulbecco, Renato. "From the Molecular Biology of Oncogenic DNA Viruses to Cancer." *Science* 192 (1976), 437–440.

Folkman, Judah. "The Vascularization of Tumors." *Scientific American,* May 1976, pp. 59–73.

Holland, J. F., and Emil Frei, III, eds. *Cancer Medicine.* Philadelphia: Lea and Febiger, 1973.

Chapter 4

Hilton, B., D. Callahan, M. Harris, et al., eds. *Ethical Issues in Human Genetics.* New York: Plenum Press, 1973.

Lerner, I. M. *Heredity, Evolution, and Society.* San Francisco: W. H. Freeman and Company, 1968.

McKusick, V. A., and R. Clairborne, eds. *Medical Genetics.* New York: H. P. Publishing Co., 1973.

Sutton, H. E. *An Introduction to Human Genetics.* New York: Holt, Rinehart and Winston, 1975.

Chapter 5
Clowes, R. C. "The Molecule of Infectious Drug Resistance." *Scientific American,* April 1973, pp. 18–27.
McCarthy, Maclyn, ed. "Host-Parasite Relations in Bacterial Diseases." In *Microbiology,* ed. B. D. David, R. Dulbecco, H. N. Eisen, H. S. Ginsberg, and W. B. Wood. 2d ed. Hagerstown, Md.: Harper & Row, 1973.
Smith, M. E. D. "Immunization: The Current Scene." *Hospital Practice,* November 1969, pp. 42–53.
Weinstein, L. "Chemotherapy of Microbial Diseases." In *The Pharmacological Basis of Therapeutics,* ed. L. S. Goodman and A. Gilman. 5th ed. New York: Macmillan Co., 1975.

Chapter 6
Green, W. *Virus Hunters.* New York: Alfred A. Knopf, 1959.
Hilleman, Maurice R., and Alfred A. Tytell. "The Induction of Interferon." *Scientific American,* July 1971, pp. 26–31.
Holland, John J. "Slow, Inapparent and Recurrent Viruses." *Scientific American,* February 1974, pp. 32–40.
Maugh, Thomas H., II. "Chemotherapy: Antiviral Agents Come of Age." *Science* 192 (1976), 128–132.

Chapter 7
Hollander, Joseph Lee, and Daniel J. McCarty. *Arthritis and Allied Conditions.* Philadelphia: Lea & Febiger, 1972.
Porter, R. R. "The Structure of Antibodies." *Scientific American,* October 1967, pp. 81–90.
Samter, M. *Immunological Diseases.* 2d ed, Boston: Little, Brown and Co., 1971.
Terne, Niels Kaj. "The Immune System." *Scientific American,* July 1973, pp. 52–60.

Chapter 8
Fieve, R., D. Rosenthal, and H. Brill, eds. *Genetic Research in Psychiatry.* Baltimore: Johns Hopkins University Press, 1975.
Kety, S. S. "Current Biochemical Approaches to Schizophrenia." *New England Journal of Medicine* 276 (1967), 325–333.
Matthysse, S., and S. S. Kety, eds. *Catecholamines and Schizophrenia.* Oxford: Pergamon Press, 1975.
Rosenthal, D., and S. S. Kety, eds. *The Transmission of Schizophrenia.* Oxford: Pergamon Press, 1968.
Snyder, Solomon H. *Madness and the Brain.* New York: McGraw-Hill, 1975.

Chapter 9
Cahalan, D. *Problem Drinkers.* San Francisco: Jossey-Bass, 1970.
Lieber, Charles S. "The Metabolism of Alcohol." *Scientific American,* March 1976, pp. 25–33.

Mello, N. K., and J. H. Mendelson. "Alcoholism: A Biobehavioral Disorder." In *American Handbook of Psychiatry*, Vol. IV, *Organic Conditions and Psychosomatic Medicine*, ed. M. Rieser. New York: Basic Books, 1975.

Mendelson, J. H. "Biological Concomitants of Alcoholism." *New England Journal of Medicine* 283 (1970), 24–32, 71–81.

Mendelson, J. H., A. M. Rossi, and R. E. Meyer, eds. *The Use of Marihuana: A Psychological and Physiological Inquiry*. New York: Plenum Press, 1974.

Musto, David F. *The American Disease: Origins of Narcotic Control*. New Haven: Yale University Press, 1973.

Scott, J. M. *The White Poppy*. London: Heinemann, 1969.

Chapter 10

Bernstein, N. R., ed. *Diminished People: Problems and Care of the Mentally Retarded*. Boston: Little, Brown and Co., 1970.

Milunsky, A. *The Prevention of Genetic Disease and Mental Retardation*. Philadelphia: W. B. Saunders Co., 1975.

Penrose, L. S., and J. B. S. Haldane. *The Biology of Mental Defect*. London: Charles Birchall & Sons, 1966.

Stevens, H. A., and R. Heber, eds. *Mental Retardation: A Review of Research*. Chicago: University of Chicago Press, 1964.

Zigler, E. "Familial Mental Retardation: A Continuing Dilemma." *Science* 155 (1967), 292–298.

Chapter 11

Geschwind, N. "Language and the Brain." *Scientific American*, April 1972, pp. 76–83.

Geschwind, N. "Late Changes in the Nervous System: An Overview." In *Plasticity and Recovery of Function in the Central Nervous System*, ed. D. Stein, J. Rosen, and N. Butters. New York: Academic Press, 1974.

Geschwind, N. *Selected Papers on Language and the Brain*. Boston: Reidel Publishing Co., 1974.

Tower, Donald B., et al., eds. *The Nervous System*. New York: Raven Press, 1975. 3 vols.

Chapter 12

Blakeslees, A. L., and J. Stamler. *Your Heart Has Nine Lives*. Englewood Cliffs, N.J.: Prentice-Hall, 1966.

Effler, Donald B. "Surgery for Coronary Disease." *Scientific American*, October 1968, pp. 36–43.

Lown, Bernard. "Intensive Heart Care." *Scientific American*, July 1968, pp. 19–27.

Spain, David M. "Atherosclerosis." *Scientific American*, August 1966, pp. 48–56.

Chapter 13

Avery, Mary Ellen, Nai-San Wang, and H. William Taeusch, Jr. "The Lung of the Newborn Infant." *Scientific American*, April 1973, pp. 75–85.

Ayres, S. M. *Cigarette Smoking and Lung Diseases: An Update. Basics of RD*, vol. 3. New York: American Lung Association, 1975.

Borgatta, Edgar F., and R. R. Evans, eds. *Smoking, Health, and Behavior.* Chicago: Aldine Publishing Co., 1969.
Brodeur, P. "The Magic Mineral." *The New Yorker Magazine,* October 12, 1968, p. 117.
Clements, John A. "Surface Tension in the Lungs." *Scientific American,* December 1962, pp. 120–130.
Goldsmith, J. R. *Health Effects of Air Pollution. Basics of RD,* vol. 4. New York: American Lung Association, 1975.
U.S. Department of Health, Education and Welfare. *The Health Consequences of Smoking.* Washington, D.C.: U.S. Government Printing Office, 1973.

Chapter 14
Merrill, John P. "The Transplantation of the Kidney." *Scientific American,* October 1959, pp. 57–63.
Merrill, John P. "The Artificial Kidney." *Scientific American,* July 1961, pp. 56–64.

Chapter 15
Asimov, Isaac. *The Living River.* London and New York: Abelard-Schuman, 1959.
Hackett, Earle. *Blood.* New York: Saturday Review Press/E. P. Dutton & Co., 1973.

Chapter 16
Dudrick, Stanley J., and Jonathan E. Rhoads. "Total Intravenous Feeding." *Scientific American,* May 1972, pp. 73–80.
Sleisenger, M., and J. Fordtran. *Gastrointestinal Diseases.* Philadelphia: W. B. Saunders Co., 1973.

Chapter 17
Maugh, Thomas H., II. "Diabetes Therapy: Can New Techniques Halt Complications?" *Science* 190 (1975), 1281–1284.
Renold, A. E., W. Stauffacher, and G. F. Cahill, Jr. "Diabetes Mellitus." In *Metabolic Basis of Inherited Disease,* ed. J. B. Stanbury, J. B. Wyngaarden, and D. S. Fredrickson. 3rd ed. New York: McGraw-Hill, 1972.

Chapter 18
Friedmann, Theodore. "Prenatal Diagnosis of Genetic Disease." *Scientific American,* November 1971, pp. 34–42.
Marx, Jean L. "Estrogen Drugs: Do They Increase the Risk of Cancer?" *Science* 191 (1976), 838.
Segal, Sheldon J. "The Physiology of Human Reproduction." *Scientific American,* September 1974, pp. 53–62.

Chapter 19
Montagna, William. "The Skin." *Scientific American,* February 1965, pp. 56–66.

Chapter 20
Brown, W. E., ed. *Oral Health, Dentistry, and the American Public.* Norman,
Okla.: University of Oklahoma Press, 1974.
Morris, A. L., and R. C. Greulich. "Dental Research: The Past Two Decades."
Science 160 (1968), 1–7.
Scherp, H. W. "Dental Caries: Prospects for Prevention." *Science* 173 (1971),
1199–1205.

Chapter 21
Claymore, C. N., ed. *Biochemistry of the Eye.* New York: Academic Press, 1970.
Heyningen, Ruth van. "What Happens to the Human Lens in Cataract." *Scien-
tific American,* December 1975, pp. 70–81.
Mueller, C. G., and M. Rudolph. *Light and Vision.* New York: Time Inc. Book
Division, 1966.

Chapter 22
Békésy, George von. "The Ear." *Scientific American,* August 1957, pp. 66–78.
Beranek, Leo L. "Noise." *Scientific American,* December 1966, pp. 66–76.
Kryter, K. *The Effect of Noise on Man.* New York: Academic Press, 1970.

Chapter 23
Bassett, C. Andrew L. "Electrical Effects in Bone." *Scientific American,* October
1965, pp. 18–25.
McLean, Franklin C. "Bone." *Scientific American,* February 1955, pp. 84–91.

Chapter 24
Cartwright, Frederick F. *The Development of Modern Surgery.* New York:
Crowell, 1967.
Earle, A. S., ed. *Surgery in America: From the Colonial Era to the Twentieth
Century. Selected Writings.* Philadelphia: W. B. Saunders Co., 1965.
Moore, F. D. *Transplant: The Give and Take of Tissue Transplantation.* Rev.
ed. New York: Simon and Schuster, 1972.
Moore, F. D. "Surgery." In *Advances in American Medicine: Essays at the
Bicentennial,* ed. John Z. Bowers and Elizabeth F. Purcell. New York:
Josiah Macy Jr. Foundation, 1976. 2 vols.

Chapter 25
Abrams, H. L. "Diagnostic Radiology in the Medical School: Quandary or
Crisis?" *Journal of Medical Education* 41 (1966), 850–859.
Gordon, Richard, Gabor T. Herman, and Steven A. Johnson. "Image Recon-
struction from Projections." *Scientific American,* October 1975, pp. 56–68.

Chapter 26
Nelson, Richard R., et al. *Technology, Economic Growth and Public Policy.*
Washington, D.C.: The Brookings Institution, 1967.
Novick, David, ed. *Program Budgeting: Program Analysis and the Federal
Budget.* Washington, D.C.: U.S. Government Printing Office, 1965.

Russell, Louise B., et al. *Federal Health Spending, 1969–1974.* Washington, D.C.: Center for Health Policy Studies, National Planning Association, 1974.

Schultze, Charles L. *The Politics and Economics of Public Spending.* Washington, D.C.: The Brookings Institution, 1968.

Chapter 27

Fox, T. *Crisis in Communication.* London: University of London, The Athlone Press, 1965.

Ingelfinger, F. J. "Medical Literature: The Campus Without Tumult." *Science* 169 (1970), 831–837.

Ingelfinger, F. J. "Peer Review in Biomedical Publication." *American Journal of Medicine* 56 (1974), 686–692.

Price, D. J. *Little Science Big Science.* New York: Columbia University Press, 1963.

Contributors

HERBERT L. ABRAMS is Philip H. Cook Professor of Radiology and Chairman of the Department of Radiology at Harvard Medical School; he is also Radiologist-in-Chief at the Peter Bent Brigham Hospital, Boston.

K. FRANK AUSTEN is Theodore B. Bayles Professor of Medicine at Harvard Medical School and Physician-in-Chief at the Robert B. Brigham Hospital, Boston.

MICHAEL J. BARZA is Associate Professor of Medicine at Tufts University and the New England Medical Center Hospitals, Boston.

JOYCE E. BERLIN is Administrative Assistant to the Department of Epidemiology, Harvard School of Public Health.

GEORGE F. CAHILL, JR., is Director of Research at the Joslin Diabetes Foundation, Inc., Boston, and is Professor of Medicine at Harvard Medical School.

TE-WEN CHANG is Associate Professor of Medicine at the Tufts University School of Medicine, Boston.

RICHARD W. ERBE is Assistant Professor of Pediatrics at Harvard Medical School and is Chief of the Genetics Unit and Associate Pediatrician at the Massachusetts General Hospital, Boston.

RASHI FEIN is Professor of the Economics of Medicine at Harvard Medical School and is Assistant Director of the Harvard Center for Community Health and Medical Care.

THOMAS B. FITZPATRICK is Edward Wigglesworth Professor of Dermatology and Chairman of the Department of Dermatology at Harvard Medical School and is Chief of the Dermatology Service at Massachusetts General Hospital, Boston.

DONALD FREDRICKSON is Director of the National Institutes of Health, Bethesda.

EMIL FREI, III, is Director of the Sidney Farber Cancer Institute, Boston, and Professor of Medicine at Harvard Medical School.

EDWARD A. GAENSLER is Professor of Surgery and Physiology at Boston University School of Medicine and is Visiting Surgeon at University Hospital, Boston.

NORMAN GESCHWIND is James Jackson Putnam Professor of Neurology at Harvard Medical School and is Director of the Neurological Unit at Beth Israel Hospital, Boston.

PAUL GOLDHABER is Dean of the Harvard School of Dental Medicine, where he is Professor of Periodontology.

W. MORTON GRANT is David Glendenning Cogan Professor of Ophthalmology at Harvard Medical School and is Director of the Glaucoma Consultation Service of the Massachusetts Eye and Ear Infirmary, Boston.

JOEL GURIN is a writer specializing in science and medicine and is a contributing Editor of *Harvard Magazine*.

FRANZ J. INGELFINGER is Editor of the *New England Journal of Medicine* and is Clinical Professor of Medicine at Boston University School of Medicine.

KURT J. ISSELBACHER is Mallinckrodt Professor of Medicine at Harvard Medical School; he is also Chairman of the Harvard University Cancer Committee and is Chief of the Gastrointestinal Unit at Massachusetts General Hospital, Boston.

RICHARD A. JOHNSON is Instructor in Dermatology at Harvard Medical School and Chief of Dermatology Associates at Massachusetts General Hospital, Boston.

SEYMOUR S. KETY is Professor of Psychiatry at Harvard Medical School and is Director of the Psychiatric Research Laboratories at Massachusetts General Hospital, Boston.

BRIAN MACMAHON is Henry Pickering Walcott Professor and Head of the Department of Epidemiology of the Harvard School of Public Health.

HENRY J. MANKIN is Edith M. Ashley Professor of Orthopaedic Surgery at Harvard Medical School and is Orthopedist-in-Chief at the Massachusetts General Hospital, Boston.

JOHN P. MERRILL is Professor of Medicine at Harvard Medical School and is Director of the Renal Service at the Peter Bent Brigham Hospital, Boston.

NANCY K. MELLO is Associate Professor of Psychology in the Department of Psychiatry at Harvard Medical School and is Psychologist and Associate Director at the Alcohol and Drug Abuse Research Center, McLean Hospital, Belmont, Massachusetts.

JACK H. MENDELSON is Professor of Psychiatry at Harvard Medical School and is Director of the Alcohol and Drug Abuse Research Center of McLean Hospital, Belmont, Massachusetts.

FRANCIS D. MOORE is Elliott Carr Cutler Professor of Surgery at Harvard Medical School and Surgeon at the Peter Bent Brigham Hospital, Boston.

HUGO W. MOSER is Director of the John F. Kennedy Institute in Baltimore and is Professor in the Departments of Neurology and Pediatrics at the Johns Hopkins School of Medicine.

DAVID G. NATHAN is Professor of Pediatrics at Harvard Medical School, Pediatrician-in-Chief at the Sidney Farber Cancer Center, Boston, and Chief of the Division of Hematology and Oncology at the Sidney Farber Cancer Center and Children's Hospital Medical Center, Boston.

KENNETH J. RYAN is Kate Macy Ladd Professor and Chairman of the Department of Obstetrics and Gynecology at Harvard Medical School; he is also Chief of Staff of the Boston Hospital for Women and Director of the Laboratory of Human Reproduction and Reproductive Biology at Harvard Medical School.

HAROLD F. SCHUKNECHT is Walter Augustus LeCompte Professor of Otology and Professor of Laryngology at Harvard Medical School and is Chief of Otolaryngology at the Massachusetts Eye and Ear Infirmary, Boston.

THOMAS W. SMITH is Associate Professor of Medicine at Harvard Medical School and is Chief of the Cardiovascular Division of the Peter Bent Brigham Hospital, Boston.

HENRY WECHSLER is Director of Research at The Medical Foundation, Inc., Boston and is Lecturer at the Harvard School of Public Health.

LOUIS WEINSTEIN is Visiting Professor of Medicine at Harvard Medical School and is Chief of the Infectious Disease Service at West Roxbury V.A. Hospital and Physician at the Peter Bent Brigham Hospital, Boston.

Index